# Roberts'

Roberts' Nutrition Work

Ethel Austin Martin and Virginia A. Beal

# Nutrition Work with Children

*Fourth Edition*

*The University of Chicago Press*
*Chicago and London*

ETHEL AUSTIN MARTIN has been on the nutrition staffs
and in the home economics departments of the
University of Illinois, the University of Chicago, and
Northwestern University. She was director of the
nutrition service of the National Dairy Council from
1929 to 1951. Her publications include *Nutrition in
Action* and *Nutrition Education in Action*.

VIRGINIA A. BEAL is associate professor of nutrition
at the University of Massachusetts. After seven years with
the growth study at the Harvard School of Public Health,
she was chief nutritionist with the Child Research
Council from 1946 to 1971. She has written extensively
on nutrition in human growth and development.

The University of Chicago Press, Chicago 60637
The University of Chicago Press, Ltd., London

© 1954, 1978 by The University of Chicago
All rights reserved. Published 1978
Printed in the United States of America

82  81  80  79  78    9  8  7  6  5  4  3  2  1

This book was first published in 1927 as *Nutrition
Work with Children*, by Lydia J. Roberts. She revised
it in 1935. In 1954 a third edition was published,
revised by Ethel Austin Martin, entitled
*Roberts' Nutrition Work with Children*.

Library of Congress Cataloging in Publication Data

Martin, Ethel Austin.
    Roberts' Nutrition work with children.

    Includes bibliographies and index.
    1. Children—Nutrition.  I.  Roberts, Lydia Jane.
Nutrition work with children.  II.  Beal, Virginia A.,
joint author.  III.  Title.  IV.  Title: Nutrition
work with children.
RJ206.M28  1978           612'.3           77-13972
ISBN 0-226-50738-6

# Contents

# Preface

The purpose of this fourth edition of *Roberts' Nutrition Work with Children* is, like the previous editions, to interpret present knowledge of nutrition in terms of principles and procedures for attaining better nutritional health for children—better in the broader sense that recognizes the interrelatedness of physical, mental, social, and emotional development.

The book is intended for college and university students of nutrition, to be used as a text and supplementary reference source. Portions of the text will be useful also to majors in related subject areas, including human development, nursing, exercise science, and education. The book assumes a basic knowledge of the science of nutrition that will serve as background for interpreting the specialized subject matter presented. In this light the book may be used by graduate students as well as by undergraduate students who have acquired the basic nutrition understandings. The text should be particularly helpful to students as they approach service in public health nutrition.

The book is also directed to practicing nutritionists in public health agencies and organizations, to pediatric dietitians, and to physicians, especially pediatricians, who are responsible for public health nutrition programs. We hope it will be useful as a source of current information and for guidance in planning and implementing nutrition education programs.

In addition, the text provides bases for communicating with professional associates in other fields—public health nurses, social workers, school administrators, and teachers—who are cooperating in the conduct of community programs involving nutrition, such as youth projects, child health clinics, comprehensive care units, and health maintenance programs. The revision will be helpful in staff education programs in public health departments designed to convey the broad concepts of nutritional care to nonnutrition trained personnel.

Many others in nutrition and related fields will find phases of the content a resource of special interest to them. For example, persons concerned primarily with the physical growth of children will find information on the history of growth studies in this country. Others may be interested in the physical and mental effects of poor nutrition or in the philosophy and techniques of nutrition education as applied to the country's school systems.

Continued call for the third edition suggests that it has met a professional need. Its in-depth consideration of nutrition as an essential factor in child development has made it particularly useful. The first two editions (1927, 1935) by Lydia J. Roberts constituted a pioneer effort in a new phase of nutrition service. The third edition by Ethel Austin Martin (1954), titled *Roberts' Nutrition Work with Children*, updated developments in the field of child nutrition over the ensuing twenty active years. Now, in 1978, there is the same need to take account of vast new accomplishments in research and education over an equally eventful period. For the fourth edition, Virginia A. Beal has joined as coauthor in the monumental task of condensing burgeoning content into a more compact volume while adhering to the purpose, general character, and approach of previous editions.

It would be impossible to name individually the many persons who have aided the revision project. We must be content to say to all of you a sincere "thank you" for providing basic material, illustrations, criticisms, ideas, and encouragement. May you feel amply rewarded by the gratitude of users of the new edition who will be the eventual recipients of your generous contributions.

# Chapter One

## The Meaning of Nutrition

## An Introduction

Nutrition is fundamental to growth and development from conception to attainment of adult size. It is essential to health and to the quality of life at all ages. The body is composed entirely of the elements present in food, water, and air. Both the quality and the quantity of body tissues and fluids therefore depend on a plentiful supply of all the nutrients needed for their formation and maintenance. This simple fact is the basis of our concern about the nutritional intake of the mother prior to and during pregnancy, of the child during infancy, the preschool years, the early school years, and adolescence. Each of these periods has its own particular growth characteristics and its own nutritional demands, but the quality of somatic growth throughout these periods lays the foundation for the health, physical fitness, and mental functioning of the adult, and for longevity.

Nutrition has been defined in a number of ways. Most simply, it is the science of food and its relation to health. A more complete definition from the American Medical Association is that "nutrition is the science of food, the nutrients and other substances therein, their action, interaction and balance in relation to health and disease, and the processes by which the organism ingests, digests, transports, utilizes and excretes food substances." Nutrition in its broadest sense is not limited to the biochemistry and physiology of the body. Food must be available before it can be eaten, so nutrition is dependent on geography, agriculture, technology, transportation, politics, and all other aspects of national and international food supply. The selection and consumption of food by the individual are tempered by his own economic, cultural, educational, social, physical, and physiological state. Therefore, while our basic concern is to provide the body with those nutrients which are essential to its optimal growth and functioning, we must take into account the many factors which determine what food is supplied to the body as well as how the body makes use of that food.

## Development of the Science of Nutrition

Nutrition is a relatively young science. The earliest records of man show his awareness of some effects of food on health and physical ability, but it is only in the past century that we have been able to identify the many components of food and to begin to understand the biochemical and physiological functions of nutrients. Our knowledge of nutrition is still far from complete, but new research findings each year add to our conviction that the quality of life is strongly influenced by the quantity and quality of nutritional intake.

By the beginning of the twentieth century, the contributions of carbohydrate, fat, and protein to total calories and the essential nature of the nitrogen in protein to body cells had been recognized, and the functions of minerals were being investigated. In the first few decades of this century the concept of "accessory food factors" began to develop. Purified diets containing all known macronutrients and minerals resulted in disease or death of animals. The 1930s brought laboratory identification of the first vitamin (ascorbic acid), and the "era of the vitamins" had begun. At the present time the chemical structures of the vitamins which have thus far been identified have been analyzed. We know the essential metabolic functions of many but not all vitamins. The clinical symptoms of deficiencies of most vitamins have been recognized. We are still uncertain about the amounts of some of the nutrients required for optimal body functioning at various stages of the life cycle. However, our knowledge is increasing at a remarkably rapid rate.

Not only has the number of national and international journals devoted to nutrition and dietetics proliferated in the past few years, but the wide-ranging applications of nutritional science to other areas of interest and its importance in allied fields have been increasingly recognized. Articles on nutrition have for many years been published in medical and nursing journals. More recently nutrition-related reports have been appearing in publications concerned with such fields as food technology, sociology, anthropology, psychology, ecology, education, and toxicology. This is an indication of the fact that as our understanding of the effects of good and poor nutrition expands, it becomes ever more obvious that those effects apply to the total functioning of the individual. His ability to learn, to work, to earn, and to adapt to a changing environment are affected by his nutritional intake during the years of his growth and development as well as during his adult life.

## Hunger and Malnutrition

*Hunger* and *malnutrition* are terms which will be used in the following chapters, so it would be well to clarify their meanings in this context. Hunger occurs when the amount of food is inadequate. This may be transient, as one is hungry if it has been several hours since food was last consumed. Hunger may be chronic, as in developing countries or economically deprived areas where food supplies are inadequate or money to obtain food is severely restricted. Chronic hunger may lead to malnutrition.

Malnutrition is a state which results from a discrepancy between the supply of calories or essential nutrients to the body tissues and the tissues' need for them.[1] Malnutrition causes impairment of the functional ability of the body, deficiency of its structural integrity, or abnormality in development. The term includes both undernutrition, which results in deficiency symptoms, and overnutrition, which results in obesity or, for some nutrients, toxicity. Malnutrition may be either primary or secondary. Primary malnutrition is caused by inadequate or excessive intake of calories or nutrients in relation to the body's requirements and may be due to faulty food selection, lack of money to buy proper foods, or actual food shortage. Secondary malnutrition results from any interference with ingestion or absorption, or from stress or other factors which increase the body's requirement or the destruction or excretion of nutrients. Secondary malnutrition may be caused by factors such as chronic diarrhea, parasitic infestation, gastric surgery, drug therapy, or infection.

High rates of illness and death in infants and young children in developing nations have, in the past few decades, focused attention on nutrition and food supply. The shortage of food and of good quality proteins results in energy-protein malnutrition and interferes with normal growth and development. One of the first signs of acute malnutrition is interference with growth. The undernourished child is also more susceptible to infections and less able to cope with infectious agents. The synergism of malnutrition and infection has caused the deaths of countless young children.[2,3]

Investigation into retardation of somatic growth has led to fundamental research toward understanding the effects of nutrition—the study of cell growth. In energy-protein malnutrition, there is interference with both skeletal growth and brain growth. Unless adequate nutrients are supplied to the brain during the critical periods of pregnancy and infancy when brain cells are proliferating, the number of cells may be reduced. Postmortem studies of children who died after being acutely malnourished showed a smaller number of brain cells than normal controls.[4] Investigation into the etiology of obesity has recently centered on the study of fat cells at various stages of the life cycle.[5,6]

In technologically underdeveloped areas of the world where undernutrition is often acute, the physical and mental handicaps of the infant may affect his capabilities for the rest of his life, if he survives the initial effects. In technologically advanced nations, undernutrition tends to be moderate by comparison, and greater concern is focused on the effects of overnutrition. Excessive caloric intake may result in obesity, characterized by large numbers or size of adipose cells, which in turn may be related eventually to degenerative diseases of adults.

### Importance of Nutrition to the Body

The body is composed of cells and fluids. The functions of nutrients in the entire body are actually the sum of the functions of those nutrients in individual cells. A constant supply of energy, amino acids, glucose, lipids, minerals, and vitamins to the cells is indispensable for cell formation and for the specific activities of each cell. During growth, cells are increasing in both number and size. At all ages cells are constantly undergoing degradation, regeneration, replenishment of cell contents, and production of enzymes or hormones. Intracellular and extracellular body fluids must maintain their own basic composition of proteins, minerals, lipids, or carbohydrates, and must also carry nutrients to the cells of various tissues. Therefore, it is at the level of the cell and its source of supply that nutrition is important to the body. The effects of inadequate nutrition occur first at the cellular level, and the clinical signs which we associate with malnutrition are the end results of cellular changes.

Good nutrition results when all body fluids and cells are supplied with the specific nutrients each needs to carry on its particular metabolic functions. From the definition of nutrition given earlier, it is obvious that a series of actions must take place before the cells can receive their nutrient supply. The foods which contain the necessary nutrients must first be selected and eaten, then digested, and the nutrients absorbed across the intestinal wall and finally transported to and taken into the cell. It is in this sequence of events that the many facets of nutrition must be considered. The diet must contain a sufficient amount of the nutrients needed. This necessitates availability of foods, income large enough to permit their purchase, knowledge of nutrient values to select the proper foods and of the methods of storage and preparation to retain maximum nutrient value, and a healthy appetite and willingness to eat the foods.

Knowledge of food values is important in guiding an individual to proper food selection. In countries with adequate total food supplies, the main deterrent to selection of an appropriate diet for some segments of the population is economic. The education of low income families should be directed toward choice of foods which provide the greatest nutrient content for the least money. At all income levels the complexity of food selection requires knowledge of food values to make intelligent choices. It has been estimated that the average supermarket in the United States contains more than 10,000 food products and that the average shopper passes nearly 300 food items per minute in the supermarket.

Data on the nutritive value of foods are usually obtained from food value tables, such as *Handbook No. 8*[7] or *Handbook No. 456*[8] of the U.S. Department of Agriculture or compilations by other workers in the field. The values presented in these tables are averages of analyses from various parts of the country[9] and may not reflect accurately the nutrient content of the food eaten by a given individual at a given time, but the tables are simple to use and are sufficiently accurate for most dietary calculations.

Nutrient requirements vary from one individual to another and vary within the same individual from time to time. Since we cannot determine accurately the specific needs of individuals, we rely on standards such as the Recommended Dietary Allowances (RDA) set by the Committee on Dietary Allowances of the Food and Nutrition Board of the National Research Council. These allowances are the best estimates of the committee after reviewing data in the literature.

They have been revised at approximately five-year intervals as new knowledge becomes available. The eighth edition RDA table (see appendix 1) lists the recommended intakes of energy, protein, six minerals, and ten vitamins for age groupings of males and females from birth to over fifty-one years, with values also for pregnancy and lactation.[10] Except for calories, the RDA levels are above the estimated requirements of most of the population within the groups. They provide a margin of safety for individual variation, for stress, and for unusual needs. They are aimed at producing the greatest dividends in health and disease prevention. Therefore one cannot assume that individuals are malnourished if their intakes are below the RDA levels, but they are useful guides toward which to aim in planning diets for groups of people.[11]

Nutrient requirements vary, not only with age, sex, and physiological state, but also with the efficiency with which the body digests, absorbs, and utilizes nutrients. Each nutrient must be supplied to the cell in adequate amounts, and the proper blend of nutrients must be available at one time for the specific metabolic functions of the cell. For example, if the cell is to produce an enzyme, all of the components of that enzyme must be present at the same time for its formation to be possible. All processes, from ingestion to excretion, must run smoothly for the cell to function properly. This is the basis of good nutrition.

Poor nutrition, on the other hand, may result from a breakdown in any phase of the sequence. If dietary intake is inadequate, necessary nutrients are not ingested. Conditions in the gastrointestinal tract may not be ideal for digestion or absorption. For example, diarrhea may cause rapid passage of food allowing inadequate time for nutrients to be absorbed. Lack of the enzyme lactase may curtail the breakdown of lactose to a molecular size which can cross the gastrointestinal wall. After absorption of nutrients, interference with transport, excessive destruction of nutrients, inability of the cell to admit and utilize nutrients or to dispose of waste products may prevent the cell from carrying out its functions. Any of these adverse factors may result in malnutrition.

If cells do not receive an adequate supply of the proper nutrients, a series of events will follow. Nutrients will be withdrawn from blood or from any available body storage sites in an effort to increase the supply to cells. When these resources are depleted, shortage of nutrients distorts metabolic functions of the cells. As a result of this distortion, clinical symptoms appear.

During childhood the demands of the body for nutrients for somatic growth are very high. However, the primary need of the body
is for energy to sustain life, and growth becomes secondary. Therefore poor growth may be the first clinical sign of malnutrition in the
child. Other clinical symptoms depend on which specific nutrients are
deficient. For example, iron deficiency limits ability to form hemoglobin, causing microcytic hypochromic anemia. Ascorbic acid deficiency distorts collagen formation, leading to capillary fragility and
other symptoms of scurvy. A diet inadequate in one nutrient is likely
to be inadequate in several other nutrients, so that clinical symptoms
of many deficiencies may occur at the same time. And, because metabolic functions of many nutrients are interdependent, a deficiency of
one may interfere with the metabolism of another. Therefore, in both
dietary supply and biochemical function, malnutrition is often a
multifaceted state.

Severe deficiency diseases, such as rickets, scurvy, and protein-
energy malnutrition, are rarely seen in the United States and other
developed countries at the present time. When they do occur, they are
usually associated with primary problems of poverty and ignorance.
These individuals should be identified and provided with proper therapy, financial support, and education. More widespread are moderate degrees of malnutrition which are not life-threatening but which
may result in less than optimal functioning of some segments of the
population.

A review of studies[12] and several surveys have provided the beginning of a composite picture of the nutritional health of the U.S.[13–16]
and Canadian[17] populations. Nutritional assessment is defined in
broad terms, including evaluation of the physical, physiological, and
biochemical state of the body as well as study of the diet. In the surveys, which will be considered in detail in chapter 2, teams of workers
from a variety of disciplines obtained clinical examinations and histories, dental examinations, anthropometric measurements, and samples of blood and urine in addition to dietary intakes. They found
little evidence of the acute malnutrition which has been of worldwide
concern in developing nations. Physical examinations revealed few
symptoms of nutritional deficiencies, but some groups and individuals in the populations had low dietary intakes of some nutrients and
low biochemical levels. Growth retardation, iron-deficiency anemia,
and dental caries were the most common findings, particularly among
ethnic minority and low income groups. Greatest risk of malnutrition
was observed among pregnant women, small children, and ado-

lescents. Obesity was recognized as a problem in some groups. These surveys, while reassuring about the infrequency of severe nutritional deficiencies, have provided specific directions for nutrition education and intervention programs.

## The Changing Dietary Patterns

The long-familiar pattern of eating has been changing rapidly in the United States. The traditional three daily meals when family members eat together are being replaced by irregularity of eating, frequent snacking, and meals away from home. In many families the evening meal is the only one for which all members are present. Midmorning, midafternoon, and late evening snacks are becoming customary. It has been estimated that families spend an average of nearly one-third of their food budget for meals eaten away from home. Since this trend is unlikely to be altered, realistic nutrition education must recognize it and adapt to it.

Preparation of food in the home has also been greatly changed. There is available an ever-increasing variety of commercially prepared food which requires minimal handling or cooking before being consumed. The introduction of formulated foods, such as fruit-flavored drinks, milk or cream substitutes, multinutrient beverages for weight control, and sugar substitutes, has complicated the calculation of nutrient intakes. Texturized protein foods and soy extenders have increased the percent of protein from plant sources. Vegetable oils have partially replaced animal fats. Methods of processing foods are constantly being revised and altering nutrient content. Enrichment and fortification programs change the nutrient content of foods.

Changes in life style and in attitudes toward some foods[18] have been caused by a diversity of reasons and have affected the dietaries of many segments of the population. Concern about the relationship of intake of saturated fats to the etiology of coronary heart disease has led many people to substitute vegetable oils for animal fats, limit intake of eggs, and replace whole milk with skim milk. Vegetarianism has become a common practice, but ranges from the single elimination of red meat to abstention from all animal products.[19,20]

Individuals concerned about land use in relation to population growth in the world have limited their meat intake since animal products return fewer calories from land than grain products. Fear of the effects of intentional and of unintentional additives to foods have altered food selections. These are examples of reasons for continuing alteration in the types of foods which are selected and consumed.

The effects of many of these changes on the nutrient content of diets have not been evaluated. Some nutrients are decreased or lost in food processing.[21] The more widespread the use of processed foods, the more likely is the possibility that nutrient intakes will decline. Formulated food substitutes may not contain all of the minerals or vitamins naturally found in the foods they replace. The wide variability of methods of cooking and of holding foods in commercial establishments may limit retention of nutrients in restaurant meals, and the types of foods available or selected may differ from foods eaten at home. Increased consumption of grains and vegetable oils concomitant with decrease in animal products alters the intake of many nutrients. Some changes may improve the quality of the diet, but some may lead to lower intakes, especially of trace elements. These changes should be carefully monitored.[22]

Studies of foods available for consumption in the United States since 1909 by the Department of Agriculture[23,24] have shown definite trends. The intake of total fat has increased, but a greater proportion of fat is now of vegetable rather than of animal origin. Carbohydrate consumption has decreased, due primarily to less use of flour and cereal products, with sugar providing a greater percentage contribution to total carbohydrate; there has been some decline in sugar since 1973. Milk and dairy products increased between 1909 and the 1940s and have decreased somewhat in the past three decades, with a shift recently toward greater use of low-fat and skim milk. The consumption of meat, fish, and poultry has risen more than 25%; the use of poultry has tripled. Citrus fruits have increased, but other fruits have decreased. Vegetable consumption increased between 1909 and the 1940s, with a slight decline in the past thirty years. Increased use of canned and frozen vegetables has been accompanied by a decrease in the use of fresh vegetables.

Changes in food consumption in the United States have been reflected in the household surveys of the U.S. Department of Agriculture between 1935 and 1965.[25] The newest survey for the 1970s is now in the initial stages and will undoubtedly provide an estimation of the effects of the changing food patterns in the country. The effects of food regulations on nutrient content of foods and the present status of the enrichment and fortification programs will be discussed in chapter 7.

Educational programs hold the greatest promise of implementing nutrition knowledge. Chapter 8 reviews briefly the background of nutrition programs in this country and presents the framework for ongoing programs. Chapters 9 and 10 concentrate on modern concepts of nutrition education as applied to school programs. Nutrition education is most effective if it starts in childhood. Once food patterns have become well ingrained they are resistant to change. If a child is taught the importance of food to his health and performance, both physical and mental, he is more apt to be receptive to the establishment of good habits. If he learns which foods will supply the nutrients he needs for optimal functioning and develops a taste for those foods in early life, he will be better able to cope with the ever-increasing complexity of food selection. Patterns formed in early life are likely to persist into adulthood. Therefore, nutrition education of children presents the greatest hope of long-term improvement of the nutritional status of a population.

## References

1   Council on Foods and Nutrition, American Medical Association. "Malnutrition and Hunger in the United States." *JAMA* 213 (1970):272–75.

2   *Pre-School Malnutrition*. Washington, D.C.: National Academy of Sciences-National Research Council, 1966.

3   Jelliffe, D. B., and Jelliffe, E. F. P., eds. *Nutrition Programmes for Pre-school Children*. Zagreb, Yugoslavia: Institute of Public Health of Croatia, 1973.

4   Winick, M.; Brasel, J. A.; and Rosso, P. "Nutrition and Cell Growth." In *Nutrition and Development*, edited by M. Winick. New York: John Wiley & Sons, 1972.

5   Hirsch, J. "Cell Number and Size as a Determinant of Subsequent Obesity." In *Childhood Obesity*, edited by M. Winick. New York: John Wiley & Sons, 1975.

6   Knittle, J. L. "Obesity in Childhood: A Problem in Adipose Tissue Cellular Development." *Journal of Pediatrics* 81 (1972):1048–59.

7   Watt, B. K., and Merrill, A. L. *Composition of Foods: Raw, Processed and Prepared*. U.S. Department of Agriculture handbook no. 8. Washington, D.C.: Superintendent of Documents, Government Printing Office, 1963.

8   Adams, C. F. *Nutritive Value of American Foods in Common Units*. U.S. Department of Agriculture handbook no. 456. Washington, D.C.: Superintendent of Documents, Government Printing Office, 1975.

9   Watt, B. K.; Gebhardt, S. E.; Murphy, E. W.; and Butrum, R. R. "Food Consumption Tables for the 70's." *Journal of the American Dietetic Association* 64 (1974):257–61.

10   Food and Nutrition Board. *Recommended Dietary Allowances*, 8th ed. Washington, D.C.: National Academy of Sciences-National Research Council, 1974.

11   Hegsted, D. M. "Dietary Standards." *Journal of the American Dietetic Association* 66 (1975):13–21.

12  Kelsay, J. L. "A Compendium of Nutritional Status Studies and Dietary Evaluation Studies Conducted in the United States, 1957–1967." *Journal of Nutrition* 99 (1969 [suppl. 1, pt. 2]):119–66.

13  U.S. Department of Health, Education, and Welfare. *Ten-State Nutrition Survey, 1968–1970.* DHEW publications no. (HSM) 72–8130, 72–8131, 72–8132, and 72–8133. Washington, D.C.: Superintendent of Documents, Government Printing Office, 1972.

14  U.S. Department of Health, Education, and Welfare. *Preliminary Findings of the First Health and Nutrition Examination Survey, United States, 1971–1972: Dietary Intake and Biochemical Findings.* DHEW publication no. (HRA) 74–1219–1. Washington, D.C.: Superintendent of Documents, Government Printing Office, 1974.

15  U.S. Department of Health, Education, and Welfare. *Preliminary Findings of the First Health and Nutrition Examination Survey, United States, 1971–1972: Anthropometric and Clinical Findings.* DHEW publication no. (HRA) 75–1229. Washington, D.C.: Superintendent of Documents, Government Printing Office, 1975.

16  Owen, G. M.; Kram, K. M.; Garry, P. J.; Lowe, J. E.; and Lubin, A. H. "A Study of Nutritional Status of Preschool Children in the United States, 1968–1970." *Pediatrics* 53 (1974 [suppl. pt. 2]):597–646.

17  Nutrition Canada. *National Survey: A Report by Nutrition Canada to the Department of National Health and Welfare.* Catalog no. H58–36–1973. Ottawa: Information Canada, 1973.

18  Frankle, R. T., and Heussenstamm, F. K.: "Food Zealotry and Youth: New Dilemmas for Professionals." *American Journal of Public Health* 64 (1974):11–18.

19  Dwyer, J. T.; Mayer, L. V. D. H.; Kandel, R. F.; and Mayer, J. "The New Vegetarians." *Journal of the American Dietetic Association* 62 (1973):503–9.

20  Brown, P. T., and Bergen, J. G. "The Dietary Status of the 'New Vegetarians.'" *Journal of the American Dietetic Association* 67 (1975): 455–59.

21  Schroeder, H. A. "Losses of Vitamins and Trace Minerals Resulting from Processing and Preservation of Foods." *American Journal of Clinical Nutrition* 24 (1971):562–73.

22  Henderson, L. "Nutritional Problems Growing out of the New Patterns of Food Consumption." *American Journal of Public Health* 62 (1972): 1194–98.

23  Friend, B. "Nutrients in the United States Food Supply: A Review of Trends 1909–1913 to 1965." *American Journal of Clinical Nutrition* 20 (1967): 907–14.

24  *Food Consumption, Prices and Expenditures.* Supplement for 1975 to Agricultural Economic report no. 138. Washington, D.C.: U.S. Department of Agriculture, 1977.

25  U.S. Department of Agriculture. *Food Consumption of Households in the United States: Seasons and Year, 1965–66.* Agriculture Research Service report no. 12. Washington, D.C.: Superintendent of Documents, Government Printing Office, 1972.

# Chapter Two

## Assessment of Nutritional Status

To be most effective, a nutrition program should address itself to the specific problems of the people for whom it is intended. Whether the program is educational, interventional, or legislative, it should be based on firm data of the needs of the population group involved. The household surveys of the U.S. Department of Agriculture have provided national data on food consumption since 1935, but until recent years little effort has been expended on evaluation of nutritional health in the country. Often the baselines for action programs have been fragmentary studies of small groups or the impressions of professional workers or lay persons. Techniques for the study of the nutritional status of large populations have been developing for several decades, but only in the past decade has federal money been allocated for surveys designed to assess nutritional status within the United States. Data from these surveys can provide the focus for effective nutrition programs.

The first classification of standards for evaluation of nutritional status of populations was compiled by Bigwood[1] for the League of Nations in 1939. As knowledge has increased and techniques have improved, a number of subsequent guidelines for obtaining and interpreting data in clinical, anthropometric, biochemical, and dietary studies have been developed, including those of the Interdepartmental Committee on Nutrition for National Defense (ICNND),[2] the World Health Organization (WHO),[3] the Ten-State Nutrition Survey (TSNS),[4] the Health and Nutrition Examination Survey (HANES) of the National Center for Health Statistics,[5,6] and the Nutrition Canada National Survey.[7]

The variations in the standards used by each of these groups are indicative of the lack of agreement of acceptable standards for rating, especially of the biochemical and dietary levels. Current knowledge of the physiological significance of marginal changes in level is inadequate. Problems of methodology and standards will be discussed in each section of this chapter because they are vital to the interpretation of survey findings and the extent of malnutrition observed. As with all developing arts and sciences, techniques need constant analysis and refinement, and errors in interpretation become evident only after the methodology has been corrected.

Component parts of nutritional assessment are community evaluation, clinical examinations and medical history, anthropometric measurements, analysis of blood and urine for selected nutrients or metabolites, and dietary intake studies. Each component contributes to the total evaluation. In developed countries where few acute deficiency diseases are likely to be found, no single area of study gives a definitive picture of the nutritional health of either an individual or a population group. The components explain and complement each other.

The sequence of development of nutrient deficiencies, adapted from Pearson,[8] is as follows:

1. Initial deficiency, either primary or secondary. In a primary deficiency the cause is inadequate dietary intake. In a secondary deficiency the contributing factors may be poor absorption, decreased utilization by tissues, impaired transport by blood or other body fluids, or increased excretion, destruction, or requirement.
2. Depletion of tissue levels of the nutrient.
3. Development of biochemical lesions with distortion of function.
4. Clinical lesion as a result of functional impairment.

This sequence of events is the basis for some of the disagreements in evaluation of findings in surveys. Most surveys in developed countries have shown poor correlation between dietary, biochemical, and clinical findings. With current methodology, the component parts of the assessment are measuring different stages of nutriture. Dietary studies, by their nature, are usually limited to present or immediate past intake, which may not be typical of long-term intake. Levels of some nutrients or metabolites in blood or urine are altered by immediate past intake, but others change only after an extended period of deficient intake and would not necessarily be related to current intake levels. Clinical lesions found on physical examination are the last to develop and reflect long-standing deficiency. These time differences decrease the likelihood of finding correlations between component parts of the assessment.

Methodology in each area is imperfect and standards for evaluation of findings are not precise. The various survey groups cited above have often used different levels for rating dietary intake, blood levels, and urinary excretions as "adequate," "low," or "deficient." In the technologically advanced countries where ranges of variation in either dietary or biochemical levels are relatively small and alterations in physiological function or physical state are minor and often difficult to differentiate, the selection of standards for rating assumes major importance in summarizing the frequency of deficiencies.

Individual variations in nutrient requirement, absorption, and utilization cause different response in blood levels and in the appearance of deficiency signs. Two persons of the same age, sex, size, and dietary intake are unlikely to have the same levels of nutrients in blood or tissues. Variations in the length of time required by different individuals to show blood changes or clinical symptoms on experimentally deficient diets have been demonstrated in many studies. The adaptation of the body to lower or higher levels of intake has long been recognized but is difficult to quantify. Previous nutrition history from conception, physiological efficiency, and body storage are difficult or impossible to measure, but they affect the current status of the body more than immediate past intake. Thus there are several explanations for the lack of correlation between component parts of nutritional assessment studies.

Surveys are designed to identify the extent and distribution of malnutrition in a given population, usually for the purpose of planning corrective programs. The type of study methods selected will depend on the geographic area, number and type of personnel available, funding, laboratory and computer facilities, and the many other factors which affect purpose and feasibility. No effort will be made here to deal with studies in developing countries. The publications of the World Health Organization are an invaluable source of information on conducting and evaluating studies in those parts of the globe. A WHO summary[3] of the types of information needed and their nutritional implications, applicable to all areas of the world, is shown in table 2.1.

## Community Assessment

A broad picture of the nutritional health of a community may be obtained indirectly from data easily available from existing sources. Nutritional health is closely related to certain characteristics of an area. If a high percentage of the population is economically, socially, educationally, and/or medically deprived, nutritional problems are likely to be found. Therefore a demographic description of a community may provide clues to possible dietary deficiencies.

Sources of information may include census figures (including age distributions), birth rates, morbidity and mortality statistics, hospital records, and data from health and welfare agencies. One may compile a profile of income, housing, sanitation, disease rates, cultural and ethnic characteristics, food supply, and availability of health programs and nutritional resources.

## Clinical Assessment

Procedures include a health history, physical examination with special attention to signs which might be associated with nutritional aberrations, and a dental examination. Body measurements are often included in the category of clinical assessment, but in the present discussion will be treated separately because of the importance of growth assessment in children.

The clinical signs indicative or suggestive of malnutrition in table 2.2, adapted from a more extensive WHO table, were included in a detailed guide to methodology and interpretation of studies of nutritional assessment prepared by a committee of the American Public Health Association.[9] These signs, however, are not frequently found in developed countries. For example, in three studies which included preschool children in the United States, cheilosis was reported in no children under six years in the HANES I survey, in 0.4% of children in the Preschool Nutrition Survey (PNS),[10] and in 0 to 4.1% in various sex, ethnic, and income groups of children under six in the TSNS. Hyperkeratosis of the arm was found in 2.3% of preschool children in HANES I, 0.3% in PNS, and 0 to 2.9% in TSNS. The

**Table 2.1**    Information Needed for Assessment of Nutritional Status

| Sources of Information | Nature of Information Obtained | Nutritional Implications |
|---|---|---|
| (1) Agricultural data<br>Food balance sheets | Gross estimates of agricultural production<br>Agricultural methods<br>Soil fertility<br>Predominance of cash crops<br>Overproduction of staples<br>Food imports and exports | Approximate availability of food supplies to a population |
| (2) Socioeconomic data<br>Information on marketing, distribution, and storage | Purchasing power<br>Distribution and storage of foodstuffs | Unequal distribution of available foods between the socioeconomic groups in the community and within the family |
| (3) Food consumption patterns<br>Cultural-anthropological data | Lack of knowledge, erroneous beliefs and prejudices, indifference | |
| (4) Dietary surveys | Food consumption | Low, excessive, or unbalanced nutrient intake |

| | | Special problems related to nutrient utilization |
|---|---|---|
| (5) Special studies on foods | Biological value of diets<br>Presence of interfering factors (for example, goitrogens)<br>Effects of food processing | |
| (6) Vital and health statistics | Morbidity and mortality data | Extent of risk to community<br>Identification of high-risk groups |
| (7) Anthropometric studies | Physical development | Effect of nutrition on physical development |
| (8) Clinical nutritional surveys | Physical signs | Deviation from health due to malnutrition |
| (9) Biochemical studies | Levels of nutrients, metabolites, and other components of body tissues and fluids | Nutrient supplies in the body<br>Impairment of biochemical function |
| (10) Additional medical information | Prevalent disease patterns, including infections and infestations | Interrelationships of state of nutrition and disease |

SOURCE: World Health Organization. Expert Committee on Medical Assessment of Nutritional Status: Report. Technical report series no. 258. Geneva: World Health Organization, 1963.

**Table 2.2**    Physical Signs Indicative or Suggestive of Malnutrition

| Body Area | Normal Appearance | Signs Associated with Malnutrition |
|---|---|---|
| Hair | Shiny; firm; not easily plucked | Lack of natural shine; hair dull and dry; thin and sparse; hair fine, silky and straight; color changes (flag sign); can be easily plucked |
| Face | Skin color uniform; smooth, pink, healthy appearance; not swollen | Skin color loss (depigmentation); skin dark over cheeks and under eyes (malar and supra-orbital pigmentation); lumpiness or flakiness of skin of nose and mouth; swollen face; enlarged parotid glands; scaling of skin around nostrils (nasolabial seborrhea) |
| Eyes | Bright, clear, shiny; no sores at corners of eyelids; membranes a healthy pink and are moist; no prominent blood vessels or mound of tissue or sclera | Eye membranes are pale (pale conjunctivae); redness of membranes (conjunctival injection); Bitot's spots; redness and fissuring of eyelid corners (angular palpebritis); dryness of eye membranes (conjunctival xerosis); cornea has dull appearance (corneal xerosis); cornea is soft (keratomalacia); scar on cornea; ring of fine blood vessels around corner (circumcorneal injection) |
| Lips | Smooth, not chapped or swollen | Redness and swelling of mouth or lips (cheilosis); especially at corners of mouth (angular fissures and scars) |
| Tongue | Deep red in appearance; not swollen or smooth | Swelling; scarlet and raw tongue; magenta (purplish color) of tongue; smooth tongue; swollen sores; hyperemic and hypertrophic papillae; and atrophic papillae |
| Teeth | No cavities; no pain; bright | May be missing or erupting abnormally; gray or black spots (fluorosis); cavities (caries) |
| Gums | Healthy; red; do not bleed; not swollen | "Spongy" and bleed easily; recession of gums |
| Glands | Face not swollen | Thyroid enlargement (front of neck); parotid enlargement (cheeks become swollen) |

| | Good | Poor |
|---|---|---|
| Skin | No signs of rashes, swellings, dark or light spots | Dryness of skin (xerosis); sandpaper feel of skin (follicular hyperkeratosis); flakiness of skin; skin swollen and dark; red swollen pigmentation of exposed areas (pellagrous dermatosis); excessive lightness or darkness of skin (dyspigmentation); black and blue marks due to skin bleeding (petechiae); lack of fat under skin |
| Nails | Firm, pink | Nails are spoon-shape (koilonychia); brittle, ridged nails |
| Muscular and skeletal systems | Good muscle tone; some fat under skin; can walk or run without pain | Muscles have "wasted" appearance; baby's skull bones are thin and soft (craniotabes); round swelling of front and side of head (frontal and parietal bossing); swelling of ends of bones (epiphyseal enlargement); small bumps on both sides of chest wall (on ribs)—beading of ribs; baby's soft spot on head does not harden at proper time (persistently open anterior fontanelle); knock-knees or bow-legs; bleeding into muscle (musculoskeletal hemorrhages); person cannot get up or walk properly |
| *Internal Systems:* | | |
| Cardiovascular | Normal heart rate and rhythm; no murmurs or abnormal rhythms; normal blood pressure for age | Rapid heart rate (above 100 tachycardia); enlarged heart; abnormal rhythm; elevated blood pressure |
| Gastrointestinal | No palpable organs or masses (in children, however, liver edge may be palpable) | Liver enlargement; enlargement of spleen (usually indicates other associated diseases) |
| Nervous | Psychological stability; normal reflexes | Mental irritability and confusion; burning and tingling of hands and feet (paresthesia); loss of position and vibratory sense; weakness and tenderness of muscles (may result in inability to walk); decrease and loss of ankle and knee reflexes |

SOURCE: Reprinted, with permission, from Christakis, G., ed. "Nutritional Assessment in Health Programs." *American Journal of Public Health* 63 (1973 [suppl.]): 19.

finding of signs of nutritional deficiency on clinical examination correlated poorly with biochemical levels and dietary intakes.[4,7,10,11]

"Clinical examinations of malnutrition are most valuable in situations where the deficiency of one or more nutrients has reached the stage of overt disease, i.e., where the health and, in fact, the life of the individual are jeopardized. The value of physical examinations is therefore extremely high for impoverished populations and diminishes in importance as the adequacy of the food supply for a population improves."[7] Many of the signs and symptoms which might be attributed to nutrient deficiencies are nonspecific and may instead be caused by nonnutritional factors, especially in countries where the overall prevalence of malnutrition is low and the symptoms relatively mild. The identification of many of the signs is subjective and inter-examiner differences are often high.[9] It is important that all physicians on the examining team have common training, with special emphasis on the nutrition-related signs.

Despite the shortcomings of the clinical examination in surveys of some population groups, it "should be an integral part of most nutrition surveys for the following reasons: A physical examination may reveal evidence of certain nutritional deficiencies which will not be detected by dietary or laboratory methods. The identification of even a few cases of clear-cut nutritional deficiency may be particularly revealing and provide a clue to other pockets of malnutrition in a community. The nutritional examination may reveal signs of a host of other diseases which merit diagnosis and treatment."[9]

For interpretation of clinical signs in relation to overall nutrition and to specific nutrients, the following list has been adapted from a WHO guide:[3]

Dietary obesity: Excessive weight in relation to height; excessive skinfolds; excessive abdominal girth in relation to chest girth

Undernutrition: Mental and physical lethargy; low weight in relation to height; diminished skinfolds; exaggerated skeletal prominences; loss of elasticity of skin

Protein-calorie deficiency diseases: Edema; muscle wasting; low body weight; psychomotor change; dyspigmentation, easy pluckability, thinness and sparseness of hair; flaky paint dermatosis; diffuse depigmentation of skin

Vitamin A deficiency: Xerosis of skin; follicular hyperkeratosis; xerosis conjunctivae; keratomalacia; Bitot's spots

Riboflavin deficiency: Angular stomatitis; magenta tongue; central atrophy of papillae of tongue; nasolabial seborrhea; inflammation of angles of eyelids; corneal vascularization

Thiamine deficiency: Loss of knee and/or ankle jerks; sensory loss and motor weakness; calf muscle tenderness; cardiovascular dysfunction; edema

Niacin deficiency: Pellagrous dermatosis; scarlet or raw tongue; fissures or atrophy of papillae of tongue; facial skin pigmentation

Ascorbic acid deficiency: Spongy and bleeding gums; petechiae; echymoses; intramuscular or subperiosteal hematoma; painful enlargement of epiphyses

Vitamin D deficiency: Epiphyseal enlargement; beading of ribs; craniotabes; muscular hypotonia; frontal and parietal bossing; knock-knees or bowed legs; deformities of thorax

Iron deficiency: Pallor of mucous membranes; koilonychia; atrophy of papillae of tongue

Iodine deficiency: Enlargement of thyroid

Excess of fluorine: Mottled enamel

The presence of any of these signs should not be taken as conclusively diagnostic of a deficiency of the nutrient indicated, but should be used for screening to indicate further study, including dietary and biochemical investigations. Other vitamins than those cited may be implicated as causes of the symptoms. A deficiency of one member of the vitamin B complex is often related to deficiencies of others, both dietarily and physiologically. Nasolabial dermatitis may be a sign of pyridoxine deficiency. Changes in color and papillae of the tongue may occur in deficiencies of folacin or cobalamin. Follicular hyperkeratosis has been reported in fatty acid or B-vitamin deficiencies. As our knowledge of nutrients and their deficiencies increases, the interpretation of clinical signs is changed and expanded.

The major purpose of including these observations in the physical examination is to indicate whether nutritional problems may exist within a population. Further confirmation by biochemical or dietary study and investigation of causes unrelated to nutrients are required before a final diagnosis can be made.

A dental examination should be included in nutritional assessment. The state of dental health may reflect dietary inadequacy during tooth formation or the carbohydrate and fluorine intakes following tooth eruption. In addition, severe dental problems may influence food intake and may be a cause of present dietary inadequacy. Screening should include a count of decayed, missing, and filled teeth and an evaluation of the status of gingival hygiene. The poor state of dental health and the obvious lack of dental care were among the major findings of the TSNS.[4]

## Anthropometric Measurements

Growth is a sensitive indicator of nutritional status in children. In developing countries, measurements of weight and height, and their ratio, are primary indexes of protein-calorie malnutrition and are especially useful for children whose ages may not be known. The smoothness of growth in the healthy, well-nourished child has been well documented and a number of growth charts are readily available (see chapter 4).

The pattern of growth over a time period and the child's progress along a consistent channel are the best measures of whether the diet is supplying sufficient nutrients for growth, energy, and other physiological needs without the excess which may lead to obesity. In surveys which provide only a single contact with the child, the one available set of measurements will provide a tentative evaluation of growth, at least by identifying the child who is very short, thin, or heavy for his age so that he may be studied further.

A large array of body measurements may be done, but for practical use measurements should be limited to those which contribute most to the evaluation of growth, of overnutrition, and of undernutrition. The choice of anthropometric measurements will also depend on the age of the child, his cooperation in the procedure, the degree of detail desired, and the skill and accuracy of the examiners. Infants and very young children are difficult to measure accurately because of crying and resistance to handling. Older children are usually more cooperative in positioning and remaining still; then the skill of the examiner is the major source of error.

Weight and height are the measurements best standardized and most reliable in the hands of semitrained personnel. Other measurements should be obtained only by skilled workers carefully trained in the techniques. If more than one examiner participates in the taking of measurements, their techniques and reliability should be standardized and compared to limit interexaminer differences and to improve the reproducibility of the measurements. Equipment and techniques for various measurements have been described in detail in survey reports.[6]

Measurements which are especially helpful in the nutritional assessment of children include the following:

Stature: Recumbent length from birth to two years of age;
standing height after two years; one may also measure stem length
(crown-rump length) to two years; sitting height after two years

imental studies of urinary excretion may provide a measure
saturation. After a known amount of a nutrient, such as
acid, has been given, a high percentage of the test dose is
if the tissues are well saturated and a lower percentage if a
cy exists. Load tests may also be used as a measure of nu-
n the body. For example, in a pyridoxine deficiency the feed-
ryptophan results in the excretion of xanthurenic acid because
nterruption of the normal conversion of tryptophan to niacin.
e deficiency a load test of histidine results in the excretion of
inoglutamic acid (FIGLU), an intermediary product. These
e rarely done in surveys, however.

nt studies have suggested that analysis of hair may provide
ce of zinc or copper deficiency, but much work must be done
dardize techniques and interpretation of results.

ction of tests for nutritional assessment has more often been
on practicality and simplicity of the analytic procedures than
significance and sensitivity of the tests. "The biochemical
rement of nutrients in the blood (serum or plasma) is at best
e indicator of the supply of these nutrients. It does not tell us
he nutrient content is in the body tissue stores, such as liver or
marrow. It is, however, the only feasible method under the cir-
ances of a field survey."[5] Many tests require elaborate equip-
or facilities which are not readily available. Reproducibility of
tests is poor, and wide variations in results from different lab-
ries have been reported. There is great need for improved meth-
gy and for simple and reliable tests which will produce com-
le results.

ere is especially need for more data on which to base the physio-
al significance of variations in blood levels. Much of the cur-
y available data have been derived from young adult males, for
n standards therefore have greater reliability. The greatest gaps
owledge occur in other age and sex groups, especially pregnant
en and children. Despite lack of adequate data, surveys have
lished standards for rating blood levels as "high," "acceptable,"
," and "deficient," as TSNS and HANES have, not always with
same cutoff points, or as "high risk," "moderate risk," and "low
" as the Canadian group did with still different levels for some of
biochemicals. Not only is the use of this terminology confusing,
the selection of different cutoff points makes difficult the com-
son of findings in the various surveys. This problem will not be
lved until we have enough data on blood levels and the accom-

Weight: Obtained on all subjects

Circumferences: Head and chest circumferences to six years;
additional circumferences for comparison with weight: waist,
upper arm, midthigh, and midcalf

Diameters: Wrist, knee, hip, and shoulder widths

Skinfolds: Triceps, subscapular, and chest skinfold thicknesses,
using specially designed calipers

An additional component of the clinical-anthropometric assessment may include a posterior-anterior roentgenogram of the wrist and
hand. The calcification of centers of ossification compared to a standard such as the Greulich-Pyle *Radiographic Atlas of Skeletal Development of the Hand and Wrist*[11] gives an estimation of skeletal
age for contrast with chronological age as an index to maturational
level.

## Biochemical Assessment

Biochemical studies which are applicable to nutrition surveys have
been summarized by WHO as shown in table 2.3. In the first category
are tests "which have been most extensively applied in nutrition surveys and have had their usefulness demonstrated. They are relatively
simple and their use is feasible in general nutrition surveys. The urine
studies include those which require only a single urine specimen. . . .
Application of methods in the second category usually involves relatively more complicated procedures."[3]

Blood studies may measure the levels of the nutrients themselves,
metabolites of nutrients, or enzymes for which nutrients are essential.
Those nutrients which can be measured directly include protein (total, albumin, or amino acids), calcium, vitamin A and carotene,
ascorbic acid, and lipids. Interpretation of the findings varies with
each nutrient, however. Measurement of plasma calcium may be of
limited value because of physiological homeostatic mechanisms which
maintain plasma calcium within a small range. Ascorbic acid levels
in serum are probably less meaningful than the levels in white blood
cells. Because of large body reserves of vitamin A, plasma levels are
poor indicators of nutritional status of the body. To minimize effects
of activity and recent intake, it is best to obtain the blood sample in
the morning when the subject is in a fasting state, but this is not often
possible in field surveys.

**Table 2.3**    Biochemical Studies Applicable to Nutrition Surveys

| Nutritional Deficiency | First Category* | Second Category |
|---|---|---|
| (1) Protein | Total serum protein<br>Serum albumin<br>Urinary urea (F)† | Serum protein fractions by electrophoresis<br>Urinary creatinine per unit of time (T) |
| (2) Vitamin A | Serum vitamin A<br>Serum carotene | |
| (3) Vitamin D | Serum alkaline phosphatase in young children | Serum inorganic phosphorus |
| (4) Ascorbic acid | Serum ascorbic acid | White blood cell ascorbic acid<br>Urinary ascorbic acid<br>Load test |
| (5) Thiamine | Urinary thiamine (F)† | Load test<br>Blood pyruvate<br>Blood lactate<br>Red blood cell hemolysate transketolase |
| (6) Riboflavin | Urinary riboflavin (F)† | Red blood cell riboflavin<br>Load test |
| (7) Niacin | Urinary N-methyl-nicotinamide (F)† | Load test<br>Urinary pyridone<br>(N-methyl-2-pyridone-5-carbonamide) |
| (8) Iron | Hemoglobin } Thin blood<br>Hematocrit } smear | Serum iron<br>% saturation of transferrin |
| (9) Iodine | | Urinary iodine (F)<br>Tests for thyroid function |

SOURCE: World Health Organization. *Expert Committee on Medical Assessment of Nutritional Status: Report.* Technical report series no. 258. Geneva: World Health Organization, 1963.
NOTE: Serum cholesterol levels vary widely in population groups with different dietary habits. The determination may

For some nutrients the blood
metabolism may indicate that a vit
the normal sequence of metabolism
of pyruvic acid occurs with incomp
result of thiamine deficiency.

The measurement of enzymes in
to the onset of malnutrition. The lev
vide a clue to the state of the body
form part of the enzyme or coenz
blood cell transketolase may be an
and glutathione reductase of riboflav
widely used or well standardized.

Other tests may include count of r
folate, serum B$_{12}$, serum magnesium,
erides. Prothrombin levels, as an ind
fected by vitamin K deficiency, and th
cells by vitamin E nutrition.

Studies of urinary excretion have
levels and therefore are less meaningfu
four-hour period would provide the
feasible. The urine specimen is usuall
time. Since urinary creatinine is deri
muscle and is a reflection of muscle m
relatively constant and is often used as
of thiamine, riboflavin, or N-methylnicc
per gram of creatinine when a single
alyzed. However, because of diurnal and
of both creatinine and vitamins, this is n
be obtained from a twenty-four-hour col

Additional urinary excretion studies n
TSNS and the Nutrition Canada Survey
goiter was not necessarily related to iodi
factors other than iodine nutrition were i
goiters. Urinary analyses may also incl
blood, more as indicators of pathology th

often be included in nutriti
ported association of serum
sclerosis.
*Urinary creatinine used a
urine measurements in first c
†Expressed per gram of creat
(F), in a single urine specime
(T), in timed urine specimens

Exper
of body
ascorbic
excreted
deficien
trients
ing of t
of the i
In fola
formim
tests a
Rec
eviden
to stan
Sele
based
on the
measu
a cruc
what
bone
cumst
ment
some
orato
odolc
paral
Th
logic
rentl
who
in k
won
esta
"lo
the
risk
the
but
par
res

panying physiological findings to provide unanimity of opinion. A table of guidelines for laboratory evaluations is given in appendix 2.

One example of the questionable interpretation of results because of inadequate age-related standards has been shown with vitamin A in three surveys.[4,5,7] In TSNS it was found that "in both low- and high-income ratio states, mean vitamin A levels increased with age. This trend was seen for both sexes and for all ethnic groups." In HANES, "The steady increase of mean serum levels with age suggests the need for a revision of standards by taking these age differences into account." However in each survey a single standard for plasma vitamin A was used for all age groups, with the obvious result that infants and young children had a high frequency of "deficient" or "low" ratings and the elderly had a low frequency of poor ratings. The use of an age-adjusted standard would have provided a very different interpretation of findings. On the basis of evidence presented, one cannot say that the young have more vitamin A deficiency than the old, but that is the superficial interpretation.

Biochemical assessment is a valuable adjunct to the evaluation of nutritional status; its value will increase as methodology and standards of judgment improve.

## Dietary Assessment

Dietary studies are an integral part of nutritional assessment. The aim is to obtain reliable information on the foods consumed by an individual or group in order to estimate the adequacy or inadequacy of intake. Since nutrient intake has long-term effects on physical growth and physiological state, it would be ideal to know the intake of an individual from conception. Obviously this is impractical. Except in longitudinal studies in which nutrition histories are repeated at intervals so that a continuous record of intake is obtained, most studies rely on the use of short-term data. Several methods have been developed, each with advantages and disadvantages, but none is totally satisfactory.

The choice of method depends on the purpose of the study, the personnel and funding available, the number of subjects and their intelligence and cooperation, and the degree of precision necessary. Information may be obtained on the diets of individuals or groups, by interview or self-recording, by estimation of amounts or weighing of foods, on complete diets or selected categories of foods, and for time periods ranging from one day to several months. The scoring of food intake or the calculation of nutrient content and the interpretation of results depend on the type of information obtained.

The purpose of the study may be:

To obtain information on food or nutrient intakes to compare different groups of people

To identify risk groups as a basis for educational or intervention programs

To screen individuals for further study of possible deficiencies

To evaluate the effects of nutrition programs

To conduct research, often multidisciplinary, on individuals for a given period of time

For each of these purposes one or more of the following dietary study methods may be adapted.

For a group of people with a common food preparation area, such as a household, boarding school, orphanage, or other institution, a record of the food used during a given period of time may be obtained. Adjustments may be made for food wasted and for food eaten elsewhere by members of the group. This provides an estimate of average consumption of the group but does not allow for the unequal distribution of food consumption by individuals within the unit. It is useful for comparing average intakes of different groups and for identifying groups which may be at risk of malnutrition.

Four basic methods are in common use for obtaining dietary information on individuals: twenty-four-hour intakes, food frequency lists, nutrition histories, and weighed intake. These methods vary in their value and use, their advantages and limitations, and in the personnel required to obtain them.

The twenty-four-hour intake is the method most commonly used in surveys of large populations. This summary of the kinds and amounts of all foods consumed by a subject in a twenty-four-hour period (usually from midnight to midnight) may be by recall on the following day or by record kept on the day of consumption. It may be obtained by interview or self-recorded with appropriate instructions. Opinions differ on the structure of the form, the number and selection of days, and the use of food models, each of which may affect the results in different ways.

An unstructured form merely has lines on which the subject records the foods eaten; often omitted are butter, cream, sugar, sauces, salad dressings, and other additions to basic foods. The structured form lists foods which might be consumed at various meals, with the additions above noted on the form; this may suggest to the subject that such foods "should" be eaten. Food portion models may be used to help the subject in estimating amounts, but may suggest responses. Usually the record is for a single day, but the period may be extended to two, three, or even seven days. The longer record gives a better average of intake, but may result in decreased cooperation and reliability in recording. Nutrient content of the food may be calculated from food value tables or ratings may be made of the intake of food groups.

The major disadvantage of the twenty-four-hour intake is that there is no assurance that intake on the day recorded is typical of usual current intake or of long-term intake. In countries with a wide choice of foods, marked variability in selection may occur from day to day. In addition, daily variation may be caused by appetite, activity, time schedules, and so on. Divergent opinions exist on whether the twenty-four-hour intake should be obtained only for a weekday, which tends to be standardized, or should include a weekend day, which tends to be variable. Median differences between the lowest and highest intakes on four recorded days of children in a longitudinal study[12] ranged from approximately 100 kcal in infants to more than 600 kcal in adolescents. Daily variations are wide in all nutrients, but the highest error is likely to be in vitamin A because of the high content of some food sources. Daily variation limits the usefulness of the twenty-four-hour intake as an index of typical intake and decreases the likelihood of meaningful correlations of intake with biochemical findings. This method should be used only with group data, and no effort should be made to seek association with other findings in the individual.

Despite its limitations, the twenty-four-hour intake method is used in most surveys because it is the least expensive dietary technique, both in time and in personnel, and may be used by semitrained workers. The recall intake is dependent on the memory of the subject, but completeness of the recall may be improved by adroit probing by the interviewer. Self-recording of food consumption is often improved by including questions on activities of the day as a framework within which to identify eating periods.

A food frequency list may be used to record how often, but not how much, of various foods have been consumed over a given period of time. The list may be extensive or may be limited to specific types of foods, such as dietary sources of fats or of ascorbic acid. The food frequency list cannot be calculated for nutrient content because sizes of servings are not determined, but it may be rated by a food-scoring system.

The detailed nutrition history is a more expensive and time-consuming method which requires a trained nutritionist. By interview the nutritionist obtains an estimation of the frequency and amounts of various foods consumed in a specified time period, usually one to three months. The interview is best conducted during a home visit, which permits measurement of serving sizes, checking content of recipes, brand names of products used, and other data to increase accuracy. Of the historical methods available, this is the only one which permits calculation of the usual nutrient content of diets of individuals and is more likely to be successful in correlating nutrient intake data with physical and biochemical findings.

The weighed food intake method is the most detailed and accurate, especially if accompanied by analysis of aliquot food samples, and is used primarily in balance studies or in controlled experiments. The methodology and expense restrict its use to few subjects and short periods of time. There have been a few reports in the literature of individuals weighing their food intake for extended periods of time, and British studies are more likely to involve weighing of foods in surveys, partially because of the common use of food scales in households.

Examples of the forms used in some of these methods are shown in appendix 3, and further details may be found in a number of publications.[9,13–16] Sometimes a combination of methods has been used. Although TSNS and HANES used a single twenty-four-hour recall, PNS obtained two twenty-four-hour records and also used a questionnaire to elicit information on who was responsible for feeding the child, where and by whom food shopping was done, and additional information of particular import to the feeding of preschool children. The Nutrition Canada National Survey obtained a twenty-four-hour recall and a food frequency questionnaire covering the previous month.

The accuracy of dietary study depends on the selection of the methodology, the skill of the interviewer, the rapport between interviewer and subject, and the intelligence, motivation, and memory of the subject. Most people have little reason to remember what they have eaten and recall may be incomplete. Advance warning or measurement of intake may cause alteration in the usual pattern of eating. For each method, one must be aware of potential errors and develop techniques to minimize such errors. Unfortunately, little effort has been expended to improve dietary study methodology. Increasing sophistication of anthropometric and biochemical methodology is too often accompanied by inadequate and inaccurate dietary data.

When the dietary data include amounts of food consumed, nutrient content may be calculated. Several techniques have been devised to limit the extensive and painstaking calculations required, usually by grouping foods of similar nutrient content. However, the present availability of computer programs for calculation of nutrient content has eliminated much of the drudgery. Calculations in the United States and Canada are usually based on U.S.D.A. *Handbook No. 8*[17] or on *Handbook No. 456.*[18] Food values in these publications represent averages from all parts of the country and practicality dictates their use despite the fact that they may not represent actual content of the foods consumed by the subjects. Food analysis is expensive and not feasible except in the most demanding balance study conditions.

The final step in dietary assessment is judging the adequacy of the diet. Standards of recommended nutrient intake have been established by FAO/WHO and by many countries in the world. Some standards reflect optimal allowances in countries with generous supplies of food, while others are intended to provide moderate levels of intake consistent with freedom from deficiencies for populations adapted to low intakes. Differences between standards also reflect incomplete knowledge and divergence of opinion. For example, the iron recommendations for females between menarche and menopause vary from a high of 18 mg daily in the United States, 15 mg in two countries, 14 mg by FAO/WHO, 12 mg in several countries, to a low of 10 mg in others. Changes in time also affect standards for evaluation. The Recommended Dietary Allowances (RDA)[19] for iron for infants and women have increased, but protein recommendations for all age groups have decreased. For example, the RDA for protein for the five-year-old child was 50 gm from 1943 through the 1958 revision, then decreased to 30 gm by 1974. The RDA for protein for the fourteen-year-old girl dropped from 80 gm to 44 gm and for the eighteen-year-old male from 100 gm to 54 gm. In comparing surveys published in the past which have used RDA levels as benchmarks, it is essential to know which RDA revision was used.

Confusion in the use of standards has been compounded in recent surveys. The TSNS[4] adopted standards for intakes of children from a variety of sources. Caloric and protein standards were expressed as a function of weight for age groups; calcium and vitamin A were considerably lower than RDA and closer to FAO/WHO standards; 30 mg of ascorbic acid was used for all age groups; the higher iron figures of the RDA were used; and thiamine, riboflavin, and niacin were expressed per 1,000 kcal, with a single standard for each vitamin for all age groups. HANES[5] used the same standards as TSNS except for ascorbic acid, which was 40 mg for children to twelve years of age and 50 mg thereafter. In contrast, the Canadian standards[7] were higher in protein for young children and lower for adolescents, higher in calcium for all ages after one year, lower in iron at nearly all ages, and lower in ascorbic acid for the child under five years. Obviously, when one compares data from the three surveys, the differences in dietary standards affect interpretation of findings.

### Selected Findings from Nutritional Status Surveys

Concern about malnutrition in technologically underdeveloped areas of the world occupied the attention of health specialists particularly during the period following World War II. In the developed countries only intermittent attention had been given to nutritional status over the years. Economics was a source of concern during the depression of the 1930s and availability of food during World War II, but in other times it was assumed that the plentiful food supply meant adequate nutrition for the population.

In the United States concern about possible malnutrition became widespread in the middle 1960s. At first this concern was an offshoot of the civil rights movement. In the winter of 1965–66, thirty-five blacks occupied an abandoned air base in Mississippi to protest inadequacy of jobs, housing, money, and food. In 1967 a subcommittee of the U.S. Senate, a group of physicians financed by a foundation, and the Child Development Group of Mississippi all reported that hunger, malnutrition, and inadequate medical care were major problems in that state.

Within the next year a number of reports of hunger and malnutrition in the United States appeared, including *Hunger, U.S.A.* from the Citizens' Board of Inquiry into Hunger and Malnutrition in the United States,[20] a television program on "Hunger in America," and a series of magazine and newspaper articles, with varying degrees of accuracy and alarm. Hunger and malnutrition were major issues in the Poor People's Campaign and March on Washington, D.C., in 1968. These concerns led to hearings by the Select Committee on Nutrition and Human Needs of the U.S. Senate and finally to the White House Conference on Food, Nutrition, and Health[21] in December 1969. It became evident that there were pockets of malnutrition in the United States, especially among blacks, migrant workers' families, Indians and Spanish-Americans of the Southwest, and whites in Appalachia, and inner city areas of the country. Scurvy, rickets, kwashiorkor, and marasmus were reported in children. The reports were fragmentary, however, and often emotionally expressed and difficult to verify. It was obvious that carefully designed surveys must be undertaken to document the type and extent of malnutrition in various population groups.

In 1968–70 two surveys were conducted: the Ten-State Nutrition Survey (TSNS) and the Preschool Nutrition Survey (PNS), both under the aegis of the U.S. Department of Health, Education, and Welfare. In 1971–72 nutrition studies were added to the continuing surveillance of health status of the U.S. population by the National Center for Health Statistics of the Department of Health, Education, and Welfare. Canada was also concerned about the nutritional health of its people, and in 1970–72 the first national survey of Canada was undertaken by the Department of National Health and Welfare following a recommendation by the Canadian Council on Nutrition. Other countries have also conducted surveys recently, but the present discussion will be limited to these four surveys on the North American continent. The reports of the surveys are extensive; only selected findings related to the nutritional health of children will be summarized here.

---

### Ten-State Nutrition Survey

This survey[4] was designed to investigate areas of the country where malnutrition might be expected to exist. The geographical areas selected had been in the lowest income quartile in the 1960 census; some middle and high income families in each area were included in the sampling. With the emphasis on economically deprived families, "the survey findings cannot be extrapolated and applied to the overall population of states from which the samples were drawn." The central program provided consultation, technical assistance, monitoring, and analysis of data, but a different survey team was recruited in each state by the state health department or a university medical school, resulting in some differences in data collection among the states.

Ten states were selected, with a separate survey of New York City. Later analysis of data showed that the states could be divided into two groups by income level: the low income ratio (LIR) states were

Texas, Louisiana, South Carolina, Kentucky, and West Virginia; the high income ratio (HIR) states were Washington, California, Michigan, Massachusetts, and New York.

Demographic data were obtained on 24,000 families comprised of approximately 86,000 persons. Approximately 40,000 individuals had clinical evaluations, which included medical history, physical and dental examinations, anthropometric measurements, wrist roentgenograms, and blood drawn for hemoglobin and hematocrit determinations. Subgroups whose risk of malnutrition might be higher were selected for more detailed dietary and biochemical evaluations and included children under three years, adolescents between ten and sixteen years, pregnant and lactating women, and persons over sixty years of age. Blacks, whites, and Spanish-Americans were ethnic groups considered separately. Two income groups were differentiated as above or below an established "poverty level."

Little clinical evidence of severe malnutrition in children was found. Most of the signs were nonspecific; skin, hair, eyes, and tongue showed a few positive findings which were generally inconclusive. Thyroid enlargement was lowest in whites and highest in Spanish-Americans but unrelated to urinary iodine excretion. In young children findings that might be related to rickets were more common in Spanish-Americans in LIR states and winged scapulae were more common in whites in all states. Bitot's spots were not found in any children under six years, and in 0 to 0.4% of all persons over six years. It was concluded that the clinical examination "did not provide a useful means of identifying specific populations at increased nutritional risk."

Dental examinations showed a high rate of decayed, missing, and filled teeth, which increased with age in all income and ethnic groups to means of six to eleven affected teeth in various ethnic and income groups by seventeen years. Differences in dental care were obvious. White children had more filled teeth; black and especially Spanish-American children had more decayed teeth. The number of filled teeth was higher in HIR states and the number of unfilled decayed teeth higher in LIR states. The state of dental health was unrelated to carbohydrates from desserts and foods that were primarily sugar eaten at meals, but was related to between-meal eating of those carbohydrates by all ethnic groups in the HIR states but only by blacks in the LIR states.

Anthropometric measurements showed marked ethnic differences. Blacks were taller than whites, regardless of income level, until adolescence, after which differences were not consistent. Black children were more advanced in skeletal and dental development, with earlier appearance of ossification centers and permanent tooth eruption, and were estimated (by extrapolation from measurements of the second metacarpal bone of the hand) to have heavier skeletons. White children, on the other hand, tended to be slightly heavier and had larger subcutaneous fat measurements. This indicated that black children had more lean body mass and white children more fat as proportions of total body weight. Differences in head circumference were not consistent. Obesity, as measured by the Seltzer-Mayer standards of triceps measurements,[22] was more common (11% to 39%) in white male adolescents than in other groups during childhood.

Aside from ethnic differences in growth, there were differences between the two groups of states. Children in HIR states tended to be taller, heavier, and fatter with earlier skeletal maturation and larger head circumferences than children in LIR states.

Evaluation of height measurements of children in TSNS raised questions about the applicability of the Stuart-Meredith standards,[23] which will be discussed in greater detail in chapter 4. The percentage frequency of children who were rated short for age was greater in the low income groups, but with little consistent difference between various sex or ethnic groups. Although poverty was associated with an excess of short-for-age children, the findings were "not fully explained in terms of income or other identifiable factors affecting nutrition," suggesting the need for development of more appropriate standards, specifically for black children.

Biochemical studies also underlined the need for improved standards for evaluation. Low serum albumin levels were found in a large proportion of pregnant and lactating women, but mean dietary protein intakes were generally above levels considered to be adequate. Plasma vitamin A levels were often low in Spanish-American children in LIR states, but there was no supporting clinical evidence of vitamin A deficiency. Iodine excretion showed no evidence of dietary deficiency despite the prevalence of goiter, which was assumed not to be a result of iodine deficiency.

The most consistently low blood levels were found for hemoglobin and hematocrit in all segments of the population. These tended to be associated with low serum iron and transferrin saturation, and to a lesser extent with low levels of serum and erythrocyte folate. There was a tendency for the lower hemoglobin levels to be associated with lower dietary intakes of iron. Two findings in relation to hemoglobin levels deserve special note. First, blood levels related to iron nutriture were lower for blacks than for whites at all ages, income levels, and dietary intakes, suggesting a difference in hematopoiesis between the two ethnic groups. Second, a high frequency of low hemoglobin levels was found in adolescent males, indicating "either that the standard for males should be revised or that there was a heretofore unappreciated problem of anemia among males." The hemoglobin standard for males above twelve years of age was 1.5 gm/100 ml blood higher than for females, and standards for serum iron, hematocrit, and transferrin saturation were also higher.

Mean dietary intakes of all nutrients except iron tended to be above the standards. However, means were elevated because of some very high intakes, and medians were lower than means, especially for iron, vitamin A, and ascorbic acid. Calorie intakes tended to be higher in HIR than in LIR states, indicating a relationship to income. More than one-half of the fifteen- to sixteen-year-olds had caloric intakes below the standard; for females this probably reflected weight consciousness. Mean intakes of calcium tended to be well above the standards for children under three years, but 6% of infants in the last half of the first year had intakes under 400 mg, and the frequency increased to 30% at two to three years, when diminished milk intake is common. Low calcium intakes of some children were observed also at older ages. Although mean calcium intakes of adolescents were generally above the standard (650 mg), 20% to 54% of ten- to sixteen-year-olds had intakes below that level.

Iron intakes were more often below the standard than any other nutrient. As noted previously, the RDA for iron was used as a standard in the TSNS and is higher during adolescence than for any other country. Iron intake was not consistently related to income. Iron intake per 1,000 kcal was often higher among the low income groups. It was concluded that the low intakes were the result of the generally low iron level of the U.S. diet.

## Preschool Nutrition Survey

This survey[10] was designed to evaluate nutritional status of a representative sample of children between one and six years of age in all sections of the country at all income levels. A total of 3,441 children were included with some data, and clinical examinations were done on approximately 2,300, from thirty-six states and the District of Columbia. Pilot studies were done in Mississippi and Ohio, followed by the national survey between November 1968 and December 1970. Unlike the TSNS, PNS used a single team of trained interviewers and examiners to conduct the entire survey; biochemical determinations were done in a single laboratory and computations by a single computer center. The variance in findings in PNS was smaller than in TSNS.

The subjects were nearly equally divided by sex and age groups and included 80% white, 14% black, 5% Latin American, and 1% American Indian or Oriental. Data were published for white and black subjects. Four categories of socioeconomic status were based on income, occupation, and housing. The lowest group had incomes less than $5,500 per year, and it was estimated that 75% of the families in TSNS were probably also in this category. Data in PNS included a medical history with retrospective prenatal and birth information as well as a health history, physical and dental examinations, hand and wrist roentgenogram, anthropometry, blood and urine studies, and dietary data based on two-day diet records and a questionnaire dealing with the feeding of the child and family attitudes and activities involving food.

Clinical examinations found relatively few of the signs which might suggest nutritional deficiencies. When abnormal physical signs were found, there was essentially no correlation with biochemical or dietary variables in individual children, but some group relationships were found. The only evidences of nutritional risk were some low dietary intakes and biochemical indexes and small physical size for age, which tended to be clustered among children of lower socioeconomic status. Since the majority of the children in the two lower socioeconomic ranks were black, an attempt was made to separate racial and genetic factors from economic factors.

Black children were lighter in weight at birth but by two years were taller and heavier with more advanced osseous development than white children. However, mean thoracic skinfold thicknesses of white children were higher than those for black children. In agreement with the TSNS data, this indicated the greater lean body mass and more rapid skeletal development of blacks and the higher body fat of white children.

Dental examinations produced results somewhat different from the TSNS data, but the PNS examinations were restricted to deciduous teeth. White children had fewer decayed, extracted, or filled teeth despite higher carbohydrate intakes, in contrast to black children. The caries attack rate was higher in the lower income groups.

Hemoglobin levels and transferrin saturation were higher in white children than in black, even when age and socioeconomic status were held constant. Other factors related to hematopoiesis showed inconsistencies. White children, but not black children, who took vitamin/ mineral supplements tended to have higher hemoglobin levels, but not necessarily an increase in transferrin saturation. The fifth and tenth percentiles of hemoglobin levels tended to rise with income, but there was little change in higher percentile levels. Transferrin saturation showed no consistent relationship to income. Within each ethnic group, taller and heavier boys tended to have higher hemoglobin levels, but no such relationship was observed in girls. PNS children in the lowest socioeconomic group had higher hemoglobin levels and higher iron intakes than TSNS children.

Children in upper socioeconomic groups had lower total plasma protein levels despite higher protein intakes. Black children had higher total plasma protein levels but slightly lower plasma albumin levels than white children. Plasma albumin levels rose with income. Cholesterol and triglyceride levels had no statistically significant relationship to intake of calories or energy-yielding nutrients. The only significant correlations between biochemical variables and the corresponding dietary nutrients were found for plasma urea nitrogen, plasma ascorbic acid, and urinary riboflavin. It appeared that when supplements of more than 125 mg ascorbic acid were taken, virtually all of the excess was excreted.

Low dietary intakes were more often found in the lowest socioeconomic group than in the upper three. Since intakes low in calories tended to be low in most other nutrients, there was little variation among the four income groups in concentration of nutrients per 1,000 kcal. Therefore it was concluded that "with the possible exception of ascorbic acid, nutritional quality of the diet correlates poorly with socioeconomic status. . . . Among the socioeconomically depressed the problem is more one of lack of sufficient quantity of food than of nutritional quality."

## Health and Nutrition Examination Survey

Whereas the TSNS and PNS were intended as single-time surveys, the purpose of HANES has been to measure the nutritional status of the U.S. population and monitor changes in status over time. Health data were intended to be used as an objective test of programs to improve nutritional status and to provide an improved basis for allocation of scarce nutrition program resources. The National Health Survey was initiated under the National Health Survey Act of 1956 and has conducted periodic examinations of representative samples of the

U.S. population in a cyclic fashion. A series of reports have been published on the health status of noninstitutionalized persons from one to seventy-four years of age. The nutritional assessment aspect of the surveys was begun with data collection for the first cycle between April 1971 and October 1972. Preliminary reports[5,6] of selected dietary, biochemical, anthropometric, and clinical findings in the first partial sample have been published and will be followed by more extensive reports. The second cycle, HANES II, was started in 1976.

As a scientifically designed probability sample of the population, HANES will permit estimates to be made for the entire U.S. population. Certain groups at high risk of malnutrition—the poor, preschool children, women of childbearing ages, and the elderly—were selected for more detailed data collection. The preliminary reports are based on thirty-five of the total of sixty-five primary sampling units in the country and include more than 10,000 persons between one and seventy-four years of age. Data are reported for whites (73%) and blacks (26%), at incomes above and below a selected poverty income level. Data summarized here are from the age groups one to five years, six to eleven years, and twelve to seventeen years.

> The clinical data show in general a fairly low prevalence of high and moderate risk signs for most nutritional deficiencies. There were a few exceptions, however, where the percent prevalence exceeds 10 percent. This is the case for follicular hyperkeratosis (vitamin A) in Negro children aged 6–11 years below poverty level, grade I goiter (iodine) in Negro youths aged 12–17 years above poverty level, a positive Chvostek's sign (calcium) in both racial and income groups of the same ages, and fungiform papillary hypertrophy of the tongue (niacin) for all Negroes. . . . Older people show generally a higher prevalence of more signs than the young do.[6]

Some signs tended to be more frequent in black than in white children, such as cheilosis, bleeding and swollen gums, bowed legs and knock-knees, but with low frequency and little or no relationship to income.

Stature was usually greater in black than in white children between one and seventeen years, but not consistently at all ages. Mean stature tended to be greater in children in the income group above poverty than in the lower group, but the differences were less than 2.5 cm in ten of the seventeen age comparisons. Mean weights and median triceps skinfold measurements were better correlated with income, especially in males between nine and sixteen years of age. Black males tended to be slightly heavier to eleven years and white males heavier thereafter; less ethnic difference was evident in females.

Mean triceps skinfolds were higher in white than in black children at almost all ages and in both sexes. Children in the higher income group had larger triceps skinfold thicknesses at almost all ages. Differences in subscapular skinfold measurements were usually not very great in relation to either ethnic group or income.

Mean caloric intakes, based on a single twenty-four-hour recall, were higher in upper income children than in lower income children. At all ages between one and seventeen years mean caloric intakes were higher for white than for black children; black mean intakes were approximately 80% of the means for white children. Mean intakes of protein, calcium, vitamin A, and ascorbic acid were well above the standards; in fact, mean intakes of vitamin A were sometimes double the standard. The high means must be considered in relation to wide individual variations. For example, 30% of black and 13% of white children between one and five years at both income levels had calcium intakes below the standard. As many as 52% of children in some age groups had vitamin A intakes below the standard. Blacks tended to have higher intakes of both vitamin A and ascorbic acid than white children, despite their lower caloric intakes. Race and income were not related to differences in mean intakes of iron, which were below the standard at nearly all ages. A relatively high standard for iron intake was met or exceeded by only 5% of one- to five-year-old children.

Blood levels of proteins, vitamin A, and iron-containing factors were included in the preliminary report. Means of total serum protein were higher for black than for white children and were also higher in the low income group than in the upper income children, possibly due to higher gamma globulin levels. Less than 5% of total plasma protein levels were considered low, and these were found more often in white children. There were no cases of low serum albumin values in children between one and seventeen years of age; mean levels tended to be higher for white than for black children.

As indicated previously, with the use of standards not adjusted for age, "low" levels of serum vitamin A were more often found in the youngest age group. Low serum values were found more often in black children of both income levels, but there was little correlation between serum vitamin A and dietary intake of the vitamin.

Similar to findings in TSNS and PNS, hemoglobin and hematocrit levels were lower for black than for white children in all age groups regardless of income. Of particular interest were observations in pre-

school children and adolescents. Low levels of iron-related blood substances were found more often in the one- to five-year-old children.
For example, 2.5% of these children had low serum iron values and
10.5% had low transferrin saturation. However, separation of this
age group by years showed that the risk decreased with age. Incidence of low serum iron values decreased from 4.2% at one year to
0.3% at five years and incidence of low transferrin saturation values
decreased from 16.9% of children at one year to 5.8% at five years.

For combined sexes in the twelve to seventeen year age group,
four to six times as many blacks had low ratings of hemoglobin and
hematocrit as did white children, regardless of income. The differences for serum iron and transferrin saturation were in the same direction but of a lower order of magnitude. The higher standards for
males resulted in marked sex differences. The percentages of "low"
values for the twelve- to seventeen-year-old males and females were
as follows: hemoglobin, 7.4% of males, 1.9% of females; hematocrit, 15.5% of males, 2.4% of females; serum iron, 2.8% of males,
1.1% of females; and saturation of transferrin, 7.7% of males and
5.3% of females. As was concluded in TSNS, either the standards
need revision or there was a high incidence of iron-deficiency anemia
among teenage males.

Further reports with additional data from the National Center for
Health Statistics and synthesis of findings from various aspects of the
survey may well provide the basis for improved evaluation of early
signs of moderate degrees of malnutrition. HANES II will provide
observation of changes in nutritional status over time.

## Nutrition Canada National Survey

More than 19,000 individuals between birth and 65+ years of age,
selected by sample designs for each of three population groups, were
surveyed to assess nutritional status according to geographic region,
two income levels, and two seasons. Medical, dental, and anthropometric examinations, a twenty-four-hour recall, and a food frequency list covering one month were obtained from all subjects; the
vast majority also had blood and urine analyses. A sample of nearly
1,000 women in the last trimester of pregnancy was included. Three
teams completed all the field work; a single laboratory was used for
all biochemical analyses; and a single center was used for all data
processing. More detailed data on food consumption patterns,[24] and
specific reports for each province, for Indians on reservations, and

for Eskimos in settlements[25] have followed the preliminary report[7] of selected data.

Age groupings for presentation of findings in the preliminary report were 0 to 4 years, 5 to 9 years, 10 to 19 years, 20 to 39 years, 40 to 64 years, and 65+ years. Sexes were combined to age nine and thereafter separated for analyses. No consistent effect of season, income (above or below a poverty level), or size of community was observed in the general population findings. The Indian and Eskimo populations indicated greater risk of malnutrition than did the general population.

Like the U.S. surveys, the Canadian survey found little clinical evidence of malnutrition. No clinical manifestations were found of deficiencies of vitamin A, thiamine, riboflavin, niacin, or folate. There was no indication of rickets in children under five years of age in any of the three population groups. Moderate risk of protein-calorie malnutrition was found in young children, based on edema, weight deficit, and hair changes. The frequency ranged from 4% to 5% in the general population, 3% to 7% in Indians, and 6% to 9% in Eskimo children under nine years of age. Only two children had body weight less than 60% of the median for age, but 5% had weights between 60% and 80% of the median.

Clinical signs indicating high risk of ascorbic acid deficiency were found in 3% to 5% of Indian adolescents and in less than 1% of the other two population groups, despite the fact that both serum and dietary levels of ascorbic acid were more often low in the Eskimo than in the Indian children. Moderate degrees of goiter were found in 7% to 10% of adolescents in the general population, which was higher than in Indian or Eskimo groups. The goiters were found more often in the prairie states, but iodine excretion levels indicated that the goiter was not due to deficient iodine intakes.

Serum levels of total protein and calcium were almost always satisfactory, as were urinary excretions of thiamine, riboflavin, and iodine. Serum vitamin A levels indicated "moderate" risk in 15% to 40% of children under nine years and in 4% to 25% of both males and females between ten and nineteen years of age; the frequency probably reflected, at least in part, the use of a standard which was not age-related. However, low serum vitamin A levels were found more frequently among Eskimos and Indians than among the general population. Serum ascorbic acid values were below the standard in 15% to 30% of children and adolescents in the general population and among Indians, but in 40% to 70% of the Eskimo children.

Hemoglobin values were below the standard for 2% to 10% of all children with the exception of ten- to nineteen-year-old males in the

Indian and Eskimo groups, for whom the frequency was 14% to 18%. Low levels of mean corpuscular hemoglobin concentration were more often observed in all groups. The largest number of children with moderate or high risk in iron-related blood factors was found for transferrin saturation, with the totals of the two risk groups ranging from 19% to 40% in the general population and 40% to 71% in Indian and Eskimo children under nineteen years of age.

The values for serum folate classified as at high risk 3% to 10% of children under nine years and 10% to 14% of adolescents in the general and Indian populations; for comparable ages the frequencies were 27% to 29% and 41% to 52% for Eskimos. Low serum folate values were not associated with clinical manifestations of folate-vitamin $B_{12}$ deficiency anemia. It was concluded that most of the anemia observed was best explained on the basis of iron deficiency.

Dietary evaluations showed the greatest number of "inadequate" ratings for ten- to nineteen-year-old girls than for any other age or sex group among the children. The frequency of inadequate ratings for these girls was protein, 4% to 12%; iron, 33% to 44%; calcium, 35% in the general population and 63% and 70% in the Indian and Eskimo girls; and vitamin A, 26% in the general population, 42% in Indians, and 69% in Eskimo girls. Ratings also tended to be lower for Indian and Eskimo children at all ages than for the general population for calories, protein, and vitamin A, and Eskimo children were most likely to have low ascorbic acid intakes. The nutrients with the fewest inadequate ratings (usually under 10%) were protein, thiamine, riboflavin, and niacin.

Iron intakes showed less variation among the population groups than did other nutrients. The frequency of inadequate ratings ranged from 11% to 38% for various age and population groups, with the adolescent girls being in the top of the range, as noted above.

---

## Lessons from Surveys

In discussing the development of a nutrition surveillance system, Lane[26] summarized the problems of assessment techniques and suggested simple and practical methods of obtaining useful data:

> Data from the major recent nutritional surveys, specifically the Ten-State Nutrition Survey, the Health and Nutrition Examination Survey of the National Center for Health Statistics, and the Preschool Child Nutrition Survey, are remarkably similar in their general conclusions. They show little or no significant amounts

of deficiencies in vitamins and most minerals. They do, however, show that a considerable proportion of the population has simple iron-deficiency anemia. They show considerable amounts of obesity, even in the poorest segments of our population. They show significant amounts of growth deficit, as measured by inappropriate developments for age determined by anthropometry. They show considerable amounts of dental caries, undoubtedly related to the overconsumption of simple sugars and carbohydrates in the American diet. With the obvious exception of dental caries, the most prevalent nutritional disorders in the United States today can be directly measured by analysis of age, height, weight, hemoglobin and/or hematocrit.

## References

1  Bigwood, E. J. *Guiding Principles for Studies on the Nutrition of Populations.* Geneva: League of Nations Health Organization, 1939.

2  Interdepartmental Committee on Nutrition for National Defense. *Manual for Nutrition Surveys,* 2d ed. Washington, D.C.: Superintendent of Documents, Government Printing Office, 1963.

3  World Health Organization. *Expert Committee on Medical Assessment of Nutritional Status: Report.* Technical report series no. 258. Geneva: World Health Organization, 1963.

4  U.S. Department of Health, Education, and Welfare: *Ten-State Nutrition Survey, 1968–1970.* DHEW publications no. (HSM) 72–8130, 72–8131, 72–8132, and 72–8133. Washington, D.C.: Superintendent of Documents, Government Printing Office, 1972.

5  U.S. Department of Health, Education, and Welfare. *Preliminary Findings of the First Health and Nutrition Examination Survey, United States, 1971–1972: Dietary Intake and Biochemical Findings.* DHEW publication no. (HRA) 74–1219–1. Washington, D.C.: Superintendent of Documents, Government Printing Office, 1974.

6  U.S. Department of Health, Education, and Welfare. *Preliminary Findings of the First Health and Nutrition Examination Survey, United States, 1971–1972: Anthropometric and Clinical Findings.* DHEW publication no. (HRA) 75–1229. Washington, D.C.: Superintendent of Documents, Government Printing Office, 1975.

7  Nutrition Canada. *National Survey: A National Priority. A Report by Nutrition Canada to the Department of National Health and Welfare.* Catalog no. H58–36–1973. Ottawa: Information Canada, 1973.

8  Pearson, W. N. "Biochemical Appraisal of the Vitamin Nutritional Status in Man." *JAMA* 180 (1962):49–55.

9  Christakis, G., ed. "Nutritional Assessment in Health Programs." *American Journal of Public Health* 63 (1973 [suppl.]):1–82.

10  Owen, G M.; Kram, K. M.; Garry, P. J.; Lowe, J. E.; and Lubin, A. H. "A Study of Nutritional Status of Preschool Children in the United States, 1968–1970." *Pediatrics* 53(1974[suppl., pt. 2]):597–646.

11  Greulich, W. W., and Pyle, S. I. *Radiographic Atlas of Skeletal Development of the Hand and Wrist*, 2d ed. Stanford, Calif.: Stanford University Press, 1959.

12  Beal, V. A. "Nutritional Intake." In *Human Growth and Development*, edited by R. McCammon. Springfield, Ill.: Charles C Thomas Co., 1970.

13  U.S. Department of Health, Education, and Welfare. *Screening Children for Nutritional Status: Suggestions for Child Health Programs.* Washington, D.C.: Superintendent of Documents, Government Printing Office, 1971.

14  Beal, V. A. "The Nutritional History in Longitudinal Research." *Journal of the American Dietetic Association* 51 (1967):426–32.

15  Flores, M. "Dietary Studies for Assessment of the Nutritional Status of Populations in Non-modernized Societies." *American Journal of Clinical Nutrition* 11 (1962):344–55.

16  Marr, J. W. "Individual Dietary Surveys: Purposes and Methods." *World Review of Nutrition and Dietetics* 13 (1971):105–64.

17  Watt, B. K., and Merrill, A. L. *Composition of Foods: Raw, Processed and Prepared.* U.S. Department of Agriculture handbook no. 8. Washington, D.C.: Superintendent of Documents, Government Printing Office, 1963.

18  Adams, C. F. *Nutritive Value of American Foods in Common Units.* U.S. Department of Agriculture handbook no. 456. Washington, D.C.: Superintendent of Documents, Government Printing Office, 1975.

19  Food and Nutrition Board. *Recommended Dietary Allowances*, 8th ed. Washington, D.C.: National Academy of Sciences-National Research Council, 1974.

20  Citizens' Board of Inquiry into Hunger and Malnutrition in the United States. *Hunger, U.S.A.* Washington, D.C.: New Community Press, 1968.

21  White House Conference on Food, Nutrition, and Health. *Final Report.* Washington, D.C.: Superintendent of Documents, Government Printing Office, 1970.

22  Seltzer, C. C., and Mayer, J. "A Simple Criterion of Obesity." *Postgraduate Medicine* 38 (1965):A101–7.

23  Stuart, H. C., and Stevenson, S. S. "Physical Growth and Development." In *Textbook of Pediatrics*, edited by W. E. Nelson. Philadelphia: W. B. Saunders Co., 1950.

24  Nutrition Canada. *Food Consumption Patterns Report.* Department of National Health and Welfare. Ottawa: Information Canada, 1977.

25  Nutrition Canada. *Provincial, Indian and Eskimo Surveys.* 12 vols. Department of National Health and Welfare. Ottawa: Information Canada, 1975.

26  Lane, J. M. "Developing a Nutrition Surveillance System." In *Nutrition: An Integral Part of a Total Health Assessment. Proceedings of a Conference Sponsored by the University of Georgia and the Georgia Department of Human Resources.* Athens: University of Georgia Center for Continuing Education, 1975.

# Chapter Three

## Measurement of Physical Growth

Growth is the increase in size of the body or of any part of the body, including both structural and functional units. Growth is a quantitative phenomenon and can be measured by a variety of techniques, direct and indirect. The initial attempts to measure growth were centered on the recording of heights and weights, but as knowledge and technology have improved, methods have been developed to measure growth at the level of tissues, organs, and cellular and even subcellular components.

The physical growth pattern of the child is one of the most useful criteria for judging nutritional status. Growth is sensitive to nutrient intake; a deficiency of any nutrient may distort biochemical function and interfere with the potential progress of growth and development. An understanding of healthy growth and of the significance of deviations from expected patterns is essential for any nutritionist working with children. The most important factors in growth are genetic inheritance, endocrine function, illness, and nutrition.

Growth of the organism proceeds in an orderly fashion and is specific to each species. From conception to maturity, increase in body size of lower animals follows a single S-shaped curve. The accelerating curve of prenatal growth is followed by a gradually decelerating curve postnatally, ending finally in mature size. Humans, however, show a double S-shaped curve for growth. The initial curve of prenatal and postnatal growth is followed by a second acceleration of growth in the adolescent period before adult size is reached. This second acceleration gives the human a longer period of growth in relation to total life span and means that man must be his own model for the study of human growth. The application of data derived from studies of animal growth can be applied to humans only with careful qualifications. It has been essential, therefore, to accumulate data on human growth.

In the past century a number of independent workers and study groups accumulated measurements of children to establish patterns and ranges of human growth. Most early reports were cross-sectional, with single measurements of children at different ages compiled to form a table or graph of body sizes of boys and girls at successive ages, mostly during the school years. These figures provide a background grid of the general growth pattern of groups of healthy children.

The differences in growth of individual children, which might be faster or slower than the average, made it obvious that a true understanding of the individuality of growth could be demonstrated only by longitudinal studies, in which a number of children could be observed with repeated measurements over an extended period of time. Every individual child has his own growth pattern which may be normal for him and yet vary considerably from the general human pattern.

> Some individuals grow slowly and always remain small and uniformly below average in their various measurements; others grow rapidly and always exceed the average. Some children pass given milestones of development early in respect to age, while others are characteristically late in arriving at successive stages. Thus a child may be large for his age, either because of strong growth impulse leading to large size at maturity, or merely because he is ahead of the usual development schedule. Large children tend to mature early, whereas small children tend to mature late. Thus, by prolonging the period of growth, small children tend to become less conspicuously small by the time growth has been completed. Likewise, by shortening the period of growth, tall children tend to avoid excessive height.[1]

The dynamic characteristics of growth in the individual cannot be observed without repeated measurements, and the significance of a single measurement of a child is limited because it shows his status at only one given moment. "How can we distinguish between the naturally small, slowly growing child and the one who is small or slow to develop because of dietary deficiency, chronic illness, emotional handicaps, or a combination of such causal factors? The answer to such a question can come only from longtime studies of individual human beings. . . . We need more emphasis on what the child is becoming, as well as on the 'how' and the 'why' of becoming."[2]

Increasing emphasis has also been placed on the realization that the child is a biologic unit with impact from many directions. Not only is his genetic inheritance unique, but his environment is different from every other child's and his response to that environment is uniquely his own. While physical growth receives major consideration in this text, it must be recognized that emotional, mental, and social growth are inextricably related to physical growth and that behavior and personality interact with physical change. The physical, cultural, economic, and emotional environment from conception affect the development of the whole child and influence his growth. Our present concepts of growth have come from all of the disciplines related to human development from anthropology to cellular biology.

## What Is Growth?

Measurements of height and weight are the most common indexes of growth. They are the simplest measurements to take and can be done with a minimum of training and expertise. However, their very simplicity masks one of the major features of growth. Each part of the body grows and develops with a rate and timing of its own. Height and weight are the sum of total body growth but are not an index of segmental growth. For example, in the embryonic-fetal period the head grows before the lower part of the body, and 90% of adult head size is achieved by the time the child is six years old. By the second month of fetal life the head is approximately half of total length; the head of the newborn comprises about one-fourth of his length; in the adult the head is only one-eighth of total height. This change in body proportions can be readily seen in the outline drawings of figure 3.1 when height is held constant.[3]

Growth occurs as a result of proliferation of cells and increase in size of those cells. Cells in some tissues of the body may be counted and their size measured by analysis of the content of deoxyribonucleic acid (DNA) and protein. DNA, the material responsible for genetic transmission, is found in a constant amount in cells of a given species.

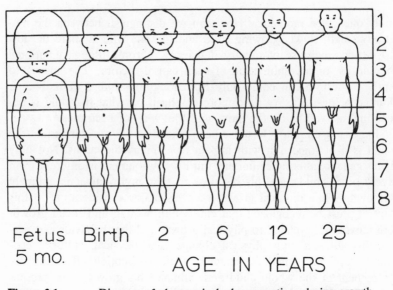

Fetus   Birth   2      6     12     25
5 mo.                  AGE  IN  YEARS

**Figure 3.1**          Diagram of changes in body proportions during growth.
                        Keeping height at a constant level, the diagram shows
                        changes from the fifth month of fetal development to
                        maturity. Adapted from Scammon, R. E., and Calkins, L. A.
                        *The Development and Growth of the Human Body in
                        the Fetal Period.* Minneapolis: University of Minnesota
                        Press, 1929.

In humans, 6.0 pg of DNA are found in each diploid cell, a cell with
normal double chromosome count.[4] The DNA is primarily in the cell
nucleus, although small amounts may be in smaller organelles of the
cell. By measuring the amount of DNA in a given weight of tissue,
the number of cells in that tissue may be calculated.

Proteins are the basic components of cell structure, and the cell re-
moves amino acids from surrounding fluids to form its own specific
proteins either for cell division or for cell growth. Therefore, the
amount of protein in the tissue increases whether the cell is dividing
(increase in number) or growing (increase in size). When cell number is increasing, both DNA and protein increase; this period has
been termed hyperplasia (fig. 3.2). This is followed by a period of
slower division, when the increment of DNA is less, but cells continue to grow in size, so the increment in protein continues. The final
stage of growth in this theoretical model is hypertrophy, when cell
division no longer occurs, as evidenced by the plateau in DNA content, but the cells are becoming larger, as evidenced by the continued
protein increase. In all nonregenerating cells which have been studied

to date, cell division, as measured by DNA, ceases before cell size has reached its maximum.[5]

Although this methodology is not applicable to adipose cells, as will be discussed later, the sequence of increase in number and size of cells seems to occur in all tissues, although the timing varies with different tissues and with a single type of tissue in different parts of the body. The importance of this concept to nutrition lies in the critical effects of overnutrition or undernutrition at different stages of cell growth. During hyperplasia the cell's need for amino acids is very high, for production of both DNA and cell proteins. Equally critical is the supply of each of the nutrients involved in protein metabolism. If amino acid supply is restricted for any reason, cell replication may be impaired.

Animal experiments, including those of Widdowson,[6] have shown that the level of intake of the suckling or weanling rat may have either a temporary or permanent effect on growth depending on the degree and timing of the dietary change. Increasing the intake of nursing rats by limiting the number of newborns in the litter resulted in faster growth and larger adult size. Inadequate intake immediately after weaning caused permanent deficits in growth, and the amount of

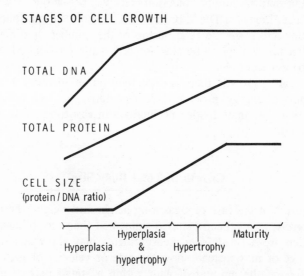

STAGES OF CELL GROWTH

TOTAL DNA

TOTAL PROTEIN

CELL SIZE
(protein / DNA ratio)

Hyperplasia          Maturity
Hyperplasia      &      Hypertrophy
hypertrophy

**Figure 3.2**    Theoretical scheme of cell growth. Changes in DNA and protein content of tissues, on which estimations of increase in cell number (hyperplasia) and cell size (hypertrophy) are based. Reprinted, with permission, from Winick, M. *Cellular Changes during Early Maturation.* Columbus, Ohio: Ross Laboratories, 1971.

deficit was greater as the period of undernutrition was extended. On the other hand, undernutrition imposed at a later age caused only a small deficit in weight which was recovered after adequate feeding was reinstituted. This implies that undernutrition during the period of cell replication (hyperplasia) may limit the number of cells formed and therefore cause a permanent deficit in growth. However, if the period of undernutrition occurs after hyperplasia is concluded, only cell size is affected and may be compensated for by later refeeding. Application of this concept to humans must consider possible moderating effects of the adolescent growth spurt.

"In the developing countries, the almost universal growth retardation is not restricted to height and weight but is also evident in other anthropometric measurements, in bone development, and in the individual's physiological function."[7] Undernutrition in children in developing countries, even when not severe enough to cause clinical signs of protein-calorie malnutrition, may result in a later adolescent growth spurt. When clinical signs are present, a growing literature has documented the alteration of physical growth. In a report on postmortem analyses of brains of South American infants who died in the first year after a period of acute malnutrition, Winick et al.[4] found that the number of brain cells was below the expected number for age. Levels of DNA, protein, cholesterol, and phospholipids in the brain were low. The relationship of the number of brain cells to intelligence remains to be elucidated, but the physical effects of undernutrition were clear.

Healthy growth, then, is dependent on an adequate and continuous supply of energy, protein, and other nutrients to all cells of the body so that they may divide and increase in size to reach their maximum potential.

## Growth in Total Body Size

Because of the ease of measuring height and weight, these dimensions of growth have been better documented than any others. The curves which are derived from measurements may show actual size related to age or may instead show the rate or velocity of growth, which is based on the amount of gain within a stated period of time. Both cross-sectional and longitudinal studies have provided data on the size of children at given ages, but true velocity of growth is available only from longitudinal studies in which the same children are measured repeatedly.

The entire period of growth from conception to maturity follows a double S-curve. The first S-curve is shown in figure 3.3, in which the acceleration of length in fetal life is followed by gradual deceleration of the curve in the first postnatal year.[8] The weight curve of the fetus has a later and more abrupt acceleration than the length curve, but the weight curve of the infant in the first year is similar to the length curve and shows the same deceleration.

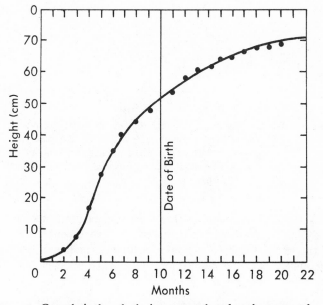

**Figure 3.3**          Growth in length during prenatal and early postnatal periods. Reprinted, with permission, from Thompson, D'A. W. *On Growth and Form*, 2d ed. Cambridge: Cambridge University Press, 1942.

After the deceleration of growth rate of the young infant, there follows a long period of slow and fairly uniform increase in size during childhood. The second acceleration is commonly called the adolescent growth spurt, which reaches a maximum velocity and then decelerates until complete cessation as adult height is attained. The pattern of growth in height is shown in figure 3.4, which is from the oldest known longitudinal study of growth. Between 1759 and 1777 Count Philibert Gueneau de Montbeillard measured the height of his son from birth to eighteen years. This was published by the French naturalist Buffon, a friend of de Montbeillard.[3]

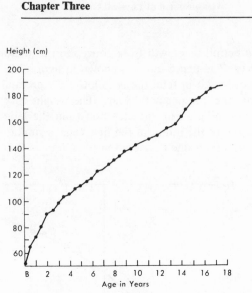

Height (cm)

**Figure 3.4**          Semiannual height measurements of his son by de Montbeillard between 1759 and 1777. Adapted from Scammon,
R. E. "The First Seriatim Study of Human Growth."
*American Journal of Physical Anthropology* 10 (1927):
329–36.

A total of more than 100 external measurements of the human
body have been established, measuring every conceivable dimension
of the body. In practical use, a relatively small number will give an
adequate numerical description of various body segments. The most
commonly used measurements are selected from the following list:

Overall dimensions: Weight, height (length), and sitting height
(crown-rump length)

Circumferences: Head, chest, waist, hip, biceps, maximum forearm,
wrist, thigh, knee, calf, ankle, and foot

Widths: Head, chest, hip, elbow, hand, knee, ankle, and foot

Lengths: Head, arm, leg, hand, and foot

Depth: Chest

Skinfold thicknesses: Triceps, subscapular, and chest

The choice of measurements from this list will be determined by the
circumstances of the observation and the need for detail. In school
health or child health clinic screening, height and weight are standard
measurements. Other measurements require a greater degree of skill
and training and are usually done only for further diagnostic evaluation or for research studies.

The ratio of one measurement to another is often of value. The ratio of head circumference to chest or hip circumference is meaningful in the child to the age of six years as an index of postnatal growth, but is of little value thereafter. The ratio of weight to height may be an index to obesity (see chapter 4). However, since weight is a composite of the bone, muscle, fat, and other organs of the body, increasing emphasis is being placed on methods of distinguishing between lean body mass and fat as components of weight.

## Growth in Stature

Linear growth is made up primarily of growth of the skeleton, with small contributions of tissues between vertebrae and other bones. Increase in height during childhood comes increasingly from growth of the legs. This may be seen in figure 3.5 from the longitudinal data of

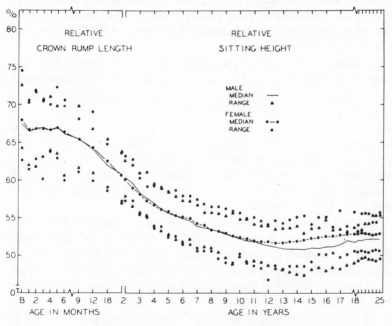

**Figure 3.5**          Sitting height as a percent of total height between birth and twenty-five years. Reprinted, with permission, from Hansman, C. "Anthropometry and Related Data." In *Human Growth and Development*, edited by R. W. McCammon. Springfield, Ill.: Charles C Thomas Co., 1970.

the Child Research Council, which shows that sitting height, which comprises about two-thirds of height in the first year, increases less rapidly than leg length. By the age of ten years sitting height is, on the average, only slightly more than half of total height.[9] This is another way of expressing the change in body proportions shown in the outline drawings of figure 3.1.

The growth of long bones of the extremities has been of particular interest in the study of human growth. The characteristics of growth of bones in width and length are somewhat different. In the central part of the bone is a cylindrical compact area, the diaphysis. At each end of the diaphysis is an area of metaphysis, which contains columns of spongy tissue, with a cartilagenous plate where most of the active growth in length occurs. The width of the cartilagenous plate is proportional to the rate of growth. The epiphysis at each end of the long bone is separated from the central part of the bone by this area of cartilage. Increase in length occurs at each end of the bone, with cartilage first being formed and gradually replaced by calcified osseous tissue, extending the length of the bone. Toward the end of adolescent growth the cartilagenous plate gradually decreases in size until finally the epiphysis is fused to the diaphysis by bone. After this fusion no further bone elongation occurs.

Increase in bone width is accomplished by the formation of new rings of osseous tissue under the periosteum, a membrane surrounding the bone. Even while new bone is being formed, there is constant change in bone already formed. Osteoclasts absorb some of the matrix of the diaphysis, creating a cavity in the center of the bone. This cavity becomes filled with marrow, which has the ability to form blood cells. The type of marrow changes with age. Marrow in the long bones loses the ability to make blood cells at about six years, although hematopoietic ability is retained by bones of the skull, face, vertebrae, ribs, and pelvis.

There is a dynamic state of balance in bone during growth. Growth of new bone occurs at the same time as resorption and modeling of old bone to adjust to changing stress. The quality of bone and the mineral density as calcium salts are deposited in the bone matrix depend on the supply of protein, calcium, phosphorus, and vitamins which are essential to bone formation and maintenance.

The appearance, size, and eventual fusion of the epiphyses and the appearance of carpal centers in the wrist may be evaluated from roentgenograms. These form the basis for the evaluation of the maturational process and, when compared to norms which have been developed from hundreds of roentgenograms of healthy children by

Greulich and Pyle[10] or by Tanner et al.,[11] a skeletal age may be assigned to the child for contrast with his chronological age. A rating of skeletal maturity is a valuable adjunct to the measurement of stature.

## Growth of Skeletal Muscle

The muscular system accounts for a considerable portion of the increase in weight. As bone increases, the supporting structure of muscle increases. The curves of increase in bone and muscle widths during childhood follow a pattern similar to that of height.[12] There is little difference between median muscle widths of boys and of girls until adolescence, although the maximum values for muscle width are usually found in boys. During adolescence the increase in muscle mass is greater in males than in females.

Muscles are responsible for the erect posture of the human, and are essential to locomotion and to the development and maintenance of body shape.

## Growth of Subcutaneous Fat

Fat may be deposited in many areas of the body. Deep fat is difficult to measure without specialized techniques, but subcutaneous fat may be evaluated by a variety of methods. There are conflicting data in the literature on the proportion of total body fat which is found in subcutaneous areas. Methods of estimating total body fat include densitometry (underwater weighing), isotope dilution (for measurement of total body water and water in intracellular and extracellular compartments), and potassium-40 counts (as measurement of lean body mass). These methods are obviously indirect and require specialized laboratory equipment. If lean body weight can be determined, the difference between that value and total body weight is assumed to be fat. Lacking simple methodology for determining total body fat, most of the emphasis has been placed on the measurement of subcutaneous fat, which is more readily accessible.

The most common measurement is by use of skin calipers. These specially designed calipers measure the thickness of a double fold of skin and subcutaneous fat, and the sites for measurement are standardized. Various sites on the trunk or extremities may be used, but most frequently triceps and subscapular sites are measured.

Roentgenograms for the study of long bone growth were taken in longitudinal studies such as those at the Harvard School of Public Health,[13] the Child Research Council,[12] and the Fels Research Institute.[14,15] As interest in body composition developed, these roentgenograms were reviewed for measurement of the shadows of bone, muscle, and fat. The sites of measurement in all studies have included the calf, and in some also the thigh, forearm, upper arm, and maximum hip bulge. The potential hazard of radiation will limit the use of nondiagnostic roentgenograms as a routine aspect of child study, but previous roentgenographic studies have provided a unique repository of serial data on several hundred children.

Both of these methods have shown similar changes in deposition of subcutaneous fat during the years of growth. Fat increases at all sites measured during the first nine months, then decreases during the preschool period. Patterns in boys and girls differ from early childhood. Boys tend to have a slow but steady decrease in subcutaneous fat widths until seven to eight years, then fat widths rise to ten years, remain on a plateau for the next year or two, then decelerate rapidly. In contrast, the median for girls is consistently higher than for boys, and while girls also increase in fat widths after seven years, their increasing curve continues to at least eighteen years of age.[16]

Measurements of subcutaneous fat layers must be interpreted with some caveats. These are measurements of thickness of layers at selected sites and are not measures of volume. For example, despite intervening changes, the median fat widths at the maximum calf site are the same for males at two months and at seven years, but since the length of the lower leg has changed appreciably, the volume of fat on the seven-year-old child's leg is obviously more than on the leg of the two-month-old infant. Individuals differ in their patterns of fat deposition in various parts of the body; some tend to add fat to the trunk or to the hips or to the legs primarily, while others may have proportional distribution in many areas. The use of a single measurement like the triceps skinfold or the calf roentgenogram may not give a true representation of total body fat. Children tend to have a larger proportion of fat on limbs than on the trunk, when compared with adults, so measurement of subcutaneous fat on the extremities is more likely to be an accurate index of body fat in children.

## Growth of Body Organs

Some body organs and tissues grow at a rate comparable to total body growth, while others have distinctively different timing. The graph by

Scammon, first published in 1930 (fig. 3.6), shows the paths by which various types of body tissue reach adult size. The general growth curve, which is typical of height and weight, is similar to those for the skeleton, muscle mass, lungs, gastrointestinal tract, blood volume, liver, spleen, heart, and kidney. In contrast, neural tissue, including the brain and therefore the skull, grows rapidly in fetal life

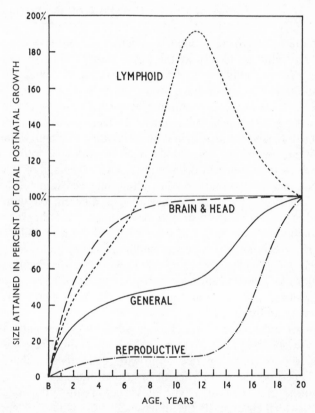

**Figure 3.6**          Growth of four types of body tissues. Adapted from Scammon, R. E. "Measurement of the Body in Childhood." In *The Measurement of Man*. Minneapolis: University of Minnesota Press, 1930.

and in the early postnatal years, with only 10% of growth not completed by six years. The reproductive organs grow very little between two years and the onset of adolescence, when there is a sudden sharp increase in the size of genital organs as the individual spurts into sexual maturity within a few years. A most unusual pattern of growth is shown by lymphoid tissue, including the thymus. By approximately twelve years the mass of lymph tissue has reached a maximum and then decreases about 50% to its adult mass. It is obvious, then, that the term *body growth* is really a composite of changes which are diverse in different organs.

## Studies of Human Growth, Past and Present

The patterns of growth which have been described have come from a variety of studies, mostly in the past century. Most of the studies, ranging from Baldwin's work to the current National Center for Health Statistics surveys, have been cross-sectional. In cross-sectional studies a large number of children at a single age or of children at different ages are each examined or measured once and the results compiled to show the distribution of findings. When different age groups are examined, the results may be compiled into a table to show distributions at consecutive ages. The advantage of this type of study is that a large number of children may be examined in a short period of time. The disadvantage is that different children are included in successive age distributions so that changes in size from one age to another may be due to the chance selection of children. However, since very large numbers of children may be included the effects of such chance selection are minimal. A further disadvantage is that the peaks in growth shown by individual children during adolescence are smoothed into an average curve which masks individual differences in velocity and timing.

The second type of study is longitudinal, in which individual children are observed for a given period of time, which may range from a few years to the full period of growth. The intensive study of individuals permits the establishment of growth increments from one age to another and shows the type of variations in timing and rate of growth which distinguish the individuality of pattern of each child. Obviously this kind of study is a lengthy undertaking and must be limited to fewer children. With one exception, each of the major U.S. growth studies has had enrollment of less than 350 subjects. These will be discussed in greater detail in this chapter.

Both types of studies are important and the data they provide complement each other. The individuality of growth of small numbers of children may be viewed against the background of the large numbers in cross-sectional studies, which provide a wider range of findings because of the diversity of large populations.

## Early U.S. Studies

Studies from those of Bowditch (1872) to Baldwin (1914) are presented chronologically in table 3.1. The major contributions of each study are summarized to show that they form the basis for much of our present knowledge. These were cross-sectional studies and chiefly confined to measurements of height and weight. Porter and Baldwin observed some of the same children over a period of years, but presented the findings cross-sectionally.

Bowditch, professor of physiology at Harvard Medical School, was the first to publish data on the size of children. He became interested in the growth of children in his own family and kept records of relatives at annual family reunions. About 1872 he did an extensive analysis of the school records of height and weight of more than 24,000 children. His questionnaires to schools asked for age in years and months; height without shoes, recorded to the nearest 0.1 inch; weight in ordinary clothing to the nearest 0.25 lb; birthplace; nationality of both parents; and occupation of both parents. He prepared tables of the average height and weight for each age, by sex and nationality as well as for the whole group. It was assumed at that time that the curves represented the normal rate of growth of children as well as if they had been secured by repeated weighings of the same children over a period of successive years.

With this pioneer investigation Bowditch earned the honor of having prepared the first tables of heights and weights of U.S. children, in addition to establishing some of the fundamental laws of growth. He showed that growth does not proceed at an even rate from five to twenty years, and that it was different for the two sexes (fig. 3.7). Bowditch believed that the difference between boys and girls in maximum growth rate was associated with puberty, which also occurs at different ages in the two sexes.

When these records of Boston children were later subjected to Galton's method of percentile ranking, another characteristic of growth appeared—that the period of adolescent acceleration occurs earlier in large children than in small children. Children who were large for their age had a growth spurt at a younger age than children who were small. Bowditch also showed important differences in the size of children of various nationalities and social groups. Children of American parentage were taller and heavier for age than those of foreign parentage. Children in private schools were also taller and heavier than children in public schools. Children of nonlaborers were taller and heavier than children of laborers at almost all ages.

Table 3.1    Early U.S. Growth Studies, 1872–1914

| Date | Reported by | Where Made | Method of Judging | No. of Subjects | Major Contributions |
|---|---|---|---|---|---|
| 1872–91 | Bowditch | Boston and suburbs; public and private schools | Height Weight | 13,715 boys, 10,516 girls 5–20 years old | Found growth did not proceed at even rate throughout growing period; nor was it same for the two sexes. Children of American parentage of the nonlaboring class and those attending private schools, at a given age, were taller and heavier than those of foreign-born parentage of the laboring class, and those attending public schools. Developed first height-weight tables. |
| 1881 | Peckham | Milwaukee public schools | Height Weight | 4,773 boys, 5,130 girls | Confirmed Bowditch findings; found superiority of girls over boys in height and weight from 12 to 15 years; superiority in height of children of American parentage over children of foreign parentage. |
| 1892–94 | Porter | St. Louis public schools | Height Weight Head length Head breadth Vital capacity Other | 33,500 boys and girls | Confirmed growth pattern and sexual difference findings of Bowditch and Peckham; found close relationship: arm span and height; sitting height and chest girth. Showed relationship between superior size and better school progress. |
| 1892 | Boas West | Worcester, Mass. schools | Height Weight | 3,250 boys and girls 5–21 years old | Found young children grew more uniformly than older children; variability increased greatly during years of adolescence, more with girls than with boys; short children grew more slowly during the early years than did tall children, but they continued growing for a longer time. |

| | | Measurements | Number | Findings |
|---|---|---|---|---|
| Barnes | Oakland, Calif. schools | | 6,000 boys and girls | Children of Oakland exceeded in height and weight children of Toronto and all other cities of the U.S. where measurements had been made. Boas computed tables for "average" children including annual increases to be expected. |
| Chamberlain | Toronto, Can. schools | | 7,608 boys, 7,411 girls | In Toronto study, relation of physical growth to mental ability (teacher's estimate) was directly opposite to that found by Porter. |
| 1899–1900 Christopher and Smedley | Chicago public schools | Height Weight Vital capacity Endurance Strength of hand Mental development | 2,788 boys, 3,471 girls<br><br>284 boys | Confirmed sex difference in growth by Bowditch and others. In addition, found boys surpassed girls at all ages in strength; were superior in vital capacity; had greater endurance at all ages. Children from favored economic group were superior in size and physical development to average American child.<br><br>Boys of jail school were inferior in all physical measurements taken, inferiority increased with age.<br><br>Confirmed Porter's conclusions of the relation between mental and physical growth. (School progress criterion of mental growth.) |
| 1914 Baldwin | Horace Mann School, N.Y. Univ. of Chicago Elem. School Francis Parker School, Chicago | Height Weight Lung capacity | 861 boys, 1,063 girls | First to follow same children through elementary and high school; confirmed earlier work regarding growth pattern. Found relation of growth to school standing in keeping with that of Porter and Smedley; tall, heavy boys and girls with good lung capacity were older physiologically and further along toward mental maturity as evidenced by school progress than short, light boys and girls. |

Sources: Reprinted, with permission, from Martin, E. A. Roberts' *Nutrition Work with Children.* Chicago: University of Chicago Press, 1954. © 1954 by The University of Chicago.

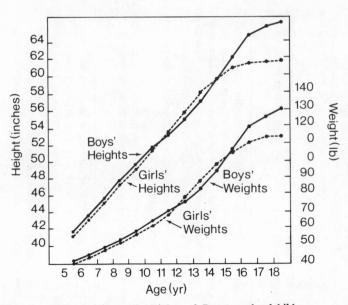

**Figure 3.7**       Mean heights and weights of Boston schoolchildren,
showing differences between sexes. Reprinted from Bowditch,
H. P. *The Growth of Children*. Annual Report to the
Massachusetts State Board of Health, no. 8, 1877,
pp. 273–323.

Bowditch's major contributions laid the foundation for our present
knowledge of growth in height and weight. He stimulated further work
in this area and provided basic tenets of growth which influenced later
research.

Peckham provided similar data on nearly 10,000 children in the
Milwaukee public schools. His study confirmed the findings of Bowditch with respect to the sex differences in the adolescent growth spurt
and to the superiority in height of children of U.S.-born parents over
children of foreign parentage.

Porter also confirmed the findings of Bowditch in his study of St.
Louis schoolchildren. In addition, he undertook to determine the laws
of normal growth in the hope that "on this firm ground may be established a system of grading which shall take into account the physical
capacity of the pupil in the apportionment of school tasks." Porter's
was the first study to record several measurements in addition to
height and weight. He found that taller children were also larger in

other body dimensions. He was also the first to suggest a relationship between size and scholastic ability. Taller and heavier children were in higher grades than smaller children of the same age.

Boas and his associates, particularly through critical summaries and evaluations of the work of others, added to the knowledge of the patterns of growth. Boas constantly stimulated others to improve methods and to use caution in the interpretation of results. A professor of anthropology at Clark University, Boas was made head of the section on anthropology for the Columbian Exposition in Chicago in 1893. To show as fully as possible the growth and development of American children, he planned studies with three collaborators in Worcester, Massachusetts; Oakland, California; and Toronto, Canada. Their major findings are summarized in table 3.1. In addition, Boas used data from his predecessors here and abroad to prepare tables of stature, weight, and annual increases at successive ages. He mathematically computed tables showing "the growth in height and weight and the absolute and proportional increases for what might be termed the average American boy or girl."

Burk is not included in table 3.1 because he reported no original work. However, his book, *The Growth of Children in Height and Weight*, published in 1898, is an excellent review and summary of all the studies which had been made until that time on the physical and mental development of children during the years commonly spent in public schools. He also published in usable form the tables of weight and height as computed by Boas on children from six American cities.

Christopher and Smedley were responsible for initiating a study on child development in the Chicago public schools about 1899. In addition to height and weight, these studies included vital capacity, endurance, hand strength, and mental development. The major findings of this study are summarized in table 3.1.

Baldwin, the final investigator in this group, published *Physical Growth and School Progress* in 1914. His study marked the first attempt to follow up consecutively the same groups of children through elementary and high schools, both in physical growth and in school standing. This study differed from previous studies in that (1) the children had superior advantages with respect to care; (2) measurements were made longitudinally; (3) weights were taken nude; and (4) measurements were made by trained people. His findings on growth, physical development, and school progress confirmed earlier studies, including those of Porter and Smedley, who had shown that precocious children tended to be taller and heavier than those of average ability at the same age. Baldwin's research continued after 1914, and his early findings were extended in later studies.

Thus a considerable body of knowledge had been accumulated by 1914 to document the heights and weights of children and to relate size to physical and mental function. These early studies laid the groundwork for the development of new techniques, refinement and extension of methodology, and realization of the need for longitudinal observations of individual children. Only with consecutive examinations and measurements of individuals can one determine growth patterns which may be masked by cross-sectional data.

## Studies since 1917

A summary of studies of growth and development of the past sixty years is difficult to encompass in a single volume. Indeed, hundreds of journal articles, monographs, and books have been published on these findings. Even a description of the methodologies used in each study would be a monumental task. As knowledge increased, it led to further questions; to answer the questions, more detailed and different kinds of procedures were added to the original protocol of each study group. The numbers of children enrolled in each longitudinal study constantly changed as mobility of the population decreased original enrollments, but new children were added each year in most studies. Even the dates when some studies were discontinued are no longer valid. With increasing interest in the health of adults and the aging process, some of the original subjects have been called back for follow-up. At present, data from different studies, past and present, are being combined to investigate specific problems which need larger numbers of cases than each study can supply alone. The discussion to follow will therefore be incomplete and the bibliography selective, but the interested reader may pursue more detailed data as desired.

Whereas earlier research had been done primarily by individuals working alone, this new era of study required teams of professionals from a variety of disciplines, including physical and physiological growth, roentgenology, biochemistry, nutrition, and psychology. The focus now became the individual child. Instead of a few measurements on thousands of children, a battery of observations were applied to a few hundred children. Some concentrated on a specific age span, but increasingly emphasis shifted to observations from birth to maturity. Many studies continued long enough to enroll second-generation subjects. Recently, with growing awareness that the problems of the middle-aged and elderly, such as hypertension, obesity, and heart disease, may have their origins in early life, some studies have been reactivated for adult examinations of subjects observed through their childhood years.

These studies have been associated with institutes, foundations, and universities. The first two studies cited here were begun in 1917 and 1922. During the 1920s the White House Conference on Children and other conferences clearly demonstrated gaps in knowledge of growth and the need for consistent tracking of individual children to determine the different patterns by which children grow. Between 1925 and 1931 eight longitudinal or semilongitudinal studies were instituted. Each study developed its own protocol and the major emphasis varied from one study to another, but each included physical measurements.

### The Iowa Child Welfare Research Station, University of Iowa

Baldwin was one of the pioneers of the movement toward more intensive growth research. He became the first director of the Iowa Child Welfare Research Station, the first organized group to study growth. Meredith later took charge of the growth studies. Height, weight, and anthropometric measurements were taken at six-month intervals on 150 children attending the Station from the age of four years; some were observed to maturity. Measurements of height, weight, and chest girth were published in 1921. The data from this study were later combined with data from the Harvard School of Public Health study to produce the Stuart-Meredith tables which have been internationally used as percentiles for evaluating physical growth of children. This study also included caliper measurements of subcutaneous tissue.

A second study at this institute concentrated on facial growth between four and twelve years, using roentgenograms, dental casts, photographs, and anthropometric measurements.

### Harvard Growth Study, Harvard University

From 1922 to 1934 this group, headed by Dearborn, obtained data at six-month intervals on approximately 1,000 children, beginning at five years. Data included weight, height, other anthropometric measurements, and wrist roentgenograms. Shuttleworth's classic analysis

of early, average, and late timing of adolescence and the growth patterns associated with different timing came from this study; these
graphic differences will be used later in this chapter.

## Institute of Child Development,
## University of Minnesota

With its primary interest in psychological development and behavior,
under the direction of Anderson, the institute collected longitudinal
data between 1925 and 1931 on approximately 100 children, with
roughly equal division between infants in the first two years and children between two and six years of age. Anthropometric measurements and illness records were obtained. Of the total 4,500 preschool
children who attended the institute and on whom some early data
were available, follow-up interviews with the parents of 300 children
were obtained in 1958.

## Berkeley Growth Study, University of California

Beginning in 1928, under the direction of Bayley, seventy-four infants were enrolled at one month of age, and examinations were done
at regular intervals until the closure of the epiphyses, at approximately
seventeen to eighteen years. Subjects were later examined at twenty-
one years, between twenty-five and thirty years, and once a decade
since then. Nearly 150 second-generation children have been examined as well. Since 1954 the study has been directed by Eichorn.
While much of the emphasis was on mental testing, consistent records
also included stature, weight, anthropometric measurements, hand-
wrist roentgenograms, photographs, physical examinations, and health
records. Subjects were white, usually with above-average incomes.

## Berkeley Guidance Study, University of California

Started in 1928 under the direction of MacFarlane, this study enrolled every third child born in Berkeley in the next two years and
observed them regularly to skeletal maturity. Many of the subjects
have since been examined at thirty years and at forty years. In addition, nearly 400 second-generation children have been examined two
to five times. The original series included approximately 250 children,
with primary emphasis on behavior and personality. Half the group
had frequent interviews and guidance; the other half, matched for

socioeconomic variables, served as controls. Physical examinations were done at twenty-one months, three years, and at regular intervals thereafter. Height, weight, and other anthropometric measurements were taken twice yearly to eighteen years, and hand-wrist roentgenograms twice yearly between eight and eighteen years. All except six subjects were white, and family incomes were assumed to be representative of the community.

### Oakland Growth Study, University of California

Under the direction, successively, of Stolz, Jones, and Clausen, this study of adolescence began in 1928 with enrollment of 212 white elementary schoolchildren at an average age of eleven years and examined them semiannually to eighteen years. At high school graduation 150 subjects were still being studied, and approximately 100 were examined later between thirty and thirty-five years and between thirty-eight and forty years. In addition, 179 offspring of the original series have been examined three times. The study protocol included health histories, physical examinations, anthropometric measurements, hand-wrist roentgenograms, photographs, and metabolic studies, as well as psychological testing and behavior studies.

### Child Research Council,
### University of Colorado School of Medicine

Between 1923 and 1930, seventy-eight children were enrolled in a study directed by Wasson with the purpose of detecting the development of disease. In 1930 Washburn became director, and emphasis shifted to the study of health with eventual addition of 256 white middle-class subjects enrolled at birth, including eighty second-generation babies. McCammon assumed the position of director in 1960. Although the original plan had been to observe subjects only to maturity, examinations were continued on the adults. At the termination of the study in 1967, 179 subjects between the ages of one and forty-five years were still actively enrolled. Procedures included health histories, physical examinations, dental examinations with head roentgenograms and casts, anthropometric measurements, roentgenograms (long bones, chest, paranasal sinuses, and hand-wrist), electrocardiograms, photographs, blood analyses, metabolic tests, nutritional intake, motor function, and psychological testing.

## Fels Research Institute, Yellow Springs, Ohio

The Fels group, directed first by Sontag and now by Falkner, has had the largest series of subjects. Since its inception in 1929, 816 individuals have been enrolled, including more than 260 second-generation children. Fels is unique in that it has endowment funds which permit continuation of its studies. The other research groups have either set specific time limitations or have had programs discontinued or curtailed due to lack of funding. The Fels study has had a central core of physical examinations, health histories, anthropometry, roentgenograms, and psychological testing done on all subjects routinely. Additional specific investigations have been conducted for varying periods of time, including metabolism, dietary intake, dental examinations, and various biochemical determinations. Most subjects are white. The oldest subjects still being examined are in their forties and provide the longest continuous records of any of the studies.

## Longitudinal Studies of Child Health and Development, Harvard School of Public Health

Between 1930 and 1956 this study enrolled approximately 300 infants, of whom 134 were observed to the age of eighteen years, under the direction of Stuart. Between 1966 and 1968, 220 subjects from the original series were recalled for follow-up examinations under the direction of Reed and Valadian. The study included health histories, physical and dental examinations, anthropometry, hematology, roentgenograms, nutrition histories, and psychological testing and observations. The nutrition history methodology for longitudinal research was developed by Burke in this study. Subjects were white and primarily in the lower middle and low income groups.

## Brush Foundation, Western Reserve University

Between 1931 and 1942, this study, directed by Todd, collected data on approximately 1,000 children by a semilongitudinal method. Subjects were entered in the study at any age from three months to adolescence and were observed for an average of 4½ years. Primary interest was in anthropometric measurements and roentgenographic evaluations. These formed the basis for Todd's *Standards for Skeletal Maturity* and later for the Greulich-Pyle *Radiographic Atlas of Skeletal Development of Hand and Wrist*.

Although some of the studies listed above have discontinued observations of subjects, they have provided a data bank which will
continue to be of use. Major blocks of data from the Child Research
Council, the Harvard School of Public Health study, the Oakland-
Berkeley studies, and the Fels Research Institute have been transferred to computer tapes for ready availability for further analysis.
The combination of data from several studies provides a larger series
for greater statistical significance. For example, ages at menarche and
growth of girls in the circumpubertal period have been collated to provide larger numbers. A study of the development of obesity, combining data from seven studies, is at present under way at Fels Research
Institute.

This discussion has been limited to the major long-term projects in
the United States. Other groups which have contributed to the understanding of growth include the Center for Research in Child Growth
at the University of Pennsylvania, which collected longitudinal data
on 600 children between seven and thirteen years of age, under Krog-
man's direction; their primary interest was in the development of the
face, jaws, and teeth, and included anthropometric measurements.
Classical metabolic balance studies of pregnant and lactating women
and of children between four and twelve years of age were done by
the Children's Fund of Michigan under the direction of Icie Macy
Hoobler, Ph.D., beginning in 1929. The data on balance studies,
pediatric examinations, anthropometry, roentgenograms, and psycho-
metric tests of children were reported in three volumes of *Nutrition
and Chemical Growth in Childhood.*

A number of growth studies have been instituted in other countries
and several of these are still continuing. They include the following:
the University of Melbourne, the Institute of Nutrition of Central
America and Panama, the Harpenden and Newcastle-upon-Tyne
studies in England, the Centre Internationale de l'Enfance in Paris,
and studies in The Netherlands and Skopje, Yugoslavia. The interest
in growth and development and the need for deeper understanding
of mechanisms and patterns of growth are increasingly concerned not
only with children but with the kinds of adults children will become.

One additional survey should be included in this discussion. The
National Center for Health Statistics of the U.S. Department of
Health, Education, and Welfare has conducted a series of surveys of
statistically selected representative samples of the noninstitutionalized
population of the country. The Health Examination Surveys (reported as Series 11 of their publications) have included physical ex-

aminations, anthropometry, roentgenograms, blood tests, and other physical and physiological measurements as well as information on health and socioeconomic status. Cycle I was done on adults eighteen to seventy-nine years of age in 1960–62; cycle II was a survey of children six through eleven years of age in 1963–65; cycle III was done on subjects twelve through seventeen years of age in 1966–70. Although one-third of the same children were examined in cycles II and III, the data are essentially cross-sectional. The method of selecting subjects was planned so that findings could be projected to the entire U.S. population. In 1970 the Center added assessment of nutritional status to its program. The first Health and Nutrition Examination Survey (HANES I) was conducted in 1971–74, and the second survey (HANES II) is to cover the period 1976–79.

## Physical Growth and Its Components

The studies listed above and other literature reports have contributed to our present knowledge of growth and the factors which influence change in body size and function. Growth is an orderly but not a uniform process. Increase in size does not follow a straight line from birth to maturity, but instead is a series of changing rates, subject to different influences at different ages. Growth is a sequence of highly interdependent events which we can describe as they occur, even though we may not know what causes them. We really do not know what initiates growth, why the rate decreases in childhood, what mechanisms provide the stimulus for the second acceleration at puberty, and why growth is self-limiting.

At any age the human pattern of growth has wide dispersion. From the preceding discussion, it is clear that much effort and time have been devoted to establishing ranges of measurements as children grow. Chapter 4 will deal in greater detail with the standards which have been developed.

Terminology tends to be confusing, whether one considers nutritional requirements, blood levels, or growth. Terms such as normal, average, healthy, deficient, retarded, and advanced are often used without precision. *Normal* is meaningless when applied to an individual child's growth unless the purpose is to identify absence of pathology. Gigantism, the excessive growth of the skeleton, and dwarfism are clearly abnormal. Obesity of an extreme degree is abnormal, but there is no consensus on the cutoff points between overweight, which may be physiologically harmless, and pathological obesity. If percentile standards are based on healthy individuals who function well in our society and are growing at consistent rates for age, even though that rate may be faster or slower than "average," it is difficult to label individuals at the extremes as "abnormal." A child below the fifth percentile in height and a child above the ninety-fifth percentile may be equally healthy. "Healthy" growth results when all of the biochemical, hormonal, and environmental factors are ideal to allow the child to reach his genetic potential. Unfortunately, we have no means of measuring his genetic potential, so even this concept is meaningless.

Average heights and weights of some population groups have increased in the past century since specific measurements have been available, and other evidence suggests that this increase has been happening for a long time. Today's soldier would have great difficulty fitting his greater size into the armor of a soldier of the middle ages. This secular change may have reached its limit, at least in economically advantaged individuals, in technically advanced nations. We may, however, question whether "bigger is better." Bigger is better only if increased size means improved health and physical and psychological functioning. There is a tendency to classify the small child or the child whose skeletal age is below his chronological age as "retarded." It is true that undernutrition and a variety of adverse physiological and environmental factors may stunt growth, but many short children are healthy. It is a truism among workers in the field of growth and development that no child is "average." While mathematical and statistical descriptions of populations are essential for orderly handling of data, the individuality of pattern within the limits of health must be kept in mind.

It is within this context of group averages and individual differences that we shall look at growth. Although growth is a continuum, we shall for convenience divide it into age periods and separate factors which are interdependent.

## Fetal Growth

The rate of growth during fetal life is faster than at any postnatal age. In 266 days, a single fertilized cell divides and grows to a full-term newborn weighing perhaps 3,500 gm and having a length of perhaps 50 cm. As seen in figure 3.3, length increase in utero is not uniform, but accelerates rapidly. Weight increase is slower in accelerating.[17] At the end of the first trimester the embryo has achieved approximately 15% of its term length, but less than 1% of its term weight. By the end of the second trimester length is 65% and weight still only 20% of newborn size. In the last two months of intrauterine life the fetus more than doubles in weight. This is consistent with the differences in body composition. Lean body mass comprises most of the weight of the embryo. At the midpoint in fetal development, less than 1% of body weight is fat, compared to an average of perhaps 16% at birth. At twenty-eight weeks the fetus contains only 40 to 45 gm of fat and will deposit more than 500 gm of additional fat by term. This discrepancy between length and weight gains is seen in the prematurely born infant, who has a greater deficit in weight than in length and has little subcutaneous fat.

The development of the embryo is cephalocaudal. That is, the head and upper part of the body differentiate and develop before the lower part of the body. The high ratios of head length to total length in the embryo and in the newborn were seen in figure 3.1. The major characteristic of early embryonic development is cell and tissue differentiation. Despite its small size, the embryo by eight to twelve weeks has all organs formed. Although the physical size at twelve weeks may be 3 inches in length and 1 oz in weight, the need for protein, minerals, and vitamins in a constant flow—both to the embryo and to the developing placenta—in the first trimester are indicated by the rapid organogenesis. The nutritional needs later in pregnancy are more related to growth in size of the fetus.

The deposition of two minerals in the fetus is of particular interest. At birth approximately 25 to 30 gm of calcium are present in the newborn's body, but the bones are still flexible to facilitate the birth process. Rapid increase in calcification and rigidity of bone occurs after delivery. On the other hand, large quantities of iron are deposited in the fetus, and the hemoglobin concentration of the term newborn is in the range of 16 to 22 gm/100 ml blood, which will provide a reserve supply of iron for blood formation in the first four to six months of extrauterine life.

### Growth in the First Year

The deceleration of growth rate which starts toward the end of fetal life (fig. 3.3) continues into postnatal life. However, the rate of growth of the young infant is faster than at any later age. The infant is likely to triple his weight and increase his length by 50% in the first year. If this rate of gain were to continue, by ten years of age he would be 96 ft tall and weigh more than 200 tons. The rapidity of growth necessitates a steady flow of nutrients, and the infant is more vulnerable to deficiencies than the older child.

The greater increase in weight than in length is consistent with the increase in body fat. Measurements of subcutaneous fat thickness increase during the first nine months faster than widths of bone and muscle.[16] Sex differences in growth of infants are not as great as during the adolescent years. The curves of length and weight for boys tend to be slightly steeper than for girls. At birth the median boy is approximately 0.5 cm longer and 0.1 kg heavier than the median girl; by one year the differences are 1.5 to 2.0 cm and less than 1 kg.

### Growth during the Preschool Period

In contrast to the smoothness of infant growth, both in group percentiles and for most individual children, changes occur during early childhood years in segmental proportions and in weight gain which may result in shift of a child's position from one percentile rank to another. Whereas median gain in length in the first year may be 25 cm, in the second year the gain drops to 10 cm, and continues to decrease to a gain of 5 to 7 cm per year until the pubertal spurt again increases the annual gain. Weight gain, which may have been approximately 6 kg in the first year, decreases to 2 to 3 kg per year. Weight gain may become erratic, and it is not unusual for the preschool child to lose weight for a brief period of time. As will be seen later, this is also a period of erratic appetite and changes in dietary components.

Relatively small changes in body proportions occur during the first six to nine months, but the rapidity of growth in the extremities in contrast to the trunk and head in the preschool period results in a drop in sitting height from 65% to 55% of total height by six years (fig. 3.5). In the Child Research Council series, nearly two-thirds of the subjects changed in percentile zones for bone lengths of the extremities relative to height and for sitting height by four years of age.[18] Body proportions show more individualistic change in the preschool period than in the early school years.

Sex differences in growth as measured by height and weight are small during this period, but body composition changes become apparent. The widths of muscle as measured by roentgenograms are similar for both sexes, but boys have progressively wider bones and girls have wider fat thickness.

## Growth in the Early School Years

In the period between five to six years and the onset of adolescent changes, which may be as early as nine years in girls and eleven years in boys, growth is relatively smooth. Boys and girls have similar gains in height, weight, sitting height, leg length, and muscle widths. However, boys have progressively wider bones and a greater increase in chest circumference while girls deposit more subcutaneous fat than boys.

## Growth in Adolescence

The dramatic changes in physical, physiological, biochemical, and hormonal characteristics of the body during this period of development have been of particular interest to workers in the field of growth and development.[19,20] This age period is sometimes divided into two stages. Puberty begins with the first appearance of secondary sex characteristics, increase in size of the breasts in females and the external genitalia in males, and the appearance of pubic hair. "Strictly, pubescence ends when sexual reproduction becomes possible; adolescence is the period from then to adulthood."[21] Most of what is called the adolescent growth spurt occurs in the pubescent period. However, the difficulty of identifying and separating consecutive and interrelated events has led to the use of *adolescence* as an all-inclusive term.

Sex differences in growth and body composition become more pronounced, and the variations in timing, magnitude, and duration of the growth spurt among children of the same sex require separate evaluation of each child for maturation, growth rate, and therefore nutrient requirements. As will be shown, the use of averages or percentiles during this age span masks the differences between children. Since it is difficult to define precisely when full maturity has been achieved, the cessation of growth in stature is usually used as the end point of the adolescent period.

Girls, on the average, enter puberty approximately two years before boys, have a slightly smaller increment in height during adolescence, and terminate growth sooner. As a result, boys have a longer period of childhood growth and enter puberty taller, gain slightly more height over a longer period of time, and are taller as adults. This is shown in figure 3.8, with data from the National Health Survey[22] in which girls were taller than boys for a total of four years.[23] The spurt in girls, as reported in various longitudinal studies, begins at an average age of 10 years, but the range may be from 7½ to as late as 14½ years.[20,24] In boys, the average age at onset is approximately 12 years, with a range from 9½ to 16 years.

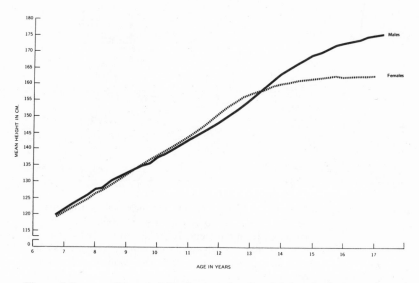

| **Figure 3.8** | Mean heights for age of males and females between six and seventeen years of age, National Health Survey Cycles I and II. Reprinted from Hamill, P. V. V.; Johnston, F. E.; and Lemeshow, S. *Height and Weight of Youths 12–17 Years, United States, 1966–1970.* Vital and Health Statistics series 11, no. 124. DHEW publication no. (HSM) 73–1606. Washington, D.C.: U.S. Government Printing Office, 1973. |

The ages at maximum growth, or peak height velocity, tend to be two years after onset of adolescent growth, or at averages of twelve years in girls and fourteen years in boys. Increments in growth during adolescence are better seen in velocity curves (fig. 3.9) for averages of boys and girls in the Brush Foundation study,[25] which are typical of curves from many longitudinal studies. However, using mean or median values over this age span obscures the variations in individual growth patterns. This was demonstrated in figure 3.10, a graph drawn

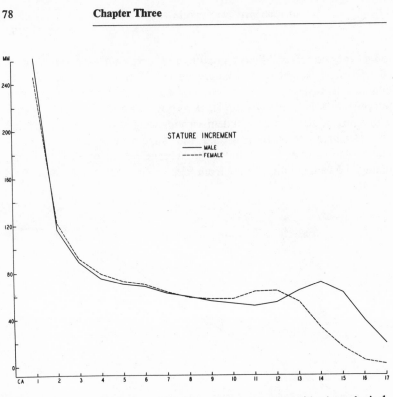

**Figure 3.9**     Increments of height of boys and girls with chronological ages (CA) from two to seventeen years. Reprinted, with permission, from Simmons, K. "The Brush Foundation Study of Child Growth and Development." *Monographs of the Society for Research in Child Development* 9 (1944): 1–87.

by Tanner[20] from data of Shuttleworth (1939) by a technique first suggested by Boas (1892). The individual velocity curves of five boys were plotted against chronological age, with the mean indicated by the dotted line. Variation in timing of maximum velocity of the individuals results in a mean with a longer and lower peak. However, when peak velocity was taken as the focus, the similarity of the curves of the five boys becomes evident and the mean velocity curve is similarly high and compressed in time.

Mean weights of boys and of girls change with curves similar to the height changes, as seen in the plotting by age of the National Health Survey data (fig. 3.11)[22] and the plotting by increments of the Brush Foundation subjects (fig. 3.12).[25] The adolescent growth spurt contributes almost one-half of adult weight, but only 10% to 15% of adult stature.[26]

Body composition changes differently for boys and for girls in adolescence. Boys develop progressively wider bones than girls. Muscle widths, similar in the sexes until adolescence, increase more sharply in boys than in girls. Therefore, lean body mass increases more rapidly in the male and his maximal lean body mass is nearly 50% higher than the female's.[27] Since lean body mass is composed of the most actively metabolizing tissues in the body, the male has higher nutrient needs both for the growth of those tissues and for their maintenance.

Fat widths increase in both sexes during early puberty, but the increase in boys is small and temporary. The increase in body fat of females is greater and is maintained. Changes in body composition are associated with changes in body shape. The increased shoulder width of boys and increased hip width of girls are particularly characteristic of adolescent changes.

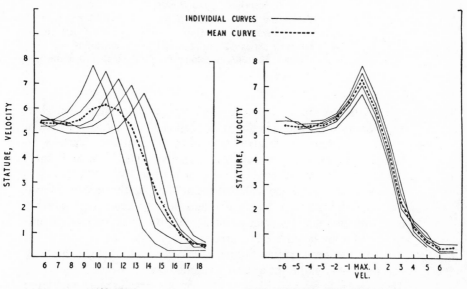

**Figure 3.10**   Individual and mean velocities of growth of girls during adolescence. Height curves plotted against chronological age (Shuttleworth 1939) in contrast to height curves plotted according to age of maximum velocity of increment. Reprinted, with permission, from Tanner, J. M. *Growth at Adolescence*, 2d ed. Oxford: Blackwell Scientific Publications, 1962.

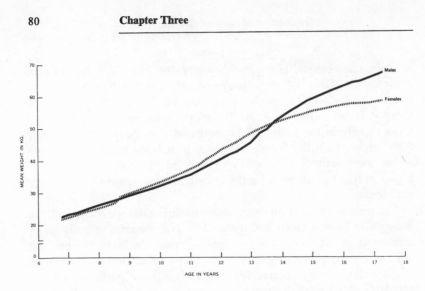

Thus far we have been concerned with chronological age. However, the wide variations in timing of adolescent changes make maturational stage more meaningful than chronological age. Various approaches to assigning maturational age have been used. Tanner[20]
graded changes in secondary sex characteristics. Skeletal age may be
evaluated by comparison of the ossification of the individual with
standards derived from roentgenograms of large numbers of children,
as shown in chapter 2. Age at menarche, the onset of menses, provides a specific landmark for girls.

Menarche occurs after the peak velocity of the height curve, so
that most of adult height has been attained before menstruation starts.
This is seen in figure 3.13, based on the data of Simmons and Greulich, in which the timing of menarche is shown in relation to the height
increment curves of groups of girls with early, average, and late
menarche. The mean age at menarche has been reported by Tanner[20]
to have decreased in the past century at the rate of four months per
decade. These data may be subject to some question, since much of
the early data were retrospective and obtained from hospital patients,
which might suggest abnormality. In addition, the use of means gives

undue weight to women with late menarche. However, there is evidence that between 1840 and 1930 there was a decrease in average age at menarche. This trend may have ceased. With careful records on age at menarche both on individual subjects and on mother-daughter combinations, the longitudinal studies of the Harvard School of Public Health, the Oakland-Berkeley group, the Fels Research Institute, and the Child Research Council have found no secular decrease in the age at menarche since 1930.

The median age at menarche found in the National Health Survey in cycles II and III was 12.77 years, with white girls having a median of 12.80 years and black girls 12.52 years.[28] The curve for distribution of ages is shown in figure 3.14. In a summary of mean ages found in eleven samples of girls, including longitudinal studies, Johnston et al.[29] found a range of means between 12.39 and 13.12 years.

Menarche is more closely related to skeletal age than to chronological age. As shown by data of Simmons and Greulich in figure 3.15, earlier menarche is associated with advanced skeletal age, indicating that the timing of events in adolescence in an individual tends to be related. Estimates of total body water and lean body mass are similar at menarche for early- and late-maturing girls.[29] Early-maturing girls

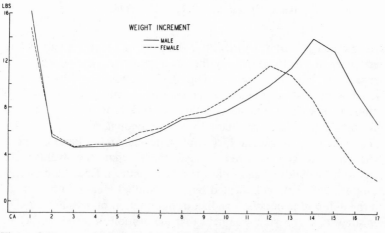

**Figure 3.12**     Increments of weight of boys and girls with chronological ages (CA) from two to seventeen years. Reprinted, with permission, from Simmons, K. "The Brush Foundation Study of Child Growth and Development." *Monographs of the Society for Research in Child Development* 9(1944):1–87.

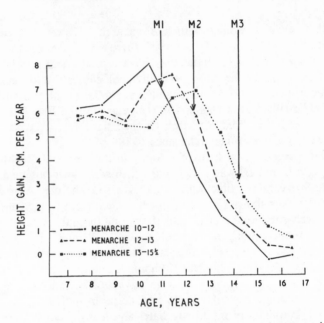

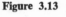

**Figure 3.13**          Peak height velocity for early, average, and late maturing
                         girls as reported by Simmons and Greulich (1943). Age
                         at menarche is indicated. Reprinted, with permission, from
                         Tanner, J. M. *Growth at Adolescence*, 2d ed. Oxford:
                         Blackwell Scientific Publications, 1962.

tend to reach menarche shortly after the peak in height velocity, while
there may be a longer delay between peak height velocity and
menarche in late-maturing girls (fig. 3.13). Theories that there is a
critical weight when menarche occurs have been disputed, and the
variations in weight indicate that this measurement is no better than
chronological age as a predictor for the individual girl.

There is a strong genetic factor in age at menarche. Parents whose
adolescent changes occurred at ages earlier than the average are
likely to have children who follow the same pattern. Racial differences
in maturation exist, as indicated by the National Health Survey data,
but the differences in either median or distribution of ages are small.[28]
For some time the view was held that maturation occurred earlier in
warmer climates, but recent data have indicated that this is not true.
For example, in recent studies the average menarcheal age in Nigeria
was 14.22 years and in Alaskan Eskimos 14.42 years.

The secular decrease in menarcheal age and the differences between populations are probably related to the same factors which
affect growth and maturation on a wider scale: socioeconomic status,

medical care, sanitation, nutrition, and other environmental factors. A variety of studies have shown that in underdeveloped countries and during periods of wartime food shortage adolescent development may be delayed. Individual variation occurs in all groups including advantaged populations; in the Child Research Council series, the range of menarcheal age was 10.5 to 15.4 years in upper middle class girls. But when environmental factors are marginal or inadequate to support potential growth, a delay in maturation is not unexpected. As environment improves, menarcheal age tends to be lower, but evidence indicates that in well-nourished and economically advantaged populations no further decrease in age is currently being seen. This is in agreement with observations that the secular increase in adult height has ceased in advantaged populations.

Assessment of skeletal maturity is another means of determining biological age as contrasted to chronological age. There is evidence that different parts of the skeleton of an individual mature at dif-

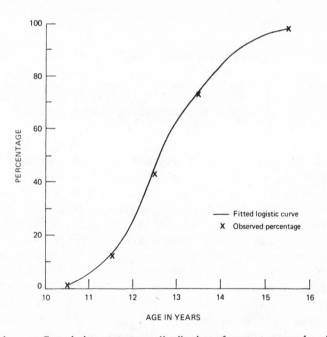

**Figure 3.14**          Cumulative percentage distribution of ages at menarche of girls in National Health Survey. Reprinted from McMahon, B. *Age at Menarche, United States.* Vital and Health Statistics series 11, no. 133. DHEW publication no. (HRA) 74–1615. Washington, D.C.: U.S. Government Printing Office, 1973.

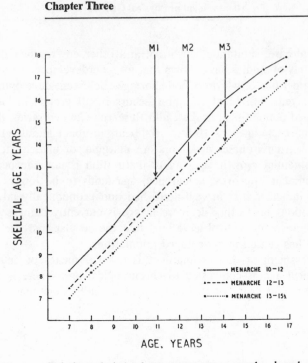

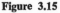

**Figure 3.15**     Relation of skeletal age to age at menarche, based on
averages of groups of girls with early, average, and late
menarche, from Brush Foundation study. Reprinted, with
permission, from Tanner, J. M. *Growth at Adolescence*,
2d ed. Oxford: Blackwell Scientific Publications, 1962.

ferent times and rates, but since total body roentgenograms are impractical, hand-wrist roentgenograms are commonly used. Figure 3.16
shows the roentgenograms of three girls at each of three ages: six,
seven, and eight years. These were selected to show maximal, average,
and minimal ossification which might be found at those ages. For
example, although the three six-year-old girls are the same chronological age, each has a different skeletal age. The most advanced of
the six-year-old girls has a bone age similar to that of the average
eight-year-old. As indicated earlier in this chapter, a skeletal age may
be assigned to each child by comparison with norms which have been
established from measurement of roentgenograms of large numbers
of children at consecutive ages.[10,11] The emergence, size, and shape of
the centers are considered in the assessment. There are thirty-one
osseous centers in the hand and wrist, but not all of them need to be
rated.

    Aside from individual variation within each sex, there are marked
differences between boys and girls. As with other maturational

changes, girls are more advanced in skeletal age than boys of the same chronological age. For example, in the Child Research Council series, all eight carpal centers were ossified in girls earlier than in boys. The first girl to have all eight centers was 5½ years old, and the latest was 11 years old. The youngest age when all eight centers were present in a boy was at 9 years and the last boy to reach that level was 14 years old.[30] The sex difference is consistent with growth rates. Early-maturing children tend to be taller at a given chronologi-

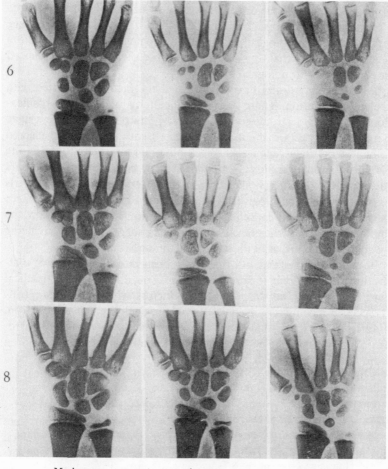

|  | Maximum | Average | Minimum |

**Figure 3.16**          Variation in carpal development of girls six, seven, and eight years of age. Courtesy of O. D. Abbott, Ph.D.

cal age than late-maturing children, whether the comparison is between boys and girls or within one sex.

Skeletal maturation may also be measured by the age at fusion of
epiphyses to the shafts of the long bones. This is a particularly useful
observation when there is concern about the amount of growth a child
may anticipate at a given age. In our society, the concern is usually
about the tall girl and the short boy. The establishment of age when
the epiphyses first ossify, intermediate changes showing progress in
maturation, and the final fusion with elimination of the cartilagenous
plate give indication of skeletal maturity. No further long bone
growth occurs after fusion; any increase in height would result from
elongation of the trunk. Therefore the short child whose skeletal age
lags behind chronological age can anticipate more growth before
reaching maturity than the short child whose skeletal age is advanced
in contrast to chronological age.

A number of studies have investigated the factors associated with
skeletal maturation. There are familial patterns of timing of ossification, indicating a strong genetic effect. Malnutrition and illness have
been shown to retard the maturation of osseous centers as measured
in hand-wrist roentgenograms. Black boys and girls were found in the
Health Examination Survey of children between six and eleven years
to be more advanced in skeletal age than were white boys and girls
at comparable chronological ages.[31] Although urban-rural differences
have been reported in other populations, none were found in the
United States. Influence of climate has been suggested but convincing
evidence is lacking, as with studies of the age at menarche.

Socioeconomic status has frequently been linked with rate of maturation. It is difficult to sort the effects of nutritional intake, medical
care, sanitation, and the many other factors which accompany differences in income and in social status, but evidence is available from
a variety of sources that low socioeconomic status is related to retardation of skeletal age. In the Health Examination Survey, children
from families with annual incomes over $10,000 were slightly more
advanced in skeletal age than children from families with annual incomes under $5,000, but the difference was not statistically signifi-
cant. Japanese and Chinese children brought up in the United States
have been reported to have more advanced skeletal ages than were
typical in the countries of their origin. Relationships between skeletal
age and socioeconomic status have been reported from the Netherlands, Tunisia, Nigeria, and Poland, but minimal or no relationship
has been found in reports from England and Belgium. Rural Jamaican
children have lower skeletal ages than blacks in Philadelphia. As

with other characteristics of growth, the differences seem to be more pronounced when the range of incomes is great, and less pronounced in those countries with smaller variations in income.

## Secular Trends in Growth and Development

Increase in body size through time has been demonstrated for a number of population groups throughout the world, as documented by Tanner.[20] This may be partially accounted for by the earlier rate of maturation and a shorter growth period. For example, maximal adult height fifty years ago was probably not reached until twenty-six years, and now in high socioeconomic groups in Western Europe and the United States mature height is more often attained by eighteen to nineteen years in males and by sixteen to seventeen years in females; reports of heights of college students or individuals of comparable ages must take into consideration the late maturation of subjects in early studies.

The growth of ten-year-old children in the United States from 1870 to 1970 is shown in figure 3.17, with a calculated regression line from data published by Meredith, on which are indicated the average heights of children in low and high income families in the 1963–65 cycle II of the Health Examination Survey[32] and the average heights of children in India and in the United Arab Republic. In the accompanying discussion and comparison of U.S. children with children in approximately fifty countries in the Meredith analysis, Hamill et al. state that the comparisons "strongly suggest that more of the factors conducive to greater size in children are available to the lowest socioeconomic groups in the United States than to all but the most highly favored few in India and to no classes at all in the underdeveloped countries such as Burma and Ethiopia. Although income and education make a very demonstrable difference, the other factors which are universally available to all classes of Americans make far more difference. This finding does not repudiate the statements of the past few years concerning 'pockets of hunger and starvation' in the United States. It does, however, emphatically limit these pockets in size, in number, and in severity."[32]

Studies of the heights and weights of college students over extended periods of time have been summarized by Hathaway and Foard [33] and by Bakwin.[34] In a seventy-year period, heights of Harvard students increased by 3 inches and weights by 9 lb. Among Amherst College freshmen, only one class prior to 1910 had as many

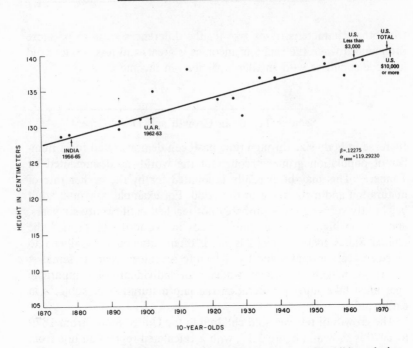

**Figure 3.17**     Regression line of growth of ten-year-old children during
the last century. Indicated are the 1963–65 Health
Examination Survey figures for the total U.S. sample of
ten-year-old children and those from families with annual
incomes above $10,000 or below $3,000, as well as heights
of children in India and the United Arab Republic.
Reprinted from Hamill, P. V. V.; Johnston, F. E.; and
Lemeshow, S. *Height and Weight of Children: Socioeconomic Status, United States.* Vital and Health Statistics
series 11, no. 119. DHEW publication no. (HSM) 73–1601.
Washington, D.C.: U.S Government Printing Office, 1972.

as 10% of men over 6 ft tall. After 1937 all but two classes had at
least 20% of its members over 6 ft, and in 1956 and 1957 more than
30% of the classes were taller than 6 ft. College records also give
evidence of the socioeconomic effect on height. Comparing students
entering Harvard in the 1930s with those entering in 1958–59, no
increase in height was observed in those from private preparatory
schools, but those from public schools were 1.5 inches taller in the
later period. The comparison of like-sexed parent and child enrolled
in the longitudinal studies in Berkeley, Denver, and Yellow Springs
show no secular increase in heights. Presumptive evidence from many
sources, then, indicates that height increases with improvement in

socioeconomic position, but that the end point has been reached in the United States for the middle and upper income groups.

In a summary of growth retardation in developing countries, Guzmán[7] stated:

Differences among races within comparable socioeconomic groups are small; those between socioeconomic groups are regularly large, an indication of the greater importance of environmental than genetic factors. Children from low socioeconomic groups, in all racial groups studied, had lower growth levels than children of high socioeconomic status; and those children in turn differed little in all measurements from accepted standards for children in industrialized countries. Retarded bone development, late initiation of the prepuberal growth spurt, later menarche, and a lesser magnitude of maximum growth during puberty all indicated an altered function associated with growth retardation.

Guzmán also stated, "Growth retardation in a population is generally accepted as being neither a fixed nor an enduring situation. Improvement occurs in the course of time as socioeconomic conditions become better, bringing enlightened health practices and progress in nutrition."

## References

1　Stuart, H. C. *Outline of Growth and Development for Medical Students and Students of Public Health*. Boston: Harvard School of Public Health, 1945.

2　Washburn, A. H. "Why Be Interested in Child Growth and Development?" *The Child* 16 (1951):50–54.

3　Scammon, R. E. "The First Seriatim Study of Human Growth." *American Journal of Physical Anthropology* 10 (1927):329–36.

4　Winick, M.; Brasel, J. A.; and Rosso, P. "Nutrition and Cell Growth." In *Nutrition and Development*, edited by M. Winick. New York: John Wiley & Sons, Inc., 1972.

5　Winick, M. *Cellular Changes during Early Malnutrition*. Columbus, Ohio: Ross Laboratories, 1971.

6　Widdowson, E. M. "Early Nutrition and Later Development." In *Diet and Bodily Constitution*. CIBA Foundation study group no. 17. Boston: Little, Brown & Co., 1964.

7　Guzmán, M. A. "Impaired Physical Growth and Maturation in Malnourished Populations." In *Malnutrition, Learning and Behavior*, edited by N. S. Scrimshaw and J. E. Gordon. Cambridge, Mass.: M.I.T. Press, 1968.

8   Thompson, D'A. W. *On Growth and Form*, 2d ed. Cambridge: Cambridge University Press, 1942.

9   Hansman, C. "Anthopometry and Related Data." In *Human Growth and Development*, edited by R. W. McCammon. Springfield, Ill.: Charles C Thomas Co., 1970.

10  Greulich, W. W., and Pyle, S. I. *Radiographic Atlas of Skeletal Development of Hand and Wrist*, 2d ed. Stanford, Calif.: Stanford University Press, 1959.

11  Tanner, J. M.; Whitehouse, R. H.; Marshall, W. A.; Heady, M. J. R.; and Goldstein, H. *Assessment of Skeletal Maturity and Prediction of Adult Height*. New York: Academic Press, 1975.

12  Maresh, M. M. "Changes in Tissue Widths during Growth: Roentgenographic Measurements of Bone, Muscle and Fat Widths from Infancy through Adolescence." *American Journal of Diseases of Children* 111 (1966):142–55.

13  Stuart, H. C., and Sobel, E. H. "The Thickness of Skin and Subcutaneous Tissue by Age and Sex in Childhood." *Journal of Pediatrics* 28(1946): 637–47.

14  Reynolds, E. L. "The Distribution of Subcutaneous Fat in Childhood and Adolescence." *Monographs of the Society for Research in Child Development* 15(1951 [no. 2]):1–189.

15  Garn, S. M., and Haskell, J. A. "Fat Thickness and Developmental Status in Childhood and Adolescence." *American Journal of Diseases of Children* 99(1960):745–51.

16  Maresh, M. M. "Measurements from Roentgenograms." In *Human Growth and Development*, edited by R. W. McCammon. Springfield, Ill.: Charles C Thomas, 1970.

17  Timiras, P. S. *Developmental Physiology and Aging*. New York: MacMillan Co., 1972.

18  Maresh, M. M. "Linear Body Proportions: A Roentgenographic Study." *AMA Journal of Diseases of Children* 98(1959):27–49.

19  McKigney, J. I., and Munro, H. N., eds. *Nutrient Requirements in Adolescence*. Cambridge, Mass.: M.I.T. Press, 1976.

20  Tanner, J. M. *Growth at Adolescence*, 2d ed. Oxford: Blackwell Scientific Publications, 1962.

21  Roche, A. F. "Some Aspects of Adolescent Growth and Maturation." In *Nutrient Requirements in Adolescence*, edited by J. I. McKigney and H. N. Munro. Cambridge, Mass.: M.I.T. Press, 1976.

22  Hamill, P. V. V.; Johnston, F. E.; and Lemeshow, S. *Height and Weight of Youths 12–17 Years, United States, 1966–1970*. Vital and Health Statistics series 11, no. 124. DHEW publication no. (HSM) 73–1606. Washington, D.C.: U.S. Government Printing Office, 1973.

23  Hamill, P. V. V. "Weight, Height and Skinfold Measurements." In *Nutrient Requirements in Adolescence*, edited by J. I. McKigney and H. N. Munro. Cambridge, Mass.: M.I.T. Press, 1976.

24   Maresh, M. M. "Variations in Patterns of Linear Growth and Skeletal Maturation." *Journal of the American Physical Therapy Association* 44 (1964):881–90.

25   Simmons, K. "The Brush Foundation Study of Child Growth and Development." *Monographs of the Society for Research in Child Development* 9(1944[no. 1]):1–87.

26   Heald, F. P. "New Reference Points for Defining Adolescent Nutrient Requirements." In *Nutrient Requirements in Adolescence*, edited by J. I. McKigney and H. N. Munro. Cambridge, Mass.: M.I.T. Press, 1976.

27   Forbes, G. B. "Biological Implications of the Adolescent Growth Process: Body Composition." In *Nutrient Requirements in Adolescence*, edited by J. I. McKigney and H. N. Munro. Cambridge, Mass.: M.I.T. Press, 1976.

28   McMahon, B. *Age at Menarche, United States.* Vital and Health Statistics series 11, no. 133. DHEW publication no. (HRA) 74–1615. Washington, D.C.: U.S. Government Printing Office, 1973.

29   Johnston, F. E.; Roche, A. F.; Schell, L. M.; and Wettenhall, H. N. B. "Critical Weight at Menarche: Critique of a Hypothesis." *American Journal of Diseases of Children* 129(1975):19–23.

30   Hansman, C. F., and Maresh, M. M. "A Longitudinal Study of Skeletal Maturation." *American Journal of Diseases of Children* 101(1961):305–21.

31   Roche, A. F.; Roberts, J.; and Hamill, P. V. V. *Skeletal Maturity of Children 6–11 Years: Racial, Geographic Area, and Socioeconomic Differentials, United States.* Vital and Health Statistics series 11, no. 149. DHEW publication no. (HRA) 76–1631. Washington, D.C.: U.S. Government Printing Office, 1975.

32   Hamill, P. V. V.; Johnston, F. E.; and Lemeshow, S. *Height and Weight of Children: Socioeconomic Status, United States.* Vital and Health Statistics series 11, no. 119. DHEW publication no. (HSM) 73–1601. Washington, D.C.: U.S. Government Printing Office, 1972.

33   Hathaway, M. L., and Foard, E. D. *Heights and Weights of Adults in the United States.* U.S.D.A. Home Economics research report no. 10. Washington, D.C.: U.S. Government Printing Office, 1960.

34   Bakwin, H. "The Secular Change in Growth and Development." *Acta Paediatrica* 53(1964):79–89.

# Chapter Four

## Standards for Evaluation of Growth

From the measurements of schoolchildren, the surveys of large populations of children, and the careful longitudinal studies of individual children, it has been clearly demonstrated that there is a pattern of human growth which has typical periods of acceleration and deceleration. Within this human growth range, each child has his own individual pattern with a level, a rate, and a timing which are distinctive for him. A single measurement of height, weight, or other body dimension may be taken to determine his position in the group at a given age. The single measurement does not tell how he reached that level nor the path he is following. Repeated measurements of a child show his individual progress in relation to the group, whether he is progressing at a pace consistent with his age and sex or is deviating from the expected curve. Deviation may be an index to his health, nutritional intake, and other environmental factors. Consecutive observations of size are a vital part of nutritional assessment of the child. Growth is sensitive to nutrient supply and is one of the simplest indexes to nutritional adequacy.

Throughout the past century, efforts have been made to develop simple but meaningful methods of evaluating growth for use in schools, in clinics, and in physicians' offices. To date, the efforts have been generally unsatisfactory. Those which are simple to use in most situations do not sufficiently describe the individual variations and may lead to erroneous conclusions. Those which are meaningful tend to be complex and require special training of the examiner. Because of the difficulty of making allowances for individuality, most available tables and graphs are norms, standards, or averages. None of the standards which have been developed has had universal acceptance, although some have been used both nationally and internationally.

Body growth is complex, with genetic and environmental factors interrelated in determining and altering the course of growth. Individuality becomes especially obvious during the adolescent period, and the early or late maturing child does not fit the average curve. There is, unfortunately, a tendency to label the slow-growing or late-maturing child as "retarded" when in truth this may be simply a variation of healthy growth. The need, so far unfilled, is for a set of standards which allow for healthy individual variations while at the same time providing a basis for identifying the child whose growth is truly deviant and indicative of pathology. As Falkner[1] has expressed it, we have a notorious affection for the norm, average, or standard, which merely describes, when ideally we need to evaluate.

The history of the study of growth, as reviewed in chapter 3, started with de Montbeillard in the eighteenth century. Quetelet (1836) was one of the first to apply a scientific approach to the study of human growth. In the United States, efforts to gather information on body measurements of children to establish tables for expected size for age began with Bowditch. A brief, but necessarily incomplete, summary of the chronological development of standards of growth in children will help to clarify the reasons why no single standard has yet been devised which allows both description and evaluation without extreme complexity.

## Historical Development of Growth Standards, United States

Bowditch (1877)[2] first established a table of average height and weight by age for boys and girls during the school years. Measurements were obtained from the schools, so were not taken by any standardized technique. Children were weighed in ordinary clothing, but heights were measured without shoes. Bowditch was foresighted in his awareness of differences due to socioeconomic level and nationality background.

Wood (1918)[3] calculated average weights for age of school children in the eastern and midwestern United States. He later collaborated with Baldwin (1923)[4] to carry the process one step further. The Baldwin-Wood tables were arranged to show the range of weights which might be expected for a given height and age of boys and girls. This gave an indication of whether the child was light or heavy in relation to his height. The measurements were taken by trained examiners on children without clothing. Many of the children had consecutive measurements, usually at yearly intervals. The Baldwin-Wood tables were more generally accepted in the United States, especially in schools, than any other tables of the time. Woodbury (1921)[5] provided the first norms for heights and weights of young children under six years of age.

The Baldwin-Wood and Woodbury tables were widely used. They created disagreement, however, about the significance of deviations from the mean. Half a century later, this disagreement has not been settled, although wider population groups and different mathematical treatments of data have been developed to expand the standards. The emphasis in much of the early publications was on the mean, or average. Deviations above the mean caused less disagreement than did deviations below the mean. The major use of these tables was as a screening technique to evaluate physical status at the time of the examination and progress in growth between examinations, and particularly to identify children who were malnourished. Health programs in many schools were based on the assumption that weight was a good criterion of nutritional status. Both in schools and in physicians' offices parents were encouraged to aim for "normal" weight for their children. A dividing line between the healthy slender child and the child who was malnourished was difficult to establish. Varying opinions selected 6%, 7%, or 10% below the mean weight for height for the younger child. Since individual variation is greater in adolescence, a cutoff point of 15% below the mean was suggested for older children. For the overweight category, a weight which was 20% or more above the mean for height and age was commonly used as the dividing line.

Franzen (1929)[6] made the first attempt to broaden the base of evaluation. He used twelve measurements, including height, weight, chest depth and width, hip width, and calf circumference. In a later publication Franzen recommended the use of a special spring caliper designed for measuring the thickness of skin and subcutaneous tissue. The appreciation that measurement of height and weight alone was not sufficient to describe health status and that body build should be part of the total evaluation was advanced by Franzen. The time required and the difficulty of obtaining accurate measurements limited the acceptance of his work.

Further advancement came with the publication of Burgess (1937)[7] of the heights of American-born children, using graphs instead of tables and percentiles instead of means. Plotting the child's measurement on a graph allowed the examiner to see at a glance the child's size in relation to other children of his age, and plotting repeated measurements showed the degree of progress and whether the increment was consistent with expected increments for his age and sex.

The use of Galton's percentiles had been applied to Bowditch's data in 1891, but seems to have been ignored in the interim. The value of percentiles versus means and standard deviations eliminated one of the problems which had made the application of growth standards controversial. The mean is the average of a group of measurements, determined by adding all the individual measurements (of height, for example) and dividing by the number of observations included. The standard deviation (S.D. or $\sigma$) is derived from a statistical formula to show the variability of values above and below the mean. Two-thirds of the cases in a distribution would fall within the range of one standard deviation above or below the mean ($m \pm 1$ SD) and 95% of cases would fall within the range of $m \pm 2$ SD. Only 2.5% of the cases would exceed $m + 2$ SD, and 2.5% would fall below $m - 2$ SD.

The use of means and standard deviations is justified if the distribution of cases is normal in the statistical sense; that is, when the frequency is plotted against the magnitude of the measurement, a bell-shaped curve results, with the distribution symmetrical and the extremes equidistant from the mean. However, many biological measurements do not have a bell-shaped distribution. Height measurements are more likely to be normally distributed than are weight measurements. The distribution of weight measurements is asymmetrical, with skewness to the right. Many values are clustered together at the lower end, while some values stretch far above the center of the distribution. The degree of overweight can obviously be much greater than the degree of underweight. Therefore mean weight is elevated by the inclusion of some very high measurements. Standard deviation falsely equalizes variability above and below the mean even though such equality is not true of the original distribution.

Percentiles depend on the distribution of values based on the number of observations rather than on the magnitude of the measurements only. To calculate percentiles, the observed measurements are arranged in order of magnitude. The fiftieth percentile (median) is the central measurement, with an equal number of measurements above and below it. Similarly, 25% of the cases fall below the level of the measurement at the twenty-fifth percentile and 25% of the cases above the seventy-fifth percentile. The expectation of the number of cases within a given range of percentiles is useful in determining the problems within a population. For example, if a survey showed that 23% of seven-year-old boys were below the fifteenth percentile for height, this would indicate an excess of short boys in that population. A discussion later in this chapter will deal with the selection of the population on whom percentile standards are based.

Because the distribution of weights is skewed to the right, there is a wider range of weight between the fiftieth and ninetieth percentiles, for example, than between the fiftieth and tenth percentiles. Similarly skewed distributions are observed in measurements of body fat, intake of most nutrients, leukocyte and eosinophil counts, and a number of other physiological measurements. The reintroduction of percentiles by Burgess was a recognition of biological variation which has become widely accepted in the development of standards.

A further attempt to include individual variation, this time in relation to body build, was the contribution of Wetzel, who devised a grid for children five through eighteen years of age (1941)[8] followed by the baby grid for ages under three years (1946).[9] The grid (fig. 4.1) was based on the principles that "1. Healthy progress prefers development along a channel of given body type on an age schedule or timetable specific for the subject and with the preservation of that subject's natural physique. 2. Each child should be considered his own standard of comparison." The grid stressed the importance of following the progress of the child in height and weight.

The grid is divided into two connected graphs. On the left, by plotting weight for height without regard for age, the child's physique may be determined. Diagonally increasing physique channels are labeled $A_4$, $A_3$, $A_2$, $A_1$, M, $B_1$, $B_2$, $B_3$, and $B_4$. The $A_4$ channel, representing the highest weight for height, indicates the fattest children. At the opposite extreme, the thinnest children follow channel $B_4$. Wetzel estimated that 60% to 70% of the children would fall within the three central channels. Crossing the channel markers are isodevelopmental lines. The child is expected to cross one isodevelopmental line per month, or twelve per year. He is not expected to shift more than one-half channel width within ten isodevelopmental lines. Such deviation in weight for height should be further investigated.

The isodevelopmental lines of the first graph extend across to the graph on the right, which introduces chronological age, to evaluate "auxodromic" progress, or developmental age. Sex differences are also introduced into the auxodrome graph. Wetzel theorized that deviation of a child from his own weight-for-height channel or from his auxodrome progress would quickly become apparent, such deviation indicating incipient disease, overnutrition, or undernutrition, earlier than in other graphic methods by showing disturbance in the child's own pattern. Two columns on the right indicate basal metabolism

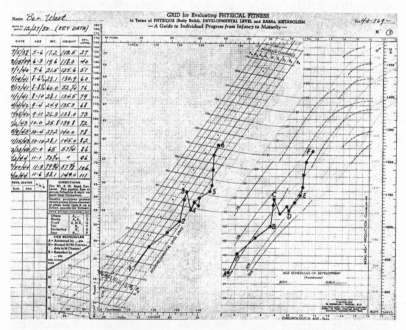

**Figure 4.1**      Wetzel grid for recording the growth of boys and girls. The record reproduced on the grid is based on a child's actual weight and height measurements, provided by Dr. Wetzel. Two episodes of growth failure (1–2) and (3–4–5) are indicated on the grid panel. Recovery responses in both cases are likewise shown: (2–3) and (5–6). Corresponding deviations from normal speed of development (A–B) and (C–D) and recovery (B–C) and (E–F) are indicated on the auxodrome panel. Wetzel, N. C. "Physical Fitness in Terms of Physique, Development and Basal Metabolism." Reprinted, with permission, from *Medical Women's Journal* 55 (1948):19.

and dietary caloric needs (the latter calculated as twice the basal calories) at each isodevelopmental level.

Criticisms of Wetzel's grid have centered around its complexity, the rigidity of allowance for deviation in channel position, and the tendency to confuse maturity with weight for height. The obese child appears on the grid to be further toward maturity than the average or slender child.

Further efforts to include body dimensions other than weight and height have been made by workers in the growth studies discussed in chapter 3. Vickers and Stuart (1943)[10] recognized that "pediatricians believe that height and weight, and at times other measurements, should be included as items in the health examination of children, but that many are in doubt as to what measurements should be taken and how they should be interpreted. There has been no standard practice as to the measurements taken, the techniques adopted, the norms used for reference, or the evaluation of the data obtained. . . . No attempt is being made at this time to settle the question as to which measurements should be used routinely and which may properly be discarded." They presented tables of weight and height and their increments, head and chest circumferences, chest and pelvic breadth, crown-rump length, and sitting height. Figures were given for the tenth, twenty-fifth, fiftieth, seventy-fifth, and ninetieth percentiles as well as means and standard deviations for boys and girls separately from birth to ten years, from data of the Harvard School of Public Health growth study. They suggested that each measurement should be evaluated as to its position in the distribution, then in relation to other measurements of the child, and finally in relation to measurements at the previous examination. Believing that measurements are of value in studying progress of growth only if they are taken in a standard way with the same technique each time, and with methods comparable to those used in the tables, they gave careful description of the equipment and techniques.

Using data from the Iowa studies of Meredith and Boyd, plus additional infant data, Jackson and Kelly (1945)[11] published sets of charts for graphing height and weight in three age groups: 0 to 1 year, 0 to 6 years, and 5 to 18 years. Heights were charted with the mean for age and the levels of the mean plus and minus one standard deviation. Weight curves were based on the sixteenth, fiftieth, and eighty-fourth percentiles on the assumption that these levels represented comparable values for the two sets of measurements. They suggested rating each child for height-age and for weight-age as deviations from the mean or median to describe body build as slender, average, or stocky in relation to height.

Stuart and Meredith (1946)[12] presented tables and graphs for the tenth, twenty-fifth, fiftieth, seventy-fifth, and ninetieth percentiles for weight, height, chest circumference, hip width, and calf girth of boys and girls from five to eighteen years for use in school health programs (fig. 4.2). These values were derived from measurements of the

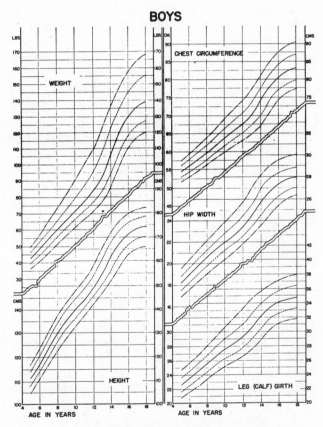

**Figure 4.2**        Stuart-Meredith graphs for plotting measurements of boys. Reprinted, with permission, from Stuart, H. C., and Meredith, H. V. "Use of Body Measurements in the School Health Program." *American Journal of Public Health* 36(1946):1365–86.

children in the Iowa growth study. Stuart and Stevenson (1950)[13] expanded the tables to include the third and ninety-seventh percentiles and added data from the Harvard School of Public Health study for the first five years of life. The Stuart-Meredith tables and graphs have been used nationally and internationally for evaluation of growth of children in many diverse populations. Their wide application meant that for the first time a single set of standards could be used for comparison of growth of children around the world. As with all standards thus far derived, questions about the applicability of values from one population to a different population group were raised.

Height and weight were the basic measurements for emphasis, and continued to be stressed, despite general agreement that these two measurements did not adequately distinguish between healthy children and those who should be more carefully examined for evidence of problems. A short child might be healthy or might be retarded in relation to his potential. A child whose weight for height was high might be obese or might simply have heavy bones and muscles. The variation in timing of adolescent changes often led to undue concern about the tall, early-maturing child or the small, late-maturing child. As we have seen, there were increasing efforts to include measurements of body build. Unfortunately, each additional inclusion of other dimensions increased the complexity and the need for careful training of examiners in taking measurements.

Bayley (1956)[14] introduced a new component in graphing growth by including an evaluation of physical maturity. Since this depended on the availability of roentgenograms of the hand and knee, widespread use of the method was unlikely, but it was an indication of the dissatisfaction with previous methods. There was, and continues to be, need for a better technique for evaluating the growth of individual children, particularly during adolescence. Bayley's data from the Berkeley Growth and Guidance Studies were used for the curves of height, weight, and their increments. Adaptation of a sample graph is shown in figure 4.3. The central curve is the average height curve. Adjacent curves, one above and one below the average curve, and following the same slope until close to the end of growth, represent children who are tall or short in their early years only because they are fast or slow in maturation. At a further distance from the average are curves representing what Bayley called constitutionally tall or small children. "Some children are large from a very early age, with a pattern of both accelerated bone age and rapid growth. They will be tall adults, and will gain this height two or three years before the average for their sex. Some children are small from an early age, and

grow and mature very slowly. They will probably attain a short adult
stature, usually after 18 (girls) or 20 (boys) years." Bayley also
added curves for annual increment. Similar curves were given for
weight. By use of maturation ratings from the roentgenograms, children could be evaluated as average, accelerated, or retarded, and
Bayley included a table to show the percent of mature height which
children in each category might be expected to achieve at ages between birth and eighteen or twenty years.

Garn (1965)[15] introduced the factor of heredity into a table of
measurements of children. Recognizing that tall parents tend to have
tall children and short parents tend to have short children, he used
data from the Ohio study to construct the Fels Parent-Specific Standards for Height (table 4.1). The heights of the mother and father

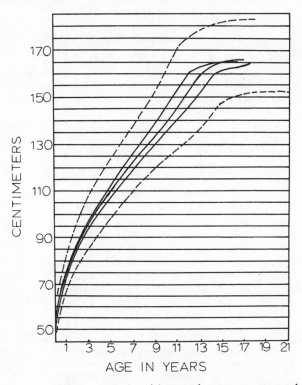

**Figure 4.3**     Height curves for girls maturing at average, accelerated,
and retarded rates. Adapted from Bayley, N. "Growth
Curves of Height and Weight by Age for Boys and Girls,
Scaled According to Physical Maturity." *Journal of
Pediatrics* 48(1956):187–94.

were averaged to give a midparent stature, divided into three groups
with average statures of 64.0, 66.5, and 69.0 inches. The mean
heights of the children of each of the three groups were calculated by
age and sex. The height of the child could then be evaluated with respect to his possible potential genetic size. Garn also recommended
the use of this technique in countries with different patterns of growth
and maturity from those observed in the United States. The tables
were later extended with additional categories of midparent size.

As growth standards have evolved, each new set has reflected the
type of data available at the time and the progress of the understanding of human growth in the past century. Until the early 1940s,
standards were based primarily on cross-sectional data, usually lim-

**Table 4.1**       Fels Parent-Specific Standards for Height: Children's
                    Stature by Age and Midparent Stature*

| Age (yr) | Midparent Stature (Inches) † | | | | | |
| | 64.0 | | 66.5 | | 69.0 | |
| | Boys | Girls | Boys | Girls | Boys | Girls |
| --- | --- | --- | --- | --- | --- | --- |
| 1 | 29.0 | 29.0 | 29.5 | 29.0 | 30.5 | 29.5 |
| 2 | 33.6 | 33.0 | 34.5 | 33.5 | 35.0 | 34.5 |
| 3 | 36.5 | 35.5 | 37.5 | 37.0 | 39.0 | 38.0 |
| 4 | 39.0 | 38.0 | 40.5 | 41.0 | 42.0 | 41.0 |
| 5 | 41.5 | 40.5 | 43.5 | 43.0 | 44.5 | 43.5 |
| 6 | 43.5 | 43.5 | 45.5 | 45.5 | 47.0 | 46.0 |
| 7 | 45.7 | 46.0 | 48.0 | 47.5 | 49.0 | 49.0 |
| 8 | 48.0 | 48.0 | 50.0 | 49.5 | 51.5 | 51.0 |
| 9 | 50.0 | 50.5 | 52.0 | 52.0 | 53.5 | 54.0 |
| 10 | 52.0 | 53.0 | 54.0 | 54.0 | 55.5 | 56.5 |
| 11 | 54.5 | 55.5 | 56.0 | 56.5 | 58.0 | 59.0 |
| 12 | 57.0 | 58.0 | 58.5 | 59.0 | 60.0 | 61.5 |
| 13 | 59.5 | 60.5 | 61.0 | 62.0 | 63.0 | 63.5 |
| 14 | 62.5 | 62.5 | 63.5 | 63.0 | 66.0 | 65.5 |
| 15 | 65.5 | 63.0 | 66.0 | 64.0 | 69.0 | 66.5 |
| 16 | 66.5 | 63.0 | 68.0 | 64.0 | 69.5 | 67.0 |
| 17 | 67.5 | 63.5 | 69.0 | 64.5 | 70.0 | 67.5 |

SOURCE: Reprinted, with permission, from Garn, S. "The
Applicability of North American Growth Standards in Developing Countries." *Canadian Medical Association Journal*
93(1965):914–19.
*Age-size tables for Ohio white children whose midparent
stature (or parental midpoint) is the average of the statures
of the two parents. All values rounded off to the nearest
half inch.
†Average of maternal and paternal statures.

ited to height and weight, most of which had been obtained from single measurements of thousands of schoolchildren. As shown in figure 3.10, grouped data do not reflect individual patterns of maturation, especially during the adolescent period. Starting in the 1940s, the longitudinal growth studies, many of which had by then collected data for twenty years, supplied tables and graphs based on consecutive measurements on samples of a few hundred children each, primarily of northern European extraction and usually within the range of middle incomes. These studies included not only a variety of anthropometric measurements but also evaluations of biological maturity. They provided data on healthy variability of growth of individual children, resulting in efforts to include body composition changes and genetic potential into the evaluation.

The wide use of growth standards based on selected groups of children enrolled in longitudinal studies has been questioned as to its applicability to other population groups, both in the United States and in other areas of the world. To replace the Stuart-Meredith charts from the 1940s, the National Center for Health Statistics (1976)[16] has constructed growth charts from a variety of sources. All charts are based on seven smoothed percentile levels (5, 10, 25, 50, 75, and 90) for each sex. Because of the lack of suitable alternative data for the first year of life, the percentiles from birth to thirty-six months were based on measurements collected between 1929 and 1975 on subjects in the Fels Research Institute study. These include weight, length, and head circumference by age. Weight-for-length charts for the first three years were based on data from birth to forty-eight months.

The NCHS growth charts for the age span from two to eighteen years were based on data collected by the Center for Health Statistics in three surveys, conducted between 1962 and 1974. The Health and Nutrition Examination Survey (HANES I) included subjects from one to seventeen years; the Health Examination Survey cycle II was conducted on subjects from six to eleven years of age; and cycle III on subjects twelve through seventeen years of age. Percentiles were calculated and smoothed for this age group for height and weight by age (see fig. 4.4). In addition, charts were made for weight for height, without regard to age, for prepubescent children. Selecting children as prepubescent for the latter graphs required judgment by the committee. No individual data were available to indicate the point of acceleration of growth since they were based on single measurements. In cycle II information was not obtained on the presence or absence of pubescent changes. The charts of weight for height

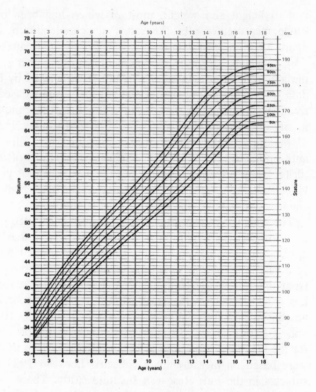

**Figure 4.4**          Percentiles of boys' stature by age, two to eighteen years.
NCHS growth charts, 1976. From Monthly Vital Statistics
Report (HRA) 76–1120, vol. 25, no. 3, suppl. Rockville,
Md.: U.S. Department of Health, Education, and Welfare,
Public Health Service, Health Resources Administration,
1976.

include data on girls to 10 years (fig. 4.5) and to 11½ years for
boys, adapted for the observed lag of nineteen months in boys as compared to girls in onset of adolescent changes in the survey data. However, without evidence to distinguish between children who had or
had not yet begun to show pubertal changes, the committee assumed
that the tallest children might have entered adolescence and eliminated from these calculations girls whose height was above the ninety-
fifth percentile by 8 years and boys at that level after 9½ years. Differences between black and white children were not considered large
enough to warrant separate racial standards.

Some differences in percentile levels appear between Stuart-Meredith and NCHS findings. For example, boys tend to be taller in the Fels sample in the first three years, although the tenth and twenty-fifth percentile levels are similar to the Stuart-Meredith values. Between two and five years, except for the ninetieth percentile, boys in the HANES survey tended to be shorter. This difference continued at all percentile levels after six years with the Health Examination Survey data, with HES boys shorter than the Stuart-Meredith levels. However, beginning with the ninetieth percentile at eleven years and progressing down the percentile range to the tenth percentile by fourteen

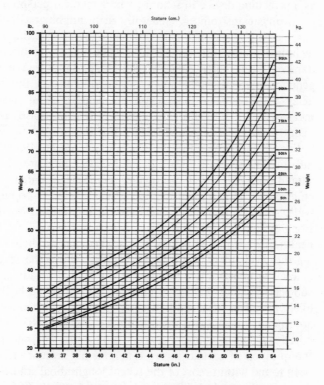

**Figure 4.5**          Percentiles of weight by stature for prepubertal girls. NCHS growth charts, 1976. From Monthly Vital Statistics Report (HRA) 76–1120, vol. 25, no. 3, suppl. Rockville, Md.: U.S. Department of Health, Education, and Welfare, Public Health Service, Health Resources Administration, 1976.

years, the levels for HES boys exceeded those in the Stuart-Meredith series. As a result, during the early and middle childhood years, fewer boys in a population sample would be considered short by the NCHS standards than by the Stuart-Meredith standards, but the reverse would be true in adolescence.

It is clear that no fully satisfactory growth standards have yet been developed. Perhaps no single standard can be developed to fit the disparate uses to which standards are applied. Graphs are more easily understood than tables, both by professional and semiprofessional workers and by parents, since they give a simple visual placement of the child's position in relation to the group. They can be readily used as a screening device in schools, where medical personnel are limited, or in physicians' offices. Generally such graphs are limited to weight and height; additional measurements require special equipment or technical ability and are of little value unless methodology is standardized. But height and weight alone do not take into account genetic potential, body build, or individuality in timing of growth. They may create a false sense of security about the child whose measurements fall into the middle range, or cause undue concern about children at high or low levels of the range.

Should the population on which standards are based be representative of the whole country, as the NCHS charts are after infancy, or should they be based on smaller numbers of intensively observed children in longitudinal growth studies? Large populations reflect wider socioeconomic and racial groups and varying degrees of health. Longitudinal study data reflect a narrower economic level but the health of the children is known. Large studies are better for establishing the levels of the outlying percentiles, above the seventy-fifth and below the twenty-fifth, because of the statistical advantage of many subjects. Smaller studies of children known to be healthy are more likely to reflect how children could grow if environmental conditions are satisfactory. Except for the infancy data, the NCHS standards are based on data obtained between 1962 and 1974 and thus eliminate the question of secular increase in size, but secular changes have not been found within most of the recent longitudinal studies (see chapter 3) and little secular change, at least at the twenty-fifth percentile and above, was observed in the decade of the NCHS studies. If secular increases have essentially ceased in the U.S. population, it is less important whether data were collected within the past ten years or within the past forty years. The definition of chronological age when measurements were taken is narrower for longitudinal studies than for national surveys. In the former, children were measured within a specified number of days around each age level; in the latter, subjects were examined at any time during the year and age brought to the nearest birthday, so "1 year" might include any age between 9 and 15 months and "12 years" any age between 11½ and 12½ years. The age adjustment may become significant during periods of rapid growth. Which of the available standards should be selected? It depends on the purpose for which standards are needed. Both types have advantages and disadvantages and each has contributed to our evaluation of how children grow.

## Classification of Body Physique

In the earlier discussion of methods of including indexes of body build in evaluation of growth, attention was centered on anthropometric and roentgenographic measurements. Physique is closely related to body composition of bone, muscle, and fat, and the ultimate description of physique must be based on measurements of those components. However, from early records of observations on the relationship of size to health and disease, a number of categories of physique have been described.[17]

Hippocrates described two types of body build: habitus phthisicus was tall and thin with increased susceptibility to tuberculosis; habitus apoplecticus was stocky and obese and more likely to have vascular disease. Galen based his four types on humors: sanguine, phlegmatic, choleric, and melancholic. Bryant described a carnivorous slender type, predisposed to hypothyroidism, anemia, and low blood pressure, and the robust herbivorous type, predisposed to obesity, pancreatic hyperactivity, and high blood pressure. Bunak had three categories: stenoplastic (vertical, slender, thin, and weak), mesoplastic (strong, with average fat), and euryplastic (broad, with average musculature and considerable fat). Roston divided people into four groups: *cerebral, digestif, respiratoire,* and *musculaire.*

Sheldon's somatotypes[18] were published in 1940 and have been widely used by anthropologists and anthropometrists. Standing nude photographs (back, front, and side views) were taken of subjects posed against a calibrated grid. These were inspected and measured. Ratings were assigned for body contours, prominence of various bony structures, fat covering, musculature, size of body segments, and other defined characteristics. Anthropometric measurements included width of the head, shoulders, and hips; circumferences of the neck, biceps, midthigh, calf, and ankle; and caliper measurements of fat layers.

Subjects were given comparative ratings for three categories: endomorphy, mesomorphy, and ectomorphy.

Endomorphy rates elements of softness, roundness, and smoothness. The endomorph has a predominance of abdominal mass and
structures derived from the endodermal embryonic layer. Although
obesity is not a necessary component, the extreme endomorph is
usually obese. Mesomorphy rates bone and muscle development and
connective tissue, derived from the embryonic mesodermal layer. The
mesomorph is likely to have a large chest, wide shoulders, and broad
hands and to be muscular. Ectomorphy rates elements of linearity.
The ectomorph is slender with delicate bone structure, long and nar-
row hands and feet, and poor muscularity.

Sheldon gave a numerical rating from 1 to 7 for each of the three
characteristics. Minimal strength of the component was rated 1, median 4, and maximum 7. For example, the extreme endomorph was
rated 7–1–1, the extreme mesomorph 1–7–1, and the extreme ectomorph 1–1–7. Any combination of ratings between these extremes was
possible. Most people have intermediate ratings for the three components with one component dominant.

To eliminate the necessity for photographs and for special training
in evaluating somatotypes, Damon[19] devised a series of mathematical
formulas based on measurements of weight, height, chest depth, upper arm circumference, and triceps and subscapular skinfolds, as well
as handgrip strength. The formulas provided calculated ratings for
the three Sheldon somatotypes.

## International Growth Standards

Whether growth standards from one country can be applied to populations in other countries has been an unresolved question. The international use of the Stuart-Meredith percentiles, sometimes referred
to as the Iowa standards, has provided a single framework against
which the growth of children in many countries has been compared.
However, many have questioned this use in view of genetic and economic differences.

In 1971, a commission of the International Union of Nutritional
Sciences formed a committee to establish specific guidelines on the
question of growth standards. The commission strongly recommended
that studies be carried out in as large a variety of countries as possible. "Each country's own standards must be derived from carefully

selected samples representing children growing in an optimal environment for that country." The committee report[20] stated that "justification for the creation of growth standards was as follows: anthropometric measures are the most important means of assessing nutritional and health status in communities, especially in children. Furthermore, appropriately developed standards can serve as a reference against which to measure change in health and nutrition of a given country and also as standards for evaluating the results of intervention programs. Properly designed, such studies will ultimately assist in evaluating true differences in genetic maxima for physical growth."

The committee felt that longitudinal study of a continuous population of children would be preferable but not practical on a nationwide or international basis, so recommended repeated cross-sectional studies within designated socioeconomic and age groups. First priority should be given to the group between birth and four years of age and second priority to ages seven to nine years, but it would be desirable to have measurements at five and six years and annually between ten and eighteen years. Samples in each country should be selected for genetic homogeneity. The first study should be done on the "modern elite group," selected on the basis of education and occupation of parents and use of medical facilities. A second group would be selected from the same ethnic stock but exposed to economic and other depriving circumstances.

Seven measurements were recommended to form the baseline for the studies: nude weight, height or length, head circumference to three years, upper arm circumference, triceps skinfold, chest circumference, and tooth eruption. Standardization of methodology was considered mandatory.

As the discussion in this chapter has shown, it is universally agreed that measurements of body size are essential to the evaluation of health and nutritional status of children and that they offer great potential for identifying children who need nutritional support. However, in view of the continued controversy both in the United States and in the international community about the selection of standards, the statement of Vickers and Stuart[10] more than three decades ago is still applicable: "Many are in doubt about what measurements should be taken and how they should be interpreted. There has been no standard practice as to the measurements taken, the techniques adopted, the norms used for reference, or the evaluation of the data obtained."

## References

1   Falkner, F. "General Considerations in Human Development." In *Human Development*, edited by F. Falkner. Philadelphia: W. B. Saunders Co., 1966.

2   Bowditch, H. P. *The Growth of Children*. Annual Report to the Massachusetts State Board of Health, no. 8, 1877, pp. 273–323.

3   Wood, T. D. *Height and Weight Table for Boys and Girls*. New York: New York Child Health Organization, 1918.

4   Baldwin, B. T., and Wood, T. D. "Tables for Boys and Girls of School Age." *Mother and Child* 4(1923[suppl.]):3–7.

5   Woodbury, R. M. *Average Heights and Weights of Children under Six Years of Age*. Children's Bureau publication no. 84. Washington, D.C.: U.S. Department of Labor, 1921.

6   Franzen, R. "Physical Measures of Growth and Nutrition." *Monograph of the American Child Health Association* 2(1929):138.

7   Burgess, M. A. "The Construction of Two Height Charts." *Journal of the American Statistical Association* 32(1937):290–310.

8   Wetzel, N. C. "Physical Fitness in Terms of Physique, Development and Basal Metabolism." *JAMA* 116(1941):1187–95.

9   Wetzel, N. C. "Baby Grid: An Application of the Grid Technique to Growth and Development in Infants." *Journal of Pediatrics* 29(1946): 439–54.

10   Vickers, V. S., and Stuart, H. C. "Anthropometry in the Pediatrician's Office: Norms for Selected Body Measurements Based on Studies of Children of Northern European Stock." *Journal of Pediatrics* 22(1943): 155–70.

11   Jackson, R. L., and Kelly, H. G. "Growth Charts for Use in Pediatric Practice." *Journal of Pediatrics* 27(1945):215–29.

12   Stuart, H. C., and Meredith, H. V. "Use of Body Measurements in the School Health Program." *American Journal of Public Health* 36(1946): 1365–86.

13   Stuart, H. C., and Stevenson, S. S. "Physical Growth and Development." In *Nelson Textbook of Pediatrics*. Philadelphia: W. B. Saunders Co., 1950.

14   Bayley, N. "Growth Curves of Height and Weight by Age for Boys and Girls, Scaled According to Physical Maturity." *Journal of Pediatrics* 48 (1956):187–94.

15   Garn, S. "The Applicability of North American Growth Standards in Developing Countries." *Canadian Medical Association Journal* 93(1965): 914–19.

16   Hamill, P. V. V.; Drizd, T. A.; Johnson, C. L.; Reed, R. B.; and Roche, A. F. *NCHS Growth Charts, 1976*. Monthly Vital Statistics report (HRA) 76–1120, vol. 25, no. 3, suppl., 22 June 1976. Rockville, Md.: U.S. De-

partment of Health, Education, and Welfare, Public Health Service, Health Resources Administration, 1976.

17   Seltzer, C. C., and Mayer, J. "Body Measurements in Relation to Disease." In Mayer, J. *Human Nutrition: Its Physiological, Medical and Social Aspects.* Springfield, Ill.: Charles C Thomas Co., 1972.

18   Sheldon, W. H. *The Varieties of Human Physique.* New York: Harper and Brothers, 1940.

19   Damon, A. "Delineation of Body-Build Variables Associated with Cardiovascular Diseases." *Annals of the New York Academy of Sciences* 126 (1965):711–27.

20   "The Creation of Growth Standards: A Committee Report." *American Journal of Clinical Nutrition* 25(1972):218–20.

# Chapter Five

## Development of Good Nutritional Status

The life cycle is a continuum which spans from one generation to another. Each individual is the product of his own history and, through inheritance of genes, the product of his parents' histories. Environmental factors become operative as soon as the ovum has been fertilized and starts to travel down the Fallopian tube to the site in the uterus where it will be implanted and grow. The embryo is dependent on the nutritional state of the maternal body for all substances needed for differentiation of tissue, for formation of body structures, for increase in size, and for developmental progress. The mother's nutritional status, which in turn depends on her own history, is vital to the healthy development of this small organism.

The physical state, maturity, and nutritional health of the neonate set the pattern for early development of the infant. Prematurity, immaturity, congenital defects, low birth weight, poor vitality—all present hazards to the newborn in his sudden adjustment to independent life. In the brief time span of delivery and severing of the umbilical cord, he must accomplish his own control of respiration, circulation, and temperature control and shortly thereafter ingestion, digestion, absorption, and elimination. The full-term newborn who has had an optimal prenatal environment in the body of a healthy, well-nourished woman is best able to achieve physiological independence.

The rapid growth in the first year requires a steady supply of nutrients. The infant is likely to triple his weight and add 50% to his length. He is setting the postnatal pattern of cell multiplication which will influence his size for the rest of his life. At the same time, he is developing psychological reactions to the giving and acceptance of food and to the social aspects of eating which may affect his lifelong food habits.

As the child progresses through his formative years, his health and development in each period are based on his achievements in the preceding phases. The adolescent may be obese due to adipocyte numbers or dietary patterns established in infancy. The timing and magnitude of the adolescent growth spurt may be affected by prepubertal health and dietary intake. The pregnant woman may have a contracted pelvis as a result of rickets in her own childhood. To evaluate a child at any given age, it is important to know his history.

Studies of animals and humans have shown that at some periods malnutrition or other interference with normal processes may result in permanent retardation. On the other hand, the phenomenon of catch-up growth has long been recognized. Studies of cell growth will help to explain why irreversible retardation occurs at some times and compensatory growth is possible at other times. If there are critical ages when cell multiplication must occur but adverse environmental conditions or undernutrition or disease prevent the body from achieving its full potential of cell numbers at that time, later adequate feeding or improvement in health may come too late to be within the period of cell replication and permanent retardation results. However, if undernutrition or illness occurs at a time when the full complement of cells has been completed or nearly completed, the adverse conditions may affect only cell size, for which later compensation may be possible.

Just as each stage of childhood has its own characteristics of growth in body size and in development of function, so each stage also has its own nutritional requirements and dietary patterns. Experimentation with inadequate diets during human pregnancy and childhood is unethical, so our knowledge comes from experiments with animals and observational studies of humans. Growth rates and nutritional requirements of animals are different from those of humans and the results of such studies are not always applicable. Much of our understanding of the effects of diet on human growth is inferential, and the figures for nutrient requirements in pregnancy, lactation, and childhood have often been established as the best guess with available data, so controversy is not unusual. Actual requirements for growth are seldom known with any degree of certainty, and recommended allowances are subject to change as knowledge expands or viewpoints change.

More than forty nutrients are known to be essential to health and growth. Many are widely distributed in commonly used foods and there is little concern about deficiencies. However, some nutrients are found in relatively few foods or may be partially destroyed in food processing. With rapid changes in food technology, in the greater availability of formulated, engineered, and textured foods, and in the replacement of home preparation of foods with commercially premixed food or with restaurant meals, the need for studies of the adequacy of food intake as sources of essential nutrients has become more pressing. In order to evaluate adequacy, standards of nutrient intake for various segments of the population are essential.

The first standards were established in England in 1862 and were designed to "prevent starvation diseases." Standards later were developed to ensure adequate diets for armies and for civilian populations in wartime. The League of Nations formulated standards in 1935 to coordinate the nutrient needs of people with agricultural production. Gradually the objective changed from prevention of disease to nutritional well-being and positive health. A number of countries have established standards, some based on estimation of requirement and some with varying margins of safety to allow for the efficiency of nutrient utilization in various foods, individuality in requirement, and adjustment for factors of size, climate, and activity within their own populations. Therefore, standards or allowances vary from one country to another, and the Food and Agriculture Organization and the World Health Organization have established still another set of standards for international use.

## Recommended Dietary Allowances

The first edition of the *Recommended Dietary Allowances* by the Food and Nutrition Board of the National Research Council was published in 1943 with the objective of "providing standards to serve as a goal for good nutrition." The origin of the RDA has been described by Lydia J. Roberts,[1] who was chairman of the first Committee on Recommended Dietary Allowances. Recommended Dietary Allowances have been revised at intervals, and the 1974 revision[2] is the eighth edition. From their original function as a guide for advising on nutrition problems in connection with national defense, their uses have expanded to include planning food supplies for groups, interpreting food consumption records, establishing standards for public assistance and nutrition education programs, developing new food products, and establishing guidelines for nutritional labeling of foods. The Board has repeatedly expressed concern about the misuse of the RDA as a standard of judging adequacy of nutrient intake of individuals and populations. As the 1974 edition stresses, two common statements are equally invalid: "RDA include a large safety factor; therefore a diet that meets two-thirds of the RDA standard should be adequate" and "The average intake meets RDA standards; therefore there is no problem of nutritional inadequacy." In view of the common misuse of the RDA, the seldom-read publication which describes the purpose and basis of the figures should be required reading for everyone who uses the widely distributed table (appendix 1).

"The Recommended Dietary Allowances are the levels of intake of essential nutrients considered, in the judgment of the Food and Nutrition Board on the basis of available scientific knowledge, to be adequate to meet the known nutritional needs of practically all healthy persons." The RDA should not be confused with requirements. Because of individual variations, there is no way of predicting whose needs are high and whose are low, so the RDAs (except for energy) are estimated to exceed the requirements of most individuals.

The RDAs for energy are estimates of the *average* needs of population groups, not recommended intakes for individuals. For other nutrients a margin of safety is added to the average requirement. When information on mean requirement and standard deviation is adequate, the RDA is established at the level of the mean plus two standard deviations; with a statistically normal distribution for the requirements of individuals, 97.5% of the population should have requirements below the RDA. For nutrients which have not been adequately studied to permit calculation of means and standard deviations, the best judgment of the Board was used to establish an allowance. That judgment may have been based on limited human studies, perhaps more extensive animal studies, dietary survey data on apparently healthy people, estimates of needs for physiological function and for growth of body tissues, and interpolation for ages for which data were lacking.

Each successive edition of the *Recommended Dietary Allowances* has had changes in levels of some nutrients and addition of nutrients to the table when sufficient data were available to estimate allow-

ances for them. Figure 5.1 shows the changing concept of the Board
in regard to protein allowances for children. Since allowances for infants are expressed in the table as grams per kilogram of body weight,
which increases rapidly in the first year, they are not included in the
graph, but they have followed the same downward trend as for older
children. The 1958 edition omitted protein allowances in the first
year because the committee failed to reach agreement on a recommended level. For children between one year and the end of adolescence, the protein allowance was unchanged from 1943 through
1958, but it has been lowered in each succeeding edition. The 1974
allowances are approximately 50% of the 1943–58 levels at most
ages.

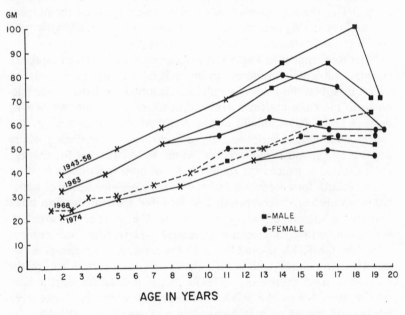

**Figure 5.1**      Recommended dietary protein allowances for children
(RDA) 1943–74.

Changes in the RDA levels of most nutrients must be taken into
consideration in interpretation of studies and surveys published in the
past thirty years if RDA levels were used in evaluating the adequacy
of dietary intakes. More diets would have been rated inadequate in
protein by 1958 allowances than by 1974 allowances, for example.
Until more complete data are available on the nutritional needs of

individuals as a basis for establishing realistic RDA levels, continual revisions of the figures may be expected.

Despite their limitations and qualifications, the RDAs do provide a framework of current thought on the levels of intake which meet the needs of all but 2½% of the population on a statistical basis. "In assessing individual dietary records, it is highly unlikely that intake is inadequate when it meets or exceeds the allowance, but as intake falls the risk of deficiency increases. Nevertheless, an intake below the allowance is not, in itself alone, evidence of nutritional inadequacy. To assess the nutritional status of an individual, records of nutrient intake must be considered in relation to the results of clinical and biochemical tests." Detailed discussion of nutritional assessment was the basis of chapter 2.

## Nutrition from Conception to Maturity

### Pregnancy

This discussion will concentrate primarily on the 266 days of pregnancy during which the fertilized ovum undergoes cell division, tissue differentiation, increased complexity, and growth to the full-term newborn. However, the state of the woman when she enters pregnancy is critical to her success in reproduction.[3-5] Her nutrition prior to pregnancy may be as important as her nutrition during gestation. The woman who enters pregnancy in an undernourished state, with minimal storage and poor tissue saturation, has little leeway in meeting the demands of her own body as well as those of the developing fetus and the increase in maternal tissues to support the fetus. Enthusiasm for weight reduction in women of childbearing age has often led to caloric restriction and to poorly balanced fad diets which may have caused depletion of some nutrients. The increased number of pregnancies in teenagers, especially in those under fifteen years, has led to a greater frequency of infants with low birth weight and risk of infant mortality. The young teenager superimposes the nutritional stress of pregnancy on a body which has just passed through a period of rapid growth and may still be growing.

Data on preconceptional dietary intakes are difficult to obtain. Retrospective data are subject to errors of memory. In the absence of such data, height of the mother has been used by some workers as an index of prior nutritional intake. However, longitudinal studies have produced some valuable records. Follow-up data on fifty-six women who had originally been enrolled in the study at the Harvard School of Public Health to eighteen years of age suggest that both childhood nutrition and height were related to reproductive performance.[6] When they were examined after a lapse of ten years or more, the fifty-six women had had a total of 209 pregnancies. Of the women whose protein intakes between eight and twelve years of age had been 70 gm daily or more, 80% had healthy babies in all pregnancies compared to 30% of those with lower intakes. Women with good reproductive performance were, on the average, 5 cm taller than those with poor performance, which included spontaneous abortions and prematurely born infants. A diet high in protein is likely to be high in most other nutrients, so the protein level of the diet is an index to total dietary adequacy.

The first trimester of pregnancy is the period of organogenesis—the differentiation of cells which have been formed from the fertilized ovum into distinct body organs. The embryo at three months may be about 3 inches long and weigh only 1 oz, but it has already developed tissues of different types so that limbs, heart, and other body components are distinguishable. Interference with nutrient or oxygen supply, viral infections, alcohol, drugs, or irradiation during this period may cause congenital defects. The added hazard of nausea and vomiting may limit food intake and absorption, so the woman who is well nourished at the start of pregnancy is more likely to have reserves to draw upon during this critical period.

The placenta begins to form soon after implantation of embryonic tissue in the uterus, and with the first heartbeat at about twenty-one days begins its task of nourishing the embryo and removing waste materials. The placenta continues to increase in its cell numbers, as measured by DNA, until the thirty-fifth week, although its protein and RNA content increase linearly to term.[7] When fully formed, it has a surface area of 40 to 45 sq ft folded into a diameter of 16 to 20 cm and a thickness of 3 to 4 cm.[8] A spongy tissue, composed largely of both maternal and fetal blood vessels, which do not connect, the placenta produces some hormones itself and transfers others from maternal to fetal circulation. Transport of nutrients may be by diffusion (especially of substances with molecular weights under 500), by carrier, or by active enzymatic transport. Amino acids, calcium, phosphorus, potassium, zinc, iodine, magnesium, folic acid, vitamin $B_{12}$, and ascorbic acid are usually higher in fetal blood than in maternal blood, indicating that the placenta selectively controls the rate of transfer. Others, such as fat-soluble vitamins, tend to be lower in fetal blood. Carbohydrate crosses the placenta as glucose and is the primary source of energy for the fetus. There is some evidence that the size of the placenta is related to the size of the fetus, but other evidence suggests that the efficiency rather than the size of the placenta or a defect in maternal circulation may be limiting factors in supply of nutrients to the fetus.[9]

Most of the growth in fetal size occurs during the last six months of pregnancy. Length increases almost linearly through most of pregnancy. Increase in weight is most marked after the fourth month. The four-month fetus may weigh approximately 125 gm; by term, weight will be about 3,500 gm on the average. The marked increase in weight is related to fat deposition. At six months the fetus contains approximately 40 gm of fat (3% to 4% of fetal weight) and by term 560 gm (16% of body weight).

The maternal body undergoes a number of physiological changes in adaptation to pregnancy. Blood volume expands approximately 32%, but not equally for plasma and cells. Plasma increases close to 40% while red blood cell volume increases only 18%.[9] This hemodilution results in a decrease in concentration of hemoglobin and red blood cells, despite the actual increase in body content of these components. Therefore, the diagnosis of anemia in the pregnant woman must be based on a different standard. For example, a hemoglobin level of 13.5 gm/100 ml blood in the nonpregnant woman may be equivalent to a hemoglobin concentration of 12 gm/100 ml toward the end of gestation. Many other blood components also have a lower concentration at the end of pregnancy as a result of dilution of blood by the greater plasma volume.

Basal metabolic rate increases approximately 15% by term as a result of the greater amount of active metabolizing tissue, but the increased caloric requirement is partially offset by a decrease in physical activity. Slower motility of the gastrointestinal tract delays the passage of food. This would provide a longer period of time for food to be absorbed from the intestinal wall, which is consistent with the observation that some nutrients are better absorbed during pregnancy.

Nutrient requirements of the pregnant woman must include allowances for maintenance of her own body, increase in maternal tissues such as the uterus and breasts, growth of the fetus and of the placenta and other tissues related to the fetus. Attempts have been made to estimate each of these needs to arrive at a total requirement. Although there are limited data on the total body composition of the healthy term newborn infant, the following estimations have been made: protein, 350 to 550 gm; calcium, 25 gm; phosphorous, 14 gm; and iron, 200 to 250 mg.

Compiling figures from several sources in the literature, a calculation of the added iron needs during pregnancy, for example, might be as follows: 200 to 250 mg for the full-term single fetus, 50 to 60 mg for the placenta, 500 mg for maternal blood increase, making a total extra need for 750 to 910 mg of absorbed iron for the entire period of gestation. There are other factors to be considered, but they may offset each other. The loss of blood at delivery, whether vaginal or caesarean, may be partially offset by the saving of iron as a result of the lack of menstrual periods. In addition, the expansion of red blood cell volume in the maternal organism during pregnancy may lead to residual retention of some of the extra iron after delivery. If adequate information were available on possible increase in absorption of dietary iron, this could be factored into the calculation of requirement. This estimation of additional iron needs for a nine-month pregnancy above nonpregnant needs for a comparable period of time permits calculation of the increase in the pregnant woman's daily requirement. Since most of the iron is needed during the last half of pregnancy, the major increase would be allocated to that period.

The RDAs for pregnancy (see appendix 1) allow for different rates of increase over nonpregnant allowances for each of the nutrients. The following percentage increases have been established: folacin, 100%; protein, 65%; calcium, phosphorous, and magnesium, 50%; zinc, ascorbic acid, thiamine, and vitamin $B_{12}$, 30% to 33%; iodine, vitamin A, vitamin E, riboflavin, and pyridoxine, 25%; calories and niacin, 15%. The RDA for iron for the nonpregnant woman has been set at 18 mg, and for pregnancy 18+ mg, with a notation that a supplement is recommended since the amount cannot be obtained from ordinary diets, and the text recommends a supplement of 30 to 60 mg per day. No allowance was set for vitamin D for adults after growth has been completed, but an allowance of 400 IU daily is set for pregnancy.

The increase of only 15% in caloric needs with an increase of 65% in protein places emphasis on the need for greater nutrient density of the diet during pregnancy. Therefore the foods which are added to meet the additional caloric allowance must be foods which supply more protein, minerals, and vitamins than carbohydrate or fat.

Historically, the changes in the extra protein allowances for the pregnant woman over nonpregnant needs have reflected the uncertainty about existing information. From the first edition of *Recommended Dietary Allowances* in 1943 through the fifth edition in 1958, the allowance for the nonpregnant woman was 60 gm daily and for pregnancy 85 gm, a difference of 25 gm. In 1964 the allowance for the nonpregnant woman was 58 gm, and of the pregnant woman 78 gm, a difference of 20 gm. In 1968 the allowance for the nonpregnant woman was lowered to 55 gm and for the pregnant woman to 65 gm, a difference of only 10 gm. In the 1974 edition, the protein allowance for the nonpregnant woman was lowered still further to 46 gm, but the allowance for the pregnant woman was raised to 76 gm, a difference of 30 gm. Another change has been in the stage of pregnancy when the additional protein is recommended. From 1943 through 1948, the higher allowance was recommended in the second half of pregnancy; in 1953 only in the third trimester; in 1958 for the latter half of pregnancy. The 1964 and 1968 editions recommended the increased protein for the second and third trimesters, and the 1974 edition recommended increasing protein from the second month to term. Therefore, not only is the differential greater, but the higher amount is recommended for essentially all of the prenatal period.

The recommendation for increased protein is consistent with the findings of the nitrogen balance studies of pregnant teenagers by Calloway and King.[10,11] The 1968 RDA protein level did not permit maximum protein storage in young primiparas. Even at an intake of 125 gm protein per day, there was no evidence that maximum storage potential had been reached.

For many years it was the practice of many physicians to limit weight gain during pregnancy. In a review of the literature on weight gain and the outcome of pregnancy, the Committee on Maternal Nutrition of the National Research Council[9] concluded: "An average gain in weight during pregnancy of 24 pounds (range of 20 to 25 pounds) is considered reasonable. This is a gain of about one pound per week during the second half of pregnancy and is commensurate with the most favorable outcome of pregnancy. Limiting the weight gain of normal women to 10 or 14 pounds is not justified; because of the possibility of adverse effects on birth weight and neurological development, weight-reduction programs and severe caloric restriction should not be undertaken." The committee also stated that the routine supplementation of the diets of pregnant women, except for iron, folic acid, and possibly iodine in areas where the soil and water are deficient, is of doubtful value and that emphasis should instead be on enhancing the nutrient intake with foods as a corrective for improper food habits.

The pattern of normal prenatal weight gain, as advocated by the National Research Council committee based on the studies of Hytten and Thomson (fig. 5.2), is increasingly used in prenatal clinics. It follows a curve of gradual increase in weight from the second month, with a gain of 3 lb in the first trimester, 11 lb in the second, and 10 lb in the third. The recommended weight gain of 24 lb during pregnancy is approximately three times the weight of the average new-

born. The additional weight is essential for the placenta, amniotic
fluid, and increases in the uterus, breasts, and blood volume of the
pregnant woman. Some of the weight gain has not been accounted for.
Increase in body fluids, both intracellular and extracellular, occurrence of some degree of edema even in healthy women, and storage
of protein and/or fat in preparation for lactation may play a role in
the additional gain.

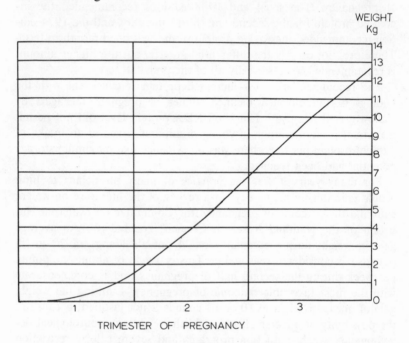

TRIMESTER OF PREGNANCY

**Figure 5.2**     Weight gain in pregnancy, based on observations of normal
primiparas. Adapted from Hytten, F. E., and Thomson,
A. M. "Maternal Physiological Adjustments." In *Maternal
Nutrition and the Course of Pregnancy*. Washington, D.C.:
National Academy of Sciences, 1970.

A gain of more than 24 lb is recommended for the teenager, who
may still be growing. This requires individual evaluation of the stage
of maturity of the teenager. Since the major increment of growth occurs before menarche, one may assume that the period of greatest
requirement for nutrients to support adolescent growth has passed
before ovulation becomes possible. However, as shown in chapter 3,
growth in the girl may continue to sixteen or seventeen years on the

average, and to eighteen or twenty years in some individuals. The allowance for weight gain during pregnancy, particularly in the girl under sixteen, should be added to the gain of her own body. An extra allowance for weight should also be given to the woman who is underweight at the start of pregnancy. Many studies have shown that the thin woman tends to retain some weight after delivery.

One reason against restriction of weight gain during pregnancy to less than twenty pounds is the relationship between inadequate weight gain and the delivery of infants whose birth weights are low for gestational age. Two categories of infants have been identified whose birth weights are less than 2,500 gm. The premature infant is born before the thirty-sixth week of pregnancy, and therefore is likely to be small because of inadequate time in utero for full development. In recent years there has been concern about infants thirty-seven or more weeks in utero who are small, often with no detectable reason. Metcoff[12] has speculated that fetal growth retardation may be one of three types. Type I results in an infant who is uniformly small with respect to weight, length, and head circumference, implying that malnutrition was present throughout gestation and the fetal growth curve was slow from the beginning. Type II is the infant whose length and head circumference are higher in percentile rank than weight, suggesting that marked deprivation of food for the pregnant woman occurred during the last trimester of pregnancy; infants of toxemic mothers may have this type of fetal growth retardation. Type III is the infant whose length and head circumference may be average and whose weight may have followed the average curve until the last three to four weeks and the fetus then sustained acute weight loss; Metcoff speculates that this may be the pattern when severe famine occurs only during the last stage of pregnancy. Whether fetal malnutrition results from fetal, placental, or maternal factors may be unknown, but evidence is strong that cell replication is somehow impaired. A variety of physical, biochemical, and behavioral characteristics of these infants deviate from normal, but not in consistent directions for all small-for-age infants, and high morbidity and mortality rates are observed.[13]

Low birth weight for gestational age has been observed more often among women with certain characteristics, including biological immaturity (under sixteen to seventeen years), short stature, low preconceptional weight for height, low weight gain during pregnancy, poor nutritional status, low protein intake, chronic heart or kidney disease, toxemia and other complications of pregnancy, viral infections, history of prior reproductive loss, multiple fetuses, smoking, and heroin addiction. Many of these characteristics indicate the nutritional inadequacy which accompanies low socioeconomic status or factors which interfere with maternal supply of nutrients to the fetus.

Meeting nutrient requirements during pregnancy without excessive caloric intake demands attention to supplementing the diet of the pregnant woman with foods which are high in protein, minerals, and vitamins. Since protein foods are usually high in minerals and vitamins of the B-complex, primary emphasis should be placed on protein. The pregnant woman should be encouraged to include 1 qt of milk, one egg, and at least 4 oz of meat, fish, or poultry in her daily diet. On a strict vegetarian diet it is difficult to include sufficient protein, and the necessity to balance vegetable proteins with their differing limiting amino acids to ensure an adequate supply of all essential amino acids to the fetus requires a detailed knowledge of food values. It is, therefore, wise to urge the vegetarian to include at least milk in her diet.

The inclusion of milk is also the most effective way to meet calcium needs. Without milk or milk products, the calcium content of the American diet rarely exceeds 300 mg/day. Dependence on calcium supplements is not recommended. Many supplements have a relatively low content of the mineral, and they do not supply the protein, vitamins, and other minerals which are supplied by milk. Women with some degree of lactase deficiency can usually consume moderate amounts of milk during the day with little or no discomfort, and most tolerate yogurt or buttermilk, which contain less lactose. Calcium is important not only for the mineralization of bones and teeth, but also for blood clotting, maintenance of muscle tone, and nerve impulse transmission. When intake is inadequate, calcium may be withdrawn from maternal bones to maintain the plasma level. It has been speculated that repeated pregnancies with low calcium intakes may be factors in the etiology of osteoporosis in elderly women.

Much controversy has centered on the high RDA level for iron, for both the menstruating woman and the pregnant woman. The usual U.S. diet contains approximately 6 mg of iron per 1,000 kcal. Unless the diet is very carefully selected, the nonpregnancy allowance of 18 mg would require an intake of 3,000 kcal, which would be excessive for most women. The Food and Nutrition Board has recommended a supplement of 30 to 60 mg of iron daily for the pregnant woman. Studies have shown that recommended supplements are not always taken, and supplemental iron is often poorly tolerated and may cause gastric distress. It is advisable to increase high-iron foods in the diet, such as liver, whole grains, meat, and green leafy vegetables.

Increase in thyroid function and in basal metabolism are normally observed in pregnancy. The use of iodized salt is recommended, especially if the intake of seafood is low.

Folacin deserves special consideration in pregnancy. It has been recognized for the past fifty years that megaloblastic anemia is more common in pregnancy, especially in underprivileged populations. There is evidence that folacin requirement is greatly increased during pregnancy. The functions of this vitamin in amino acid metabolism, synthesis of nucleic acids, and the formation and maturation of normal red and white blood cells indicate its importance in fetal development. However, studies on the effects of folacin deficiencies or supplementation of the diet on obstetric complications and fetal damage have produced conflicting results. The RDA for folacin is twice the level for the nonpregnant woman and a folacin supplement of 0.4 to 0.8 mg/day is sometimes recommended.[14] Dietary sources of folacin include liver, green leafy vegetables, meat and fish, nuts, legumes, and whole grains.

With special attention to the nutrients which have added significance in formation of the fetus and maintenance of health in the mother, the diet during pregnancy should include a variety of foods. There is no single selection of foods which must be taken to meet nutrient requirements. Adaptation of usual cultural or ethnic patterns of eating should be based on calculation of the nutrient content of the diet, followed by addition of acceptable foods which will fulfill the needs for pregnancy. For the most common pattern of food consumption in the United States, the following list will supply nutrients to ensure meeting the needs of the mother and fetus:

Milk: One quart daily. Part of the milk may be replaced by cheese, yogurt, or ice cream. Some may be used in cooking or on cereal or other foods. The milk may be whole, low-fat, buttermilk, or skim.

Meat: At least 4 oz daily. Liver and other organ meats, fish, and poultry are included in this category. Nuts or legumes may be substituted for meat.

Egg: One daily.

Fruits: At least one citrus fruit and one other fruit daily.

Vegetables: Two to four servings daily. A green leafy or yellow vegetable should be included at least three to four times per week.

Butter or fortified margarine: One to two tablespoons daily.

Bread or cereal: Two to four servings daily, preferably whole grain or enriched. Enriched pasta may be used as a substitute.

Additional foods to meet energy needs.

Infancy

There is a wealth of scientific evidence that human milk is the best food for the infant in the first six to twelve months. Both the quantity and quality of breast milk from a well-nourished mother are ideally suited to the needs of the growing baby.[15] Human milk is used as the reference standard for nutrient needs of the young infant.[16] In developing countries, poor sanitation and the high cost of formulas make breast feeding essential for infant survival. The inadequacy of substitutes has resulted in protein-energy malnutrition. Unfortunately, the practice of breast feeding is now decreasing in urban areas of many developing countries. In Western countries a higher standard of living and protection against bacterial contamination have allowed women to choose whether or not to nurse their infants. Formulas are easily available, bottle feeding is socially accepted, and increasing numbers of women are employed outside the home. The practice of breast feeding in the United States decreased with the availability of safe formulas for infants, but within the past decade more women have appreciated the values of lactation and have chosen to nurse their babies.

At the turn of the century, almost all infants in the United States were breast fed. In the 1920s more than 50% of infants were still breast fed at one year of age.[17] In 1948, Bain[18] found that only 38% were totally breast fed at hospital discharge and an additional 27% were on breast feeding with supplementary formulas. By 1958[19] those numbers had dropped to 21% and 16%, and in 1961[20] the number totally breast fed was 24% and partially breast fed 6%. The recent increase in breast feeding among higher income and well-educated mothers was seen in the Preschool Nutrition Survey[21] of 1968–70. In that survey, 21% and 23% of mothers in the two lowest income groups breast fed their infants in the first week and 9% and 12% in the second week; in the two upper income groups, 29% and 39% of infants were breast fed in the first week and 15% and 20% in the second week. However, breast feeding is too often discontinued within the first month.

Early success in breast feeding depends on a number of factors, including the attitude of the mother. Newton and Newton[22] found in a study of ninety-one mothers that 74% of those with a positive attitude toward lactation had enough milk by the fifth day to make formula supplementation unnecessary, but only 26% of the mothers with a negative attitude produced sufficient milk by the fifth day. A

New Haven group[23] observed the nursing characteristics of newborn infants. Some babies were eager and vigorous in nursing from the start; some were slow in nursing for the first few days. Some newborns nursed consistently until satisfied, while others nursed and rested alternately. The approach of each infant to the nursing situation and the response of the mother are important in the initiation of lactation.

Both physiological and psychological factors are related to nursing performance. Hormones, reflex actions, and relaxation of the mother are essential. Prolactin initiates milk production. On contact with the infant, a nerve in the breast stimulates the pituitary to release oxytocin, which in turn stimulates contraction of the cells of the mammary gland, forcing milk down the ducts to the sinuses behind the nipple, where it becomes available to the infant. The rooting reflex of the infant causes him to turn his head in the direction of a touch on the cheek. When his cheek touches the breast, his head turns toward it and he seeks the nipple. The sucking reflex and then the swallowing reflex continue the nursing process.

Tension, embarrassment, or any negative emotion or trauma may inhibit letdown, particularly during the first few weeks. It is important for the mother to be relaxed and comfortable in pleasant surroundings during the period when milk production is becoming established. The baby should be awake and hungry when he is brought to the breast. The strength of his sucking and the emptying of the breast stimulate milk production. Feeding water, with or without glucose, or other milk within an hour or two before the nursing period may limit the vigor of his sucking.

The major physiological advantage to the mother is that nursing causes contraction of the uterus, speeding involution to normal and decreasing the danger of hemorrhage. Physiological advantages to the infant are many. Breast milk forms small, soft curds in the stomach, facilitating digestion and resulting in fewer digestive upsets than cow's milk. Stools of the breast-fed infant are soft and constipation is unlikely. The composition of breast milk is suited to the human infant, and the transition from colostrum to mature milk meets the needs of the neonate and later of the growing infant. Bacterial contamination and allergenicity are minimal. Recent studies of the transfer in human milk of secretory immunoglobulin A, lactoferrin, lysozyme, antibodies to polio virus, and the bifidus factor have stressed the value of breast feeding in protection of the infant from infections, especially gastrointestinal and respiratory.[24,25]

Colostrum is a thick yellow alkaline liquid produced by the breast in the first few days. It is higher than mature breast milk in protein, ash (especially sodium and potassium), vitamin A, and carotene. This gradually changes in content and by ten days mature milk is produced.

Because of easier digestibility and faster clearance of breast milk from the stomach, the breast-fed infant is likely to want to be fed at shorter time intervals than the formula-fed infant. At first he may prefer feeding every two or three hours, but the interval gradually becomes longer. Until the mother's nipples become adapted to the sucking, she may be more comfortable if she limits the length of the nursing period. A baby who nurses well may obtain 90% of the milk within the first seven minutes, so prolonged feeding time has little advantage. If the breast is too full at the onset of nursing, and the infant cannot grasp the nipple, manual expression of a small amount of milk will help to relieve the pressure. Until the milk flow has become well established, it is wise not to substitute a bottle for a nursing. Once milk supply is stabilized, formula may be substituted for a breast feeding on occasion. Breast milk may also be expressed and frozen for use when the mother is away.

A problem frequently encountered, and often mismanaged, may occur between three and eight weeks, when a spurt in the infant's appetite and a lag in milk production cause the baby to be dissatisfied after nursing or become hungry in a short time. The mother or physician may decide that lactation is no longer successful and that the infant should be weaned to bottle feedings. However, this inequity between the infant's increased demand and the mother's inability to meet it is very likely to be temporary. With continued sucking and emptying of the breasts, milk flow is likely to increase spontaneously within twenty-four or forty-eight hours. In the interim, the mother may offer milk or formula at the end of a nursing; if the baby is fully satisfied he is likely to sleep longer, allowing time for the mother to build up a greater milk supply for the next feeding. La Leche League, an organization of women who have banded together for mutual support of breast feeding,[26] recommends more frequent nursing during this period. The increased vigor of sucking and more frequent nursing may stimulate greater production of prolactin. Patience and a few days of persistence will usually result in a new balance of supply and demand and continued success in lactation.

Dietary requirements of the mother increase both to provide the nutrients in the milk and for the process of manufacturing milk.

When the mother's diet is inadequate, the quantity of milk produced may diminish. The RDA provides for an increase of 500 kcal daily over nonpregnant, nonlactating needs. However, Widdowson has estimated that 450 additional calories daily are needed by the average woman in the first month, increasing to more than 800 kcal by the sixth month, assuming 90% efficiency in the conversion of energy. The nutrient content of breast milk suggests that the RDA increases in ascorbic acid and vitamin A would not be adequate to provide the content of those vitamins in 950 ml of breast milk.[27]

The content of some minerals and especially of vitamins reflects the adequacy of the mother's diet. The RDA levels for calories, iodine, zinc, vitamin A, ascorbic acid, riboflavin, and niacin are higher than those for pregnancy. For a plentiful supply of milk and protection of the mother's nutritional state as well as to supply the optimal quality of milk, it is important for the woman to pay special attention to foods with high nutrient density. The nursing mother has a greater leeway than the pregnant woman in calorie allowance to provide the additional protein, minerals, and vitamins, but she should include close to 1 qt of milk daily for its calcium and riboflavin, more yellow and green leafy vegetables for vitamin A, and citrus fruit for ascorbic acid. Other dietary needs are similar to those recommended for pregnancy.

Breast milk supplies all of the nutrients needed by the infant for the first four to six months, with the possible exception of vitamin D and fluorine. It is customary to provide a supplement containing vitamin D beginning at one to two weeks of age, but the finding of a water-soluble conjugate of vitamin D with sulfate in breast milk[28] may explain the protection of the breast-fed infant from rickets. Many physicians include ascorbic acid supplement or orange juice to the young infant as insurance. By four to six months the infant needs an exogenous source of iron, and semisolid foods may be offered. The introduction of solid foods will be discussed later in this chapter.

Breast-fed infants are less likely to become obese than formula-fed infants. This may be due to the probability that the nursing mother allows the infant's appetite to regulate his intake in contrast to mothers who encourage finishing bottles. Weights of infants before and after nursing indicate wide variations in breast milk consumption from one feeding to another. At one feeding the infant may be content with 1 oz and at another take 5 oz.

The milk of each species of animal is specific for its young. Throughout the world milk of different animals may be fed to infants; cow's milk is customarily used in the United States. Human milk is slightly higher in calories, 20% higher in fat, and 40% higher in lactose than cow's milk. Human milk is five times higher in linoleic acid and twice as high in oleic acid, while cow's milk contains more saturated fatty acids. Despite differences in fatty acids, serum cholesterol levels of infants fed cow's milk are similar to those of infants fed breast milk.[29] Cow's milk contains approximately three times as much protein and ash (including calcium) and seven times as much phosphorus as human milk. Human milk is higher in vitamin A, niacin, ascorbic acid, and vitamin E, while cow's milk is higher in other vitamins for which analyses have been done. Despite the lower content of nitrogen, calcium, and phosphorus, percentage retention of those nutrients from human milk is greater than from cow's milk.

Adaptation of cow's milk for human infants includes dilution with water to lower the nitrogen and ash content to decrease the renal solute load. Newborn infants may have immature kidney function with poor ability to concentrate urine and consequent loss of water; in most infants kidney function rapidly matures so the dilution may gradually be decreased. Carbohydrate is usually added to increase caloric value, but should be eliminated when the infant accepts semisolid foods well.

In the past fifty years, the types of milk fed to infants, sometimes unwisely, have included evaporated milk, whole milk, skim or low-fat milk, condensed milk, and commercially premodified infant formulas (powdered, liquid concentrate, or ready-to-feed). For infants allergic to cow's milk, goat milk and formulas based on meat or soy are also available.

From the 1920s, when it became available, to the 1950s evaporated milk was the basis of most formulas on hospital discharge for infants who were not breast fed. This formula is adapted to the individual infant, at a level of 1 oz of evaporated milk per pound of body weight. In the first two to four weeks, 2 oz of water are usually added per ounce of evaporated milk. The water is gradually decreased until four to six months, when equal parts of evaporated milk and water may be given, or whole milk substituted. Carbohydrate, such as corn syrup or sucrose, is usually added. At first 2 to 3 tablespoons may be added to the total day's formula; the amount is gradually decreased as semisolid foods are well taken, and by four to six months may be eliminated entirely. Some infants are fed whole milk from birth, at first diluted with 1 oz of water for each 2 oz of milk, with added carbohydrate. However, the heat treatment necessary for evaporation increases digestibility and decreases allergenicity of cow's milk.

Skim milk should not be recommended for the infant during the first year of life. With removal of fat from milk, the renal solute load is increased due to the higher percentage of nitrogen and ash, and dehydration becomes a danger. The lack of fat may result in deficiency of fatty acids and inhibit absorption of fat-soluble vitamins. Some infants fed skim milk develop diarrhea or eczema; both symptoms may be cured by the addition of fat. Physicians sometimes recommend skim milk during periods of illness; this is not advisable except under specific conditions. Condensed milk is also not suitable for infant feeding. Because of added sugar, its carbohydrate content is seven times that of evaporated milk and its caloric content nearly three times as high, with lower percentage content of other nutrients.

Commercially premodified infant formulas were introduced in the 1920s, first as a powdered concentrate which was difficult to dissolve in water to a smooth consistency. The marketing of liquid concentrate around 1950 and its vigorous sales promotions led to increased use of premodified formulas. Many hospitals adopted their use for newborn infants and eliminated formula preparation rooms. By 1965, 90% of formulas recommended at hospital discharge were commercially premodified, and the use of evaporated milk had decreased to 10%. In the late 1960s, ready-to-feed formulas were marketed, with water added so that no further dilution was necessary. By 1973, one-third of premodified formulas sold were ready-to-feed. Fortification with iron also increased, and by 1973 more than one-third of formulas sold in the United States were iron-fortified.[29] The cost of premodified formulas is higher than for evaporated or whole milk formulas mixed at home, and the ready-to-feed formulas cost two to three times as much in most retail markets.

Modifications of cow's milk in these formulas include decrease in the protein, calcium, and phosphorus content to approximately 50% of the content of whole milk, replacement of butterfat with vegetable oils, and addition of carbohydrate. The vegetable oils have often included coconut oil, which is highly saturated. Recently lactose has been used in addition to or in place of other added sugars. Lactose, the sugar naturally present in human and cow's milk, improves absorption of calcium, magnesium, and nitrogen, lowers intestinal pH, and encourages the growth of fermentative rather than putrefactive bacteria in the intestinal flora.

Vitamins have also been added. The first added were vitamins A and D and ascorbic acid. In the early 1950s, a new method of heat treatment of one commercial formula led to destruction of pyridoxine, causing convulsive seizures in infants,[30] so pyridoxine is now routinely added. Concern about increased need of vitamin E on high intakes of polyunsaturated fatty acids led to the addition of vitamin E.

The small infant who has no source of nutrients except formula is uniquely vulnerable to the adequacy of a single food. Changes in formulation or processing have not always been adequately tested,[31] as indicated by the pyridoxine deficiency. When carbohydrate is an integral part of the formula, it cannot be eliminated as solid foods are introduced into the diet, and the infant who is taking both solid foods and premodified formula may have a very high carbohydrate intake.[32]

After hospital discharge, many mothers, especially in low income families, discontinue the use of premodified formulas because of the high cost, frequently without professional advice, and substitute other forms of milk.[33,34] In 1971, Rivera found that by two months more than 70% of infants under the care of physicians in private practice were taking premodified formulas, while at the same age only 40% of infants seen in city clinics were taking premodified formulas and an equal number were on evaporated milk formulas.[35] By four months whole milk had replaced formula in more than half of both groups. The transfer to whole or skim milk at an early age is common but may be harmful to the infant.

Until the 1920s, infants were occasionally given beef broth, mashed potato, or cooked cereal toward the end of the first year. With the marketing of commercially puréed foods and special infant cereals, the age when these foods are introduced into the diet has become progressively earlier. In 1954, a survey of 2,000 pediatricians revealed that 66% of infants were taking semisolid foods by two months and 90% by three months, although heads of departments of pediatrics showed little support for such early feeding. A typical comment: "It is the result of empiricism and competition, not of sound nutritional principles."[36] Infants are often unwilling to accept spoon feeding until the age of 2½ to 4 months,[37] creating problems for the conscientious mother struggling to feed a baby who resists. Despite the repeated comments of professionals that the early introduction of solid foods is "an example of a widespread dietary practice which offers little in the way of nutritional advantage,"[38] most infants in the United States have been offered solids in the first month, sometimes as early as two to three days of age.[39]

One reason for the resistance of infants to spoon feeding is the protrusion, or extrusion, reflex which causes the infant to push with his tongue against anything placed in the front of his mouth. The infant with a weak reflex may accept solid foods well, but the infant with a strong reflex vigorously rejects the food. According to Bakwin, "The optimal time to introduce solid food is when the musculature of the infant is ready to accept it, generally between 3 and 4 months. . . . Young infants push vigorously with the tongue against a spoon or solid food placed between the lips. At about 3 to 4 months, a change takes place. When food is brought to the child's mouth, the lips part, the tongue carries the food to the back of the mouth, and swallowing follows."[40] The early introduction of solids may precede the production of salivary amylase, often at two to three months, to handle the complex carbohydrate of starch, and may also be harmful to the potentially allergic child whose gastrointestinal tract is too immature to handle proteins other than those in milk.

Physiologically, the nutrient needs of the infant can be met by milk with the addition of vitamins C and D and possibly fluorine, until four to six months, when exogenous iron should be supplied. High iron storage in the last trimester of intrauterine life of the full-term infant results in a high concentration of hemoglobin at birth, in the range of 16 to 20 gm/100 ml blood. Since the life span of the red blood cell is approximately 120 days, the normal breakdown of erythrocytes in the first two months results in a hemoglobin level close to 11 gm and storage of the released iron. As the infant grows and his blood volume expands, storage iron is gradually depleted. By four to six months an additional supply is necessary. There is conflicting evidence on the benefits of iron fortification for the term infant prior to three months, since the iron may not be absorbed.

The order of addition of solid foods varies, but most commonly iron-fortified cereal is followed by fruits, vegetables, meat, egg yolk, and desserts. Some physicians delay the introduction of fruit because of its sweet taste; some offer meat earlier because of its iron content. Only one new food should be offered at a time, and the quantity should be limited to not more than 1 teaspoon per serving, so that if an allergic reaction occurs, the problem food may be readily identified. Home-prepared foods may be puréed or mashed and offered in place of the commercial products, but care should be taken to limit the addition of salt and to ensure bacteriological safety.

Foods for chewing should be offered when the baby indicates by chewing motions that he is ready for them or when tooth eruption begins. The transition from puréed to chopped foods may be gradually accomplished between six and fifteen months. Most children are content with table foods after one year, but the mother may find baby foods a convenient substitute when the family meal is unsuitable for the infant.

The cup should be offered for practice before the mother intends to wean the baby from breast or bottle. Coordination of lips, tongue, and swallowing requires time to master. Weaning to the cup may be started at any age after six months but should be gradual and geared to the infant's willingness. Some infants voluntarily relinquish the bottle or breast; others enjoy sucking and the comfort of breast or bottle for a longer period of time, especially at nap time or at bedtime. Once teeth have erupted, a bottle for sweetened formula or other liquid containing sugar should be discouraged because prolonged bathing of the teeth with sweet liquids may cause caries.

In the last few months of the first year the child is likely to decrease milk intake.[41] Some children limit milk intake on weaning from the bottle, but more often the mother discontinues the use of a bottle because the child has already shown a lack of interest in it. This change heralds the alteration in feeding behavior which is characteristic of the preschool child.

## Preschool Period

The growth rate of the child slows during the first year, as shown in chapters 3 and 4, and continues to decrease until the pubertal spurt. In the first year average gain in weight is 6 kg and in height 25 cm. In the second year average gain is closer to 3 kg and 10 cm, and in the third year 2 kg and 8 to 9 cm. As a result, the need for nutrients for growth is not as demanding as in the first year. At the same time learning to walk expands the range of the child's environment and broadens his interests. Speech allows him to express his reactions in words, and he learns the power of the word *no*, which he may apply to even his favorite foods. He is developing psychological as well as physical independence. This maturation and development of new skills and the excitement of exploration of his wider world place food in a secondary position in his interests. He has reached the "Johnny won't eat" period.

Changes in appetites of the children in the longitudinal studies of the Child Research Council are shown in figure 5.3. A mother's rating of her child's appetite is subjective, and not necessarily correlated to actual changes in caloric intake. However, the fact that these data were based on the same mothers rating the same children over this age span showed that the mothers perceived alterations in their children's interest in food. At six months, 85% of the children had good or excellent appetites, 10% fair, and 5% poor or very poor. Between three and four years of age, only 20% had good or excellent appetites, 60% fair, and 20% poor. After four years there was improvement so that by seven years a majority of the children again had good or excellent appetites.[37] During the period of lowered appetite, the child often becomes erratic about food likes and dislikes. He might eat poorly at one meal and well at the next, or might have several

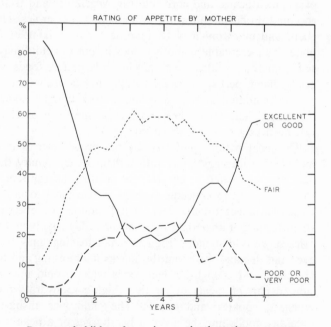

**Figure 5.3**          Percent of children from six months through seven years whose appetites were rated by their mothers as (1) excellent or good, (2) fair, or (3) poor or very poor. Reprinted, with permission, from Beal, V. A. "On the Acceptance of Solid Foods and Other Food Patterns of Infants and Children." *Pediatrics* 20(1957):448–57.

days of disinterest in food. Dinner is most often a time for fussiness. The child is tired at the end of the day, easily distracted by household activities, and often discouraged at the appearance of a large meal in which he has little interest.

Despite a decrease in appetite, caloric intake does not decrease for the average child, but progresses along a plateau for a period of time. However, some children have a real decrease in caloric intake and may lose weight for a few months. Protein intake is unlikely to increase, but carbohydrate intake rises.[42] The major decrease is in milk consumption, and therefore in calcium intake.[42,43] Daily milk intake may drop to an average of 1 pt daily, with individual children consuming only 4 oz a day while a few maintain intakes close to 1 qt.

There are characteristic eating behavior patterns during this period. Cooked vegetables may be refused, with the exception sometimes of peas, green beans, and corn, but raw vegetables and fruit are usually accepted. Food mixtures are unpopular as casseroles, although spaghetti and macaroni may be favorite foods. Mixing of food on the plate is unacceptable if mother does it, but the child may do it himself, sometimes to delay eating. The child prefers foods which he can eat by hand, perhaps because he may not have the manual dexterity and wrist motion to keep a spoon or fork upright from the plate to his mouth. The young preschool child may tire of feeding himself and need help to finish the meal.

The meal pattern preferred by the preschooler is more likely to include five feedings a day rather than the customary three meals.[43] This may be related to his constant need for energy replenishment or to his inability to consume enough at one meal to last to the next. Recent evidence on the decreased likelihood of obesity on several small feedings rather than three meals a day supplying the same calories suggests that more frequent small feedings may be wise. However, this demands care that the snacks midmorning and midafternoon are composed of high-nutrient foods which would normally be considered part of meals rather than high-carbohydrate foods such as crackers, cookies, and sweets. The child who dislikes customary breakfast foods may be given a hamburger or a peanut butter sandwich instead.

Although milk consumption may be reduced, cheese is often accepted. Meat is usually well tolerated if it is hamburger, chicken, or frankfurters, but not as roast meat. Eggs are usually accepted, although there may be periods of eating only the yolk or only the white. Fruit is usually liked and may be supplemented with raw vegetables.

The preschool child may refuse salad served at the meal, but be happy to have pieces of the salad to eat while his mother is preparing the meal. With his diminished appetite, it is important to ensure his nutrient needs by offering a variety of foods, mainly those of high nutrient value.

If the child continues to be energetic, has relative freedom from infections, recovers quickly from illness, and does not have a prolonged weight loss, there is little need for undue concern. As the findings from the Preschool Nutrition Survey indicated, despite some low intakes of calcium and vitamin C, no frank deficiency symptoms were observed.[21] The major adverse finding among children in this age group was iron-deficiency anemia, which will be discussed in chapter 6.

### Early School Years

This is a period of rather steady growth, with a gain of 2 to 3 kg in weight and 5 to 7 cm in height each year in most children. It has been called by psychologists the "latent" period because there are few dramatic changes in the child. This is true also for nutritional intake. The risk of malnutrition is greater for the child under five years of age and for the adolescent than for the child in intermediate ages.

The anorexia of the preschool child is replaced by a gradually increasing appetite. The finicky attitude toward food usually disappears, and the schoolchild is more likely to increase the range of foods he willingly accepts. Slower growth in this period places less stress on the physiological requirement of nutrients. In the HANES I survey, median intakes of children between six and eleven years were more likely to be at or above the RDA than for either younger or older children.[44] The percentage of children with blood levels indicative of iron-deficiency anemia is also less at this age.

In evaluating the nutritional status of the school-age child, certain characteristics of health and appearance should be observed. As stressed in earlier chapters, growth in weight and height consistent with age is one of the most sensitive indexes of nutritional adequacy. Firm muscles aid in good posture. Hair should be shiny and elastic, and eyes and skin clear. A healthy, well-nourished child is most likely to be alert and energetic. Although infectious diseases are readily transmitted among schoolchildren, a well-nourished child is apt to have a milder degree of illness and a faster recovery.

Dental health should be stressed during early school years, especially in view of the findings of the Ten State Nutrition Survey[45] and the National Health Survey[46] of the high frequency of decayed, missing, and filled teeth in adolescent children. Caries susceptibility is partially genetic, but the formation of healthy teeth depends on the supply of protein, calcium, phosphorus, fluorine, and vitamins A, D, and C during pregnancy and early childhood. After tooth eruption, the consumption of carbohydrates which may be fermented by mouth bacteria has been shown to increase caries. In the TSNS, particularly in the high income ratio states, poor dental status was more closely related to between-meal snacks of candy, soft drinks, and pastries than to carbohydrates consumed during meals.

With the improvement in eating behavior commonly observed in the school-age child, it is important to stress the establishment of good eating patterns. Milk intake tends to increase, although more in white than in black children.[47] Fruit continues to be more popular than vegetables, but vegetables become more readily acceptable, and the variety of vegetables the child will eat increases. Intakes of meat and of eggs rise. As the child advances in age, and as his growth continues in a relatively steady linear fashion, his greater caloric requirements usually result in increased appetite and greater total food consumption. Participation in sports and other outdoor activities should be encouraged to establish a pattern of physical exercise, both to stimulate appetite and to limit the hazard of obesity. Care should be taken that most of the child's food has high nutrient density and that foods which contain primarily carbohydrate or fat are kept to a minimum. The importance of the school programs as a source of nutrients and as a medium for nutrition education will be stressed in chapter 7.

Toward the end of this age period, the still greater appetite and enthusiasm for food which are characteristic of the adolescent begin to become evident.

## Adolescence

Acceleration of growth during adolescence is accompanied by a variety of physical, hormonal, emotional, and cognitive changes. Nutrient requirements increase to support the expansion of body mass and the need is especially high for protein, minerals, and vitamins essential to cell proliferation. At the same time, the adolescent's food selection is affected by social pressures, the desire for peer acceptance, emotional instability, and the drive toward greater independence from home and parental influences.

The teenager becomes concerned about his body image. His concept of himself, his health, and his size are important determinants of his eating patterns. In the Health Examination Survey of youths twelve to seventeen years of age, attitudes of both the children and their parents toward the health, weight, and height of the teenagers were investigated.[48] Unfortunately the data were not differentiated by sex. Parents tended to give better health ratings to their teenage children than did the children themselves. Ten percent of the black and 4% of the white youths rated their own health as fair or poor. The rest of the black teenagers were nearly equally divided between good ratings and very good or excellent ratings. In contrast, 34% of white youths rated their health good and 62% described their health as excellent. Health ratings increased with income. The lowest income group were more concerned about being underweight and the highest income group more concerned about being overweight. Parents were somewhat less likely than the children themselves to describe the children as overweight or underweight.

In a study of high school students in California, Huenemann et al.[49] explored the students' attitudes toward their own size and shape and found marked differences between boys and girls.

The predominant attitude that these students expressed was dissatisfaction—with their weight, fatness or leanness, height, and certain body dimensions. More than half the girls expressed concern about overweight, about matching the number of boys who were concerned about being underweight. Boys generally wanted to be taller, while girls seemed to be content with their height. Nearly all the boys expressed a desire for larger biceps, and almost all the girls wanted smaller waists. The number of girls who described themselves as too fat increased from 43 percent in the ninth grade to 56 percent in the twelfth grade. And some who did not feel they were too fat still wanted to lose weight because 70 percent of the girls desired a weight loss. Less than one-fourth of the boys felt they were too fat.

Nutrient requirements during this age span are dependent on the timing and amount of growth, physical activity, and other factors in body development and maintenance, but food selection is determined not only by appetite but also by the social, cultural, economic, and psychological factors in the life of the teenager.

The customary use of chronological age as a basis for determining dietary allowances is unsatisfactory during this stage of development.

The RDA tables have divided age groups into the eleven-to-fourteen year group, representative of junior high school, and fifteen to eighteen years, representative of senior high school.[50] This is an arbitrary division, and each group includes individuals at different stages of development. The span from eleven to eighteen years includes the prepubescent whose requirements are still those of the younger child, the very rapidly growing midadolescent, and the mature individual whose nutrient needs are those of the adult. The nutritionist working with the teenager needs to individualize, taking into consideration some estimation of the stage of development and of the rate of growth of each boy or girl. Although maturation ratings based on Tanner's five stages of sexual maturity[51] have been used in some centers for evaluation of nutrient intake and biochemical status,[52] their use is not widespread and requires more time and information about the individual than is usually available. Despite the general concensus that biological age is preferable to chronological age in nutritional evaluation of the adolescent, no simple frame of reference has yet been devised.

Few studies have been done on the nutrient requirements of adolescents. "The RDA data base for adolescents is meager and totally inadequate."[50] The RDAs have been either interpolated for age or estimated from adult maintenance requirements with an arbitrary allowance for growth. Allowances for nutrients when their need is related to calorie intake have been based on the ratio of the nutrient to calories. With so little definitive basis for RDA levels, the conservative decision of the Food and Nutrition Board to err on the high rather than the low side in establishing RDAs has resulted in controversy. Some of the final values are "difficult to scientifically support."[50]

A secondary result of the scarcity of data for dietary assessment of the adolescent is that dietary intakes in this age period have often been "viewed with alarm" by some nutritionists and other professionals. The omission of breakfast or lunch, irregularity of meals, and frequent consumption of snacks have often been observed. In the Berkeley study[49] the high school students reported eating breakfast four to six times a week, lunch five to six times a week, and dinner six to seven times a week, on the average. Daytime snacks were reported four to nine times a week, and evening snacks two to five times a week for various age and weight groups.

The assumption that between-meal eating spoils the appetite for meals and supplies calories but little else has been reinforced by the prominent advertising of potato chips, pretzels, soft drinks, and candy and has led to the suggestion that snacks should be fortified with minerals and vitamins. However, studies of the nutrient intakes of adolescents show that between-meal eating can be nutritionally beneficial.[53] In the twenty-four-hour recalls in the Ten State Nutrition Survey slightly more than three-fourths of the ten- to sixteen-year age group reported eating between meals. For various age, sex, and ethnic groups, food between meals supplied 12% to 20% of calories, 7% to 19% of protein, 14% to 30% of calcium, 7% to 20% of iron, 4% to 55% of thiamine, 8% to 28% of riboflavin, and 15% to 50% of ascorbic acid for the day. When calculated per 100 kcal, between-meal food met or exceeded the RDA ratio for protein, riboflavin, ascorbic acid, and thiamine.[47] Therefore it is obvious that the teenager may obtain an appreciable proportion of his nutrient intake from foods consumed between meals. Although some adolescents may consume foods low in protein, minerals, and vitamins, the need to fortify snacks does not seem indicated. Guidance in the choice of foods consumed between meals so that they contain a high concentration of nutrients should be provided by parents, nutritionists, and school personnel.

The increased need for nutrients to support faster growth usually results in a larger appetite than is observed in a younger child. Indicative of the greater appetite was the finding in the Berkeley study[49] that nearly one-half of the boys and approximately one-third of the girls in the ninth grade reported that they were hungry all or most of the time. In contrast, approximately 10% of girls and even fewer boys said that they were hardly ever or never hungry. The degree of hunger also varied during the day. Few were hungry in the morning, consistent with the lower frequency of breakfast consumption. Girls were more hungry at noon, and boys equally hungry at noon and at dinner time.

The growth spurt begins at an average age of 10 years in girls (range 7½ to 14½ years) and 12 years in boys (range 9½ to 16½ years), as shown in chapter 3. Increased need for nutrients to support the increased lean body mass has the same sex differences and varies with each individual depending on the timing of the spurt. The period of greatest nutrient need corresponds to the maximum growth velocity, usually about two years after the onset, and then declines for most nutrients as the rate of growth slows. At the termination of growth, nutrient requirements approach those of the mature adult; this occurs at an average of sixteen years for girls and eighteen years for boys, but the range of variation among individuals is wide.

The adolescent spurt in growth, as shown in chapter 3, is usually more clearly defined than is a corresponding increase in food intake. It is difficult to define a spurt in caloric intake, as seen in figure 5.4,

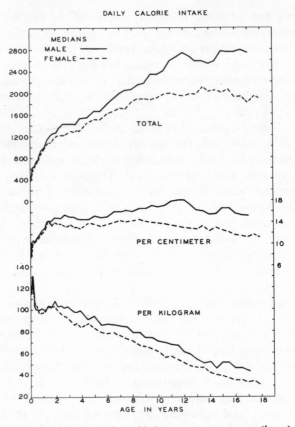

DAILY CALORIE INTAKE

MEDIANS
MALE ——
FEMALE ————

TOTAL

PER CENTIMETER

PER KILOGRAM

AGE IN YEARS

**Figure 5.4**     Calorie intakes from birth to seventeen years (boys) and
eighteen years (girls). Reprinted, with permission, from
Beal, V. A. "Nutritional Intake." In *Human Growth and
Development,* edited by R. W. McCammon. Springfield,
Ill.: Charles C Thomas Co., 1970.

from the longitudinal data of the Child Research Council. These un-
smoothed values do not show a sudden increase in the intake of girls
and only a suggestion of a spurt in intake of boys, whether considered
as total calories, calories per centimeter of height, or per kilogram of
body weight.[42] Caloric intake continues to show a pattern of change
similar to that seen in preadolescent children. Similar patterns were
observed in the studies of the Harvard School of Public Health,[54] although the caloric intake of the adolescents was higher in the Harvard
study (fig. 5.5) than in the Denver study.

The age when intake declines later in adolescence has been better described for girls than for boys. Most longitudinal studies have been continued past the age when girls begin to eat less, but many studies have terminated at or before eighteen years, when males may not yet have reached their peak intake. In the Denver and Boston studies the peak intake of girls occurred between twelve and fourteen years, and then intake declined, as shown in figures 5.4 and 5.5, but the intake of males was still increasing at seventeen or eighteen years.

Cross-sectional studies have shown varying ages at maximum intake. Widdowson[55] reported on seven-day weighed intakes of children

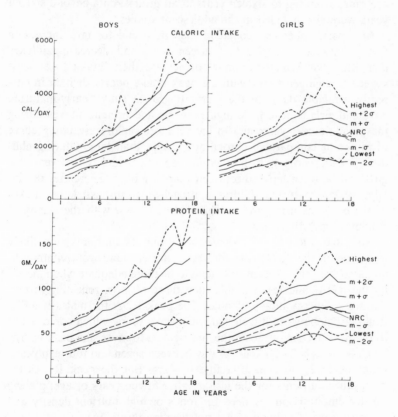

**Figure 5.5**      Distributions of calorie and protein intakes of boys and girls from one to eighteen years of age, compared to the 1958 RDA. Reprinted, with permission, from Burke, B. S.; Reed, R. B.; van den Berg, A. S.; and Stuart, H. C. *Pediatrics* 24(1959[suppl., pt. 2]):922–40.

in England between 1935 and 1939 and showed a peak intake at fourteen years in girls, and at both fifteen and eighteen years in boys, followed by declines. A collaborative study of State Agricultural Experiment Stations in thirty-nine states between 1947 and 1958[56] reported a peak caloric intake of girls at 11½ years and of boys at 16 to 17 years. In the Ten State Nutrition Survey[47] girls in the low income ratio states reached a peak in calorie and protein intakes at twelve to fourteen years and had lower intakes at fifteen to sixteen years, but girls in the high income ratio states tended to have higher intakes with increasing age. Intakes of boys increased throughout the age range from ten to sixteen years in all groups; data beyond sixteen years were not included in the adolescent studies.

In general, one may conclude that girls tend to have increasing dietary intakes to twelve to fourteen years and decreasing intakes thereafter, while boys continue to increase their intake to at least sixteen to eighteen years, with the peak intake poorly defined in currently available data. In the Harvard growth study, early-maturing boys and girls tend to have higher calorie and protein intakes during the preadolescent years and to have a more rapidly ascending curve of intake at comparable chronological ages than late-maturing children.[57] Differences were marked between eight and twelve years for girls and between ten and fourteen years for boys. Thereafter the intakes of late-maturing children approached or surpassed the intakes of the early-maturing group. This was consistent with the timing of maximum growth velocity.

Repeated studies[43,44,56,58] have shown that the nutrients most likely to be low in the diet of the adolescent are calcium, iron, vitamin A, and ascorbic acid. Diets of boys tend to be more adequate when judged by the RDA[2] and less variable than those of girls, reflecting in part the higher energy intake of boys. The peak RDA for males is 3,000 kcal per day between fifteen and twenty-two years, which corresponds to the peak RDAs of most other nutrients. However, the peak energy RDA for girls is 2,400 kcal per day between seven and fourteen years, dropping to 2,100 kcal after fifteen years. But the peak RDAs for most other nutrients for the girl are after fifteen years of age, placing greater emphasis on the need for foods of high nutrient density and increasing the likelihood of her not meeting the RDAs.

The calcium intake of girls tends to be lower than that of boys from early childhood but the difference becomes more pronounced after eight years and particularly during the adolescent years, as shown in figure 5.6 from data of the Child Research Council[42] in which the median intake of girls was only slightly above the tenth percentile of intake of boys after ten years. The lower calcium intake of girls reflects decreasing milk consumption, often related to increasing weight consciousness and desire to lose weight at this age.

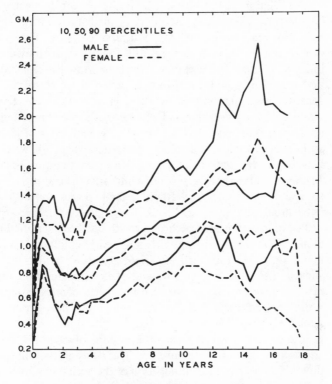

**Figure 5.6**          Calcium intakes from birth to seventeen years (boys) and eighteen years (girls). Reprinted, with permission, from Beal, V. A. "Nutritional Intake." In *Human Growth and Development*, edited by R. W. McCammon. Springfield, Ill.: Charles C Thomas Co., 1970.

The RDA for iron has been set at 18 mg per day for males during the years of rapid growth, primarily because of the marked increase in muscle mass[59] which requires greater blood volume. The need for iron by the adolescent girl is less for increase in lean body tissue but greater for replacement of menstrual losses, and the RDA of 18 mg continues throughout the reproductive years of the woman. Since most diets in the United States contain approximately 6 mg of iron per 1,000 kcal, the RDA is unlikely to be reached except with extremely careful selection of foods on intakes of 2,100 to 2,400 kcal. As will be shown in chapter 6, the wide variations in menstrual losses necessitate individual assessment of iron needs of females.

The relationship of nutrient intake to growth has been repeatedly demonstrated, especially the effect of inadequate nutrition on inhibition of increase on stature. Mitchell reported on the increasing stature of children in Japan between 1900 and 1960, attributed to increase in protein intake.[60] These data have been extended to 1970 (fig. 5.7) and show further advances in the stature of Japanese children at all ages. Of particular interest in these graphs is the effect of food restrictions during World War II, when growth was limited more during adolescence than at any other age. The growth rates of girls at twelve and fourteen years and of boys at fourteen years were more adversely affected than at other ages from six years to eighteen years. Just as the infant and very young child are sensitive to undernutrition, so also is the adolescent. Rapid growth places special demands on nutrient supply.

The impetus toward catch-up growth has been reported by Dreizen et al.,[61] who observed sixty girls from early childhood to early adulthood. Half the group had experienced chronic undernutrition which slowed their rates of growth and skeletal maturation and delayed menarche, in contrast to the well-nourished control group. However, a prolonged growth period of the undernourished group resulted in adult heights which were not significantly different from the faster-growing well-nourished girls. Other reports of catch-up growth during adolescence have been reported.[59] The delay in the onset of maturational changes and the prolongation of the period of adolescent growth have been shown in the secular trends discussed in chapter 3. Catch-up growth may under some circumstances be a compensatory mechanism during adolescence.

Pregnancy imposes further nutritional stress on the adolescent girl. More than 50% of girls between fifteen and nineteen years of age in the United States are married, and pregnancies in unmarried girls, especially under fifteen years of age, have been increasing. At the present time, approximately 8,000 live births per year are reported for mothers under fifteen years of age. Since menarche, and presumably ovulation, follow the period of maximum growth velocity, growth of the girl is decelerating at the time when pregnancy becomes possible. There is, however, continued growth after menarche which must be supported, in addition to the higher requirements of pregnancy.

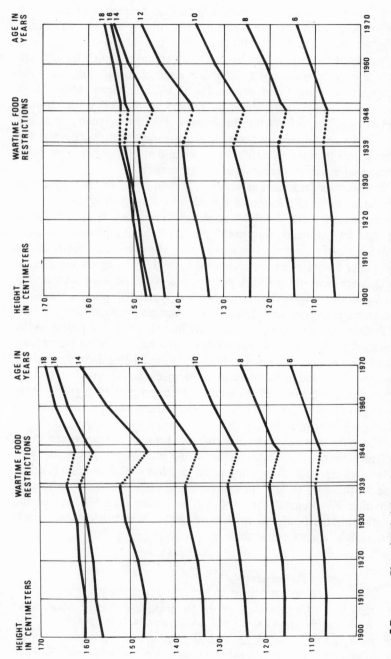

**Figure 5.7**    Changing heights of Japanese boys and girls at seven age levels between six and eighteen years since 1900. Courtesy of Helen S. Mitchell, Ph.D.

The younger teenager is more likely to have toxemia and may have higher risks of both maternal and infant mortality and of delivering a baby weighing less than 2,500 gm.[62]

Nutrient requirements for the pregnant teenager should be adjusted for her chronological age and for her stage of maturation, requiring individual evaluation and advice. The RDA table allows for addition of the pregnancy needs for each nutrient to the RDA for chronological age. The RDAs for the female over fifteen years, as noted previously, are higher for most nutrients except calories, despite the slower growth after menarche, in recognition of the need for good nutritional status in preparation for pregnancy.

Special consideration was given to protein needs of the teenager in pregnancy in the discussion of the basis for the RDA levels.[2] For the nonpregnant female, the RDA at eleven to fourteen years is 1.0 gm/kg body weight, decreasing to 0.9 gm at fifteen to eighteen years and to 0.8 gm after nineteen years. However, the pregnancy needs of the girl under fifteen years are estimated to be 1.7 gm/kg, of the fifteen- to eighteen-year-old girl 1.5 gm/kg, and of the mature woman 1.3 gm/kg body weight. Therefore the recommended protein intake is increased proportionately more for the younger girl than for the adult.

Weight gain during pregnancy may include tissue increment in the maternal body as well as that related to the pregnancy, so the recommended gain should be greater than the 20- to 24-lb gain of the mature woman. The additional calorie allowance should provide for increased nutrient needs of the younger teenager, but even greater care must be taken to select foods of high nutrient content than for the adult pregnant woman.

The risks during pregnancy of the younger teenager are compounded by the probability of her being unmarried. She is likely to delay seeking medical care and to be in a low socioeconomic bracket. The attitudes of society have been changing and there is increasing provision for prenatal care and further educational facilities of the young unmarried girl, but these have not yet been made widely available with adequate outreach.

## References

1   Roberts, L. J. "Beginnings of the Recommended Dietary Allowances." *Journal of the American Dietetic Association* 34(1958):903–8.

2   Food and Nutrition Board. *Recommended Dietary Allowances*, 8th ed. Washington, D.C.: National Academy of Sciences-National Research Council, 1974.

3   Tompkins, W. T. "Nutrition in Pregnancy." In *Modern Nutrition in Health and Disease*, edited by M. G. Wohl and R. S. Goodhart. Philadelphia: Lea & Febiger, 1955.

4   Stearns, G. "Nutritional State of the Mother Prior to Conception." *JAMA* 168(1958):1655–59.

5   Gold, E. M. "Interconceptional Nutrition." *Journal of the American Dietetic Association* 35(1969):27–30.

6   Valadian, I., and Reed, R. B. "Influence of Nutritional Factors during Early Adolescence on Reproductive Efficiency." In *Congenital Defects: New Directions in Research*. New York: Academic Press, 1974.

7   Winick, M., and Noble, A. "Cellular Growth in Human Placenta: I. Normal Placental Growth." *Pediatrics* 39(1967):248–51.

8   Timiras, P. S. *Developmental Physiology and Aging*. New York: MacMillan Co., 1972.

9   Committee on Maternal Nutrition, Food and Nutrition Board. *Maternal Nutrition and the Course of Pregnancy*. Washington, D.C.: National Academy of Sciences-National Research Council, 1970.

10  Calloway, D., and King, J. "University of California (Berkeley) Study." In *Nutritional Supplementation and the Outcome of Pregnancy: Proceedings of a Workshop*. Washington, D.C.: National Academy of Sciences, 1973.

11  Calloway, D. H. "Nitrogen Balance during Pregnancy." In *Nutrition and Fetal Development*, edited by M. Winick. New York: John Wiley & Sons, 1974.

12  Metcoff, J. "Biochemical Markers of Intrauterine Malnutrition." In *Nutrition and Fetal Development*, edited by M. Winick. New York: John Wiley & Sons, 1974.

13  Winick, M., ed. *Nutrition and Fetal Development*. New York: John Wiley & Sons, 1974.

14  Committee on Nutrition. *Nutrition in Maternal Health Care*. Chicago: American College of Obstetricians and Gynecologists, 1974.

15  Laupus, W. E. "Feeding of Infants." In *Nelson's Textbook of Pediatrics*, edited by V. C. Vaughn, R. J. McKay, and W. E. Nelson. Philadelphia: W. B. Saunders Co., 1975.

16  American Academy of Pediatrics Committee on Nutrition. "Commentary on Breast Feeding and Infant Formulas Including Proposed Standards for Formulas." *Pediatrics* 57(1976):278–85.

17  Woodbury, R. M. *Causal Factors in Infant Mortality*. Children's Bureau publication no. 142. Washington, D.C.: U.S. Government Printing Office, 1925.

18  Bain, K. "The Incidence of Breast Feeding in Hospitals in the United States." *Pediatrics* 2(1948):313–20.

19  Meyer, F. F. "Breast Feeding in the United States: Extent and Possible Trends: A Survey of 1,904 Hospitals with Two and a Quarter Million Births in 1956." *Pediatrics* 22(1958):116–21.

20  Robertson, W. O. "Breast Feeding Practices: Some Implications of Regional Variation." *American Journal of Public Health* 51(1961):1035–42.

21  Owen, G. M.; Kram, K. M.; Garry, P. J.; Lowe, J. E.; and Lubin, A. H. "A Study of Nutritional Status of Preschool Children in the United States, 1968–1970." *Pediatrics* 53(1974[suppl., pt. 2]):597–646.

22  Newton, N. R., and Newton, M. "Relationship of Ability to Feed and Maternal Attitudes toward Breast Feeding." *Journal of Pediatrics* 31 (1947):415–19.

23  Barnes, G. R., Jr.; Lethin, A. N., Jr.; Jackson, E. B.; and Shea, N. "Management of Breast Feeding." *JAMA* 151(1953):192–99.

24  Gerrard, J. W. "Breast Feeding: Second Thoughts." *Pediatrics* 54(1974): 757–64.

25  Jelliffe, D. B. "World Trends in Infant Feeding." *American Journal of Clinical Nutrition* 29(1976):1227–37.

26  La Leche League International. *The Womanly Art of Breast Feeding.* Franklin Park, Ill.: Interstate Printers and Publishers, 1974.

27  Widdowson, E. M. "Nutrition and Lactation." In *Nutritional Disorders of American Women*, edited by M. Winick. New York: John Wiley & Sons, 1977.

28  Lakdawala, D. R., and Widdowson, E. M. "Vitamin-D in Human Milk." *Lancet* 1(1977):167–68.

29  Fomon, S. J. *Infant Nutrition*, 2d ed. Philadelphia: W. B. Saunders Co., 1974.

30  Coursin, D. B. "Convulsive Seizures in Infants with Pyridoxine-Deficient Diets." *JAMA* 154(1954):406–8.

31  Lowe, C. U. "The Responsibility of a Professional Society." *American Journal of Clinical Nutrition* 25(1972):1–5.

32  Beal, V. A. "Breast- and Formula-Feeding of Infants." *Journal of the American Dietetic Association* 55(1969):31–37.

33  Fomon, S. J., and Anderson, T. A., eds. *Practices of Low-Income Families in Feeding Infants and Small Children, with Particular Attention to Cultural Subgroups.* Rockville, Md.: U.S. Department of Health, Education, and Welfare, Maternal and Child Health Service, 1972.

34  Vihljalmsdottir, L. B.; Beal, V. A.; Ferris, A. G.; and Pellett, P. L. *Study of Nutritional Status of Infants in Western Massachusetts: Length, Weight and Milk Intake.* Northeast Regional Research publication 73. College Park, Md.: Maryland Agricultural Experiment Station, 1976, pp. 1–9.

35  Rivera, J. "The Frequency of Use of Various Kinds of Milk during Infancy in Middle and Lower Income Families." *American Journal of Public Health* 61(1971):277–80.

36  Butler, A. M., and Wolman, I. J. "Trends in the Early Feeding of Supplementary Foods in Infants, and Analysis and Discussion Based on a Nationwide Survey." *Quarterly Review of Pediatrics* 9(1954):63–85.

37  Beal, V. A. "On the Acceptance of Solid Foods and Other Food Patterns of Infants and Children." *Pediatrics* 20(1957):448–57.

38  "Solid Foods in the Nutrition of Young Infants." *Nutrition Reviews* 25 (1967):233–35.

39  Sackett, W. W., Jr. "Use of Solid Foods Early in Infancy." *General Practitioner* 14(1956):98–102.

40  Bakwin, H. "Feeding Programs for Infants." *Federation Proceedings* 23 (1964):66–68.

41  Beal, V. A. "Calcium and Phosphorus in Infancy." *Journal of the American Dietetic Association* 53(1968):450–59.

42  Beal, V. A. "Nutritional Intake." In *Human Growth and Development*, edited by R. W. McCammon. Springfield, Ill.: Charles C Thomas Co., 1970.

43  Eppright, E. S.; Fox, H. M.; Fryer, B. A.; Lamkin, G. H.; Vivian, V. M.; and Fuller, E. S. "Nutrition of Infants and Preschool Children in the North Central Region of the United States of America." *World Review of Nutrition and Dietetics* 4(1972):269–332.

44  U.S. Department of Health, Education, and Welfare. *Preliminary Findings of the First Health and Nutrition Examination Survey, United States, 1971–1972: Dietary Intake and Biochemical Findings.* DHEW publication no. (HRA) 74–1219–1. Washington, D.C.: Superintendent of Documents, Government Printing Office, 1974.

45  U.S. Department of Health, Education, and Welfare. *Ten-State Nutrition Survey, 1968–1970: III. Clinical, Anthropometry, Dental.* DHEW publication no. (HSM) 72–8131. Washington, D.C.: Superintendent of Documents, Government Printing Office, 1972.

46  Kelly, J. E., and Harvey, C. R. *Decayed, Missing, and Filled Teeth among Youths 12–17 Years, United States.* Vital and Health Statistics series 11, no. 144. DHEW publication no. (HRA) 75–1626. Washington, D.C.: Superintendent of Documents, Government Printing Office, 1974.

47  U.S. Department of Health, Education, and Welfare. *Ten-State Nutrition Survey, 1968–1970: V. Dietary.* DHEW publication no. (HSM) 72–8133. Washington, D.C.: Superintendent of Documents, Government Printing Office, 1972.

48  Roberts, J. *Examination and Health History Findings among Children and Youths, 6–17 Years, United States.* Vital and Health Statistics series 11, no. 129. DHEW publication no. (HRA) 74–1611. Washington, D.C.; Superintendent of Documents, Government Printing Office, 1974.

49  Huenemann, R. L.; Hampton, M. C.; Behnke, A. R.; Shapiro, L. R.; and Mitchell, B. W. *Teenage Nutrition and Physique.* Springfield, Ill.: Charles C Thomas Co., 1974.

50  Mueller, J. F. "Current Recommended Dietary Allowances for Adolescents." In *Nutrient Requirements in Adolescence*, edited by J. I. McKigney and H. N. Munro. Cambridge, Mass.: M.I.T. Press, 1976.

51  Tanner, J. M. *Growth at Adolescence*, 2d ed. Oxford: Blackwell Scientific Publications, 1962.

52  Gaines, E. G., and Daniel, W. A., Jr. "Dietary Iron Intakes of Adolescents: Relation of Sex, Race and Sex Maturity Ratings." *Journal of the American Dietetic Association* 65(1974):275–80.

53  Thomas, J. A., and Call, D. A. "Between Meal Eating: A Nutrition Problem among Teenagers?" *Nutrition Reviews* 31(1973):137–39.

54  Burke, B. S.; Reed, R. B.; van den Berg, A. S.; and Stuart, H. C. "Caloric and Protein Intakes of Children between 1 and 18 Years of Age." *Pediatrics* 24(1959[suppl., pt. 2]):922–40.

55  Widdowson, E. M. *A Study of Individual Children's Diets*. Medical Research Council special report series no. 257. London: His Majesty's Stationery Office, 1947.

56  Morgan, A. F., ed. *Nutritional Status U.S.A.* California Agricultural Experiment Station bulletin 769. Berkeley: University of California, 1959.

57  Mitchell, H. S.; Reed, R. B.; Valadian, I.; and Hoff, M. "The Adolescent Growth Spurt and Nutrient Intake." In *Proceedings of the Seventh International Congress of Nutrition*, vol. 4. Basel: S. Karger, 1966.

58  Kelsay, J. L. "A Compendium of Nutritional Status Studies and Dietary Evaluation Studies Conducted in the United States, 1957–1967." *Journal of Nutrition* 99(1969[suppl. 1, pt. 2]):119–66.

59  Hepner, R. "Discussion on Iron Requirements." In *Nutrient Requirements in Adolescence*, edited by J. I. McKigney and H. N. Munro. Cambridge, Mass.: M.I.T. Press, 1976.

60  Mitchell, H. S. "Protein Limitation and Human Growth." *Journal of the American Dietetic Association* 44(1964):165–72.

61  Dreizen, S.; Spirakis, C. N.; and Stone, R. E. "A Comparison of Skeletal Growth and Maturation in Undernourished and Well-nourished Girls before and after Menarche." *Journal of Pediatrics* 70(1967):256–63.

62  Thomson, A. M. "Pregnancy in Adolescence." In *Nutrient Requirements in Adolescence*, edited by J. I. McKigney and H. N. Munro. Cambridge, Mass.: M.I.T. Press, 1976.

# Chapter Six

## Causes and Effects of Poor Nutrition

As we have followed development from conception to maturity, we have considered food in relation to its supply of nutrients for the anabolic processes of growth. Nutrient intakes of the individual are determinants of the quality of his somatic development, but food patterns are also the bridge to nutrition education. The aim of nutrition education is to ensure that food intake will provide the optimal amount of nutrients for the child to reach his genetic potential for health and growth. However, motivation for change is basic to effective education. The educator must first understand what food means to the individual and appreciate the complex factors involved in his acceptance and consumption of food. The principles of good nutrition must be adapted to the individual's own pattern of eating. Only then can motivation for dietary change be stimulated and the individual become receptive to nutritional improvement.

The basic purpose of food is to satisfy hunger. But food has much wider meanings for each person, encompassing economic, cultural, sociological, and psychological as well as physical components. Not only does food supply physiological nourishment, but it also fills emotional and social needs. Seldom is the choice of food intellectual; rather it is based on culture, religion, familiarity, childhood associations, family patterns, status, and life style. Food has unique significance for each individual, and food patterns have complex roots. An appreciation of these factors is a prerequisite to understanding why malnutrition exists and to developing programs to prevent or cure malnutrition.

## Reasons for Food Selection

### Availability of Food

This is obviously the first necessity. For many populations of the world, food availability is limited by geography, soil, weather, and water because of dependence on local agriculture. In technologically advanced countries, extensive use of food processing, preservation, transportation, and distribution has limited dependence on local supplies and has greatly increased year-round availability of most foods. It has been estimated that between 1945 and 1975 the number of food products in U.S. supermarkets rose from 1,500 to more than 10,000 and that nearly two-thirds were processed or convenience foods requiring minimal preparation time in the home. Many fresh fruits and vegetables are transported long distances and may be bought at any season. The consumer has a wide choice of all categories of foods, and availability is rarely a restrictive factor in food selection.

### Income

Ability to purchase needed or desired foods is a major factor in food choice, particularly for some segments of the population. The Preschool Nutrition Survey[1] found that 40% of gross family income was spent for food in the lowest of four income categories, compared to only 16% in the highest income group. More than one-third of the lowest income families spent more than 50% of their income for food.

The Office of Economic Opportunity reported in 1970 that 60% of people below the poverty level were white. Low income families were more often found in large cities than in rural areas. However, annual family incomes of some Indian tribes[2] and of migrant workers[3,4] tend to be well below the poverty level. The median income of blacks in the United States has risen in the past few decades, but it is still less than two-thirds as high as the median income of white families. The number of black children in single-parent families below the poverty level has shown a steady increase in the past decade.

During periods of inflation and high unemployment, limitation of food purchases to inadequate levels is more common, and the use of food stamps and other programs for income maintenance increases. When income is low, a greater proportion of the diet is made up of less expensive carbohydrate foods; as income rises, households buy more meat, poultry, and fish and fewer cereal products.[5]

## Family Food Patterns

Food patterns have their roots in cultural and ethnic origin, religious practices, and preferences of family members. Hamburgers, apple pie, and ice cream often seem to be easily identifiable as national foods, but many families have maintained characteristics of the diets of their original homeland. German food is associated with Pennsylvania, collard greens and grits with the South, and tacos and tortillas with the Southwest. Concepts of "hot" and "cold" foods persist in some ethnic groups. Although nationwide communication and transportation have limited differences between regions of the country, New England clam chowder and Rocky Mountain trout are still considered local foods.

The life style of the family often determines which foods are eaten, at what time meals or snacks are served, in what room they are eaten, and even the order in which foods are eaten during a meal. Lewin[6] has shown that the attitude of the "gatekeeper" in each family determines the kinds and amounts of food purchased and therefore available to the rest of the family. The food purchaser may choose according to his or her own preferences, likes and dislikes of family members, or concepts of what foods ought to be eaten. Religious practices may designate feast days, periods of fasting, or proscription of specific foods. Customs and habits are often transmitted from one generation to another since people prefer foods with which they are familiar. In this respect, childhood food patterns persist into later life.

## Social Values of Foods

The offering and consumption of food have become an integral part of interpersonal relationships. Food is a symbol of hospitality and friendship as well as of status and snob appeal. Providing meals or refreshment to guests, either in the home or in a restaurant, is a means

of entertainment for both personal and business reasons. The kind of
food served and the place of eating may be different with guests than
when only the family is present. Steak with elaborate accompani-
ments may be served in the dining room to guests instead of hamburgers in the kitchen to the family alone. Holidays and special occasions have their own significance, such as turkey at Thanksgiving or
cake with candles at a birthday.

### Psychological Values of Foods

Highly personalized and sometimes difficult to identify, the origin of
psychological values of foods may be in the newborn's earliest association of food as a means of gratification or of frustration. To the
young infant, feeding represents not only relief from hunger pains,
but also security and comforting physical contact. His association
with food may be pleasant if he is fed soon after he signals his need,
or unpleasant if he has to wait for a period of time before he is fed.
This may be a factor in the sometimes-disputed psychological advantages of breast feeding, which requires no waiting for a bottle to
be heated. Permissiveness and rigidity in infant feeding have been
described in many anthropological studies as cultural determinants of
psychological development. Fashions in infant feeding have changed
in the United States. For several years a rigid schedule of feeding
every four hours was recommended so that babies would not be
"spoiled." A baby who woke early was allowed to cry until the hour
for his feeding. This was replaced by the practice of demand feeding,
which allowed for variations in hunger and was adapted to the infant's changing needs.

A child learns the social acceptability of behavior through foods.
Training often involves giving sweets or some special treat for good
behavior or withholding food for punishment. In the Preschool Nutrition Survey mothers in the lowest income group were more per-
missive in catering to food preferences of the child and in allowing
greater freedom for meals and snacks, but at the same time tended to
use food to reward or punish their children more than did parents of
higher socioeconomic levels.[1] The "good" and "bad" qualities of foods
are taught when the child is told that eating spinach is good for him
but that candy will ruin his teeth. This inconsistency between making
sweets desirable as rewards and creating guilt for eating them is a
common parental practice. Offering food to pacify a child who is fret-
ful or upset to make him feel better, even though hunger is not his

problem, may establish a pattern of eating as compensation for tension, boredom, or loneliness at a later age.

Not only do parents use food for many purposes in child training, but the child himself also learns to use acceptance or rejection of food as a sign of his independence or his power over his parents. This behavior is not uncommon during the preschool period when the child may be uninterested in food and is struggling to establish his own identity. It may recur in the adolescent who rejects family food patterns or parental advice as a form of protest against the family or even against the current practices of society. Selection of food is an expression of the individual's concept of himself as a certain kind of person. Although the teenager may resist family influence, his need for peer approval and acceptance may change his food patterns to adapt to the present culture of his age group.

Among some populations which have been subjected to discrimination or deprivation, a plentiful supply of food has a special meaning of security and prosperity. The eating of food and the offering of food to others provide great enjoyment. A slender baby is not admired, and extra weight on children or adults is a sign of financial success and a comfortable life.

The foods a child particularly likes may have a pleasant association with a specific person or event. Disliked foods may be related to an unpleasant experience or a stomach upset. Often the episode occurred so early in life that it has long since been forgotten. It is very difficult to find reasons for personal tastes.

## Physiological Factors

Food acceptance begins with appetite. During periods of rapid growth, especially pregnancy, lactation, early infancy, and adolescence, appetite usually increases and food consumption satisfies a hunger which may be frequent and demanding. In the preschool period appetite may be lower and the drive for food less persistent. A temporary decrease in appetite may accompany infection or any minor illness, but this is usually compensated for upon recovery. However, poor food habits may develop as a result of poor appetite or of inappropriate parental reaction to food refusals. In the healthy individual appetite is a guide to physiological need. Distortion of normal appetite signals may occur in obesity or in anorexia nervosa so that usual controls of hunger and satiety do not operate properly.

Appeal of food to the senses of taste and smell as well as the esthetic appearance and palatability of food may evoke eager acceptance, indifference, or rejection. The comfort of the gastrointestinal tract after ingestion of specific foods varies from one person to another; experience leads the individual to avoid those foods which upset him. For example, intestinal discomfort as a result of lactase insufficiency usually leads to limitation or avoidance of milk. Needless to say, allergy or diseases which require special diets also affect the choice of foods.

### External Factors

Particularly in our present society, external factors alter food selection. Advertising, placement of products on supermarket shelves, color and size of package, and the amount of time spent in shopping all affect the purchase of foods. The advice, approval, or disapproval of family and friends, currently popular books on nutrition, and magazines or newspaper articles have an impact, temporary or permanent.

Nutrition education must fit into this complex of reasons why individuals choose to eat or avoid certain foods. The introduction of new foods must fit into the present intake pattern. The preference for familiar foods within the culture of the recipient of nutrition teaching must be recognized in giving dietary advice. If the necessary improvement can be accomplished by increasing foods which are already a part of the customary diet or by adding foods which are acceptable within the context of the culture, such recommendations are more likely to be followed. Attempts to change the individual's diet to conform to an alien pattern will probably be unsuccessful. Restriction or elimination of foods should be considered only after developing an appreciation of the meaning of those foods to the individual. Unless he is highly motivated, he is unlikely to follow dietary advice which deprives him of foods he likes and is accustomed to eating.

In discussing the need to combine the science of nutrition with the systematic study of relevant human behavior, Mead[7] stated that during the 1940s it was presumed that people would be ready to change their "bad" food habits if and when they were told how to do so, but it became obvious that the nutritional value of foods they chose to eat were neither its most important aspect nor the reason for their choice.

The question to be asked today, therefore, is not "How do you change food habits?" but "How do food habits change?" We want to know also how the habits are established in each generation,

how the child learns what to eat and what to avoid, and how much
of certain foods should be eaten, how the learning of food habits
is sustained by other aspects of community life, where the flexible
points are, whether people accept scientific knowledge at all, and
if so in what form, how a new pattern can be developed that will
be nutritionally sound, strong enough to replace elements now
nutritionally useless, and flexible enough to change when necessary,
and what can be learned from past experience that will guide us
in our efforts to improve food habits now.[7]

Findings from surveys of the nutritional status of populations in
the United States and Canada were summarized in chapter 2. We are
concerned here with some of the specific problems of undernutrition
and overnutrition revealed in those surveys and in other studies. In
order to adapt nutrition education to current problems, we must first
analyze causative factors and determine which may be amenable to
education, to intervention programs, or to increased enrichment or
fortification of foods. Later chapters in this book will deal with preventive and therapeutic measures applicable to children.

### Malnutrition in Children

Malnutrition is a state of impaired functional ability or deficient structural integrity or development.[8] It is caused by a discrepancy between
the supply of energy and essential nutrients to the tissues and the
specific demands of the tissues. Primary malnutrition is the result of
either inadequate or excessive intake of nutrients and may be caused
by faulty food selection or lack of money to purchase foods of high
nutritional value. It may be eliminated or minimized by effective nutrition education or by programs of income supplementation or food
fortification. Secondary malnutrition is the result of interference with
ingestion, absorption, or utilization of nutrients or of factors which
increase requirement, destruction, or excretion of nutrients. This requires medical evaluation and treatment of the underlying cause. It
may involve treatment of the individual for specific problems or initiating a mass program such as the eradication of intestinal parasitic
infestation[9] to reduce the incidence of anemia. With the present state
of our knowledge, it is not always possible to identify specific causes
of malnutrition, and there is often disagreement on the best programs
for improvement of nutritional status.

Classical deficiency diseases are rarely seen in the United States,
and severe forms of malnutrition have become less common. Reports
of marasmus and kwashiorkor among Navajo children in Arizona in

1969[10] stimulated establishment of infant and child feeding programs, resulting in marked decrease in the incidence of both diseases.[11] Counterculture life styles of some young adults have been related to rickets and poor growth in their children who were given little or no milk or other animal protein foods. These acute problems require identification and treatment of the specific causes. Preventive measures are obvious for some, but difficult for others.

Major concerns about undernutrition in this country have recently centered on anemia and growth retardation. More subtle effects of malnutrition on intellectual potential and school performance have been investigated primarily through indirect evidence.[12] The high incidence of dental caries may result from inadequate supply of nutrients during tooth formation or to low fluorine or high sugar intake following eruption. Increasing attention has been devoted to overweight and its associated health hazards.

These problems have demanded the involvement of diverse health professionals in efforts to reevaluate traditional approaches to nutrition education. Changes have been made in the delivery of services to mothers and children, with new programs of food supplementation. Levels of enrichment and fortification of foods have been subjected to new thinking, and the bioavailability of commonly used iron supplements has been questioned. The identification and eradication of malnutrition as it now is found in the United States require continuous adaptation of educational and public health measures and demand new and innovative methodology.

### Iron-Deficiency Anemia

Iron-deficiency anemia is recognized as a risk especially to pregnant women, children between six and thirty-six months of age, and menstruating women. Recent survey findings suggest that the adolescent male may perhaps be added to the risk category. The balance of intake and absorption to increased needs may be tenuous for these groups for different reasons.

Blood levels in pregnant women must be viewed in relation to normal hemodilution. By the seventh month of pregnancy the percentage increase in plasma is approximately four times the increase in erythrocyte volume,[13] resulting in lower hemoglobin concentration despite an actual increase in total circulating hemoglobin. The well-nourished woman may maintain satisfactory hematologic indexes in pregnancy.[14] However, many women enter pregnancy with inadequate iron storage. The added need of iron for the fetus and for increment in maternal blood volume may result in the typical microcytic hypochromic anemia of iron deficiency. The hemoglobin level in the neonate appears to be independent of maternal hemoglobin concentration.[15]

The drop in maternal blood values during the third trimester may be minimized by administration of supplemental iron, especially if initial blood levels were low, and supplemental iron may result in higher postpartum values.[16,17] The Food and Nutrition Board of the National Research Council has recommended a daily supplement of 30 to 60 mg of iron.[18] Since orally administered iron is not well tolerated by some women and supplements may not be taken regularly, recommendation of an iron supplement should not replace dietary improvement. Foods high in iron, such as meat (especially liver), green leafy vegetables, dried fruits, and whole grain or enriched bread and cereal, also provide other minerals and vitamins, raising nutrient intake in many respects.

The infant and preschool child present a different pattern of risk. Some infants have particular susceptibility to anemia and probably should be given prophylactic iron: infants with birth weight under 2,500 gm, whether prematurely born or small for gestational age, infants with low hematologic indexes at birth, and infants who suffer blood loss. With their low iron reserves and rapid growth, hematopoiesis may not keep pace with increase in blood volume. These infants have been reported to absorb and utilize iron for hemoglobin formation more efficiently during the first three months than healthy term infants.

Hemoglobin concentration at birth is approximately 18 to 20 gm/ 100 ml in the healthy term infant. Since the average life of the red blood cell is approximately 120 days, normal destruction of these cells causes a drop in hemoglobin concentration to a mean of approximately 10 to 11 gm in the second month. Iron released from hemoglobin is held in storage for hematopoiesis as blood volume expands to serve tissue growth. It has been estimated that the iron reserve is sufficient for new hemoglobin formation until four to six months of age. Thereafter absorption of exogenous iron is necessary to maintain hemoglobin levels of 11 to 12 gm or more.

Risk of iron-deficiency anemia increases after six months, reaches a peak at eighteen months, and then diminishes. Peak incidence of hemoglobin levels under 10 gm or hematocrit values less than 31% has been reported in 10% to 65% of children in low income families in various studies, while peak incidence is rarely as high as 10% in children of middle income families.[19] In the Preschool Nutrition Survey (PNS) transferrin saturation ranged from 13% to 18% in the second year but increased with age to stabilize at 23% to 24% by four years, reflecting increased iron storage.[1] It seems, then, that the child in the second year is more susceptible to iron-deficiency anemia but that his risk diminishes after three years.[19,20]

Racial differences in hemoglobin concentration need to be identified separately from income differences. In the PNS and in the Ten-State Nutrition Survey (TSNS)[21] hemoglobin levels of black children were an average of 0.5 gm lower than those of white children. In the PNS this difference persisted even when age, socioeconomic level, and transferrin saturation were held constant. These findings suggest that a lower cutoff point should be used in diagnosing anemia in black children and that the true incidence of iron-deficiency anemia may be less than reported.

In analysis of the TSNS data, Garn and Clark[22] found that children with higher hemoglobin levels tended to be taller and heavier than children with lower levels. In the PNS data a similar relationship between size and blood levels was found in boys but not in girls. Since the iron level in the diet may be an index to total dietary adequacy, one may speculate that an intake sufficient to support rapid growth will also supply adequate protein and iron for satisfactory hemoglobin synthesis.

The most effective measure for preventing iron-deficiency anemia in the preschool child is inclusion of iron-containing foods in the diet beginning not later than six months of age. The amount of iron needed has stimulated much controversy in recent years. Until 1960 the usual recommendation for infants in the first year was 0.8 mg of iron per kilogram of body weight per day. In 1960, the Committee on Nutrition of the American Academy of Pediatrics[23] increased the recommendation to 1.5 mg/kg, but in 1969 lowered it again to 1.0 mg/kg for the healthy full-term infant.[24] Meanwhile the RDA rose from 0.8 mg to 1.0 mg in 1963 and to 1.67 mg/kg in 1968 and 1974. Although the 1974 table recommended 1.67 mg/kg, the accompanying text stated that "the normal-term infant can maintain optimal hemoglobin levels with an iron intake of 1 mg/kg/day, starting about the third month of life."[18] The latter figure would be an average allowance of 6 mg of iron per day in the first six months and 9 mg per day in the last half of the first year. After a review of the literature, Fomon concluded that "there appears to be no reasonable basis for advising an intake greater than 7 mg daily during the first year (8 mg daily between one and three years) if the infant will receive this intake virtually every day beginning no later than age four weeks."[25] The 1974 RDA for the child between one and three years is 15 mg per day. The evaluation of the adequacy of iron intake would obviously vary with the standard used.

The bioavailability of iron used for fortification of formula and cereals as well as for supplements has recently been intensively investigated.[26-28] The form of iron most readily available for absorption has not necessarily been the form added to foods, largely because of technological difficulties. New methodology can be expected to provide iron in a form more easily absorbed.

Infants who are very likely to become anemic as they advance toward the second year are those whose diets are composed largely of milk with few or no solid foods. Dependence on iron-fortified formulas or cereals is unlikely to solve the problem because these foods are often discontinued about the age when the infant's iron needs increase.[29,30] The most effective long-term program for eliminating iron-deficiency anemia in young children is education of mothers in the essentials of a well-balanced diet high in iron-containing foods. A diet low in iron is likely to be low in other nutrients as well, so general dietary improvement would result in greater benefits than iron fortification alone.

Meat has the greatest hematopoietic potential of the commonly used foods[31] and should be included in the infant's diet along with vegetables, fruits, eggs, and grain products. Both the TSNS and the PNS found that the iron content per 100 kcal in the diets of children in low income families was similar to or higher than that of children in higher income families, suggesting that the total quantity of the diet was a more limiting factor than iron intake itself. Therefore, emphasis should be placed on the adequacy of calories for all children. The slower growth rate of children with anemia implies that their total dietary intake is inadequate and that attention should be paid to more than iron content. Dietary improvement could be expected to increase both hemoglobin levels and growth rate.

During adolescence increased growth requires additional iron, both for myoglobin in muscle and for hemoglobin in increased blood volume. It has been estimated that 46 mg of iron is incorporated in each kilogram of muscle tissue. Males gain more weight, more muscle, and less fat than do females during adolescence. Blood volume of the male is likely to double from 2.5 or 3.0 liters to 5 or 6 liters, while the female's increases from 2.5 liters to 3.5 liters. Therefore the iron needs of the male for body growth are higher. His production of testosterone is associated with increased hemoglobin concentration,[32] adding further iron stress.

A theoretical calculation of the iron needs of the fifteen-year-old male was made by Hepner[33] as follows: with a weight gain of 19 gm per day, of which 92% is lean body mass with iron content of 46 mg/kg, and assuming 10% absorption of intake, iron needs for growth would be 8 mg per day; allowing 100% margin of safety would raise the level to 16 mg of iron per day. Hepner further calculated that a boy whose height is at the ninety-seventh percentile would require twice as much iron as a boy at the third percentile. Nutrient requirements during adolescence depend on the timing, amount, and duration of increased growth, as discussed in chapter 3. The peak iron need would coincide with peak growth velocity in the male, and the degree of need would be related to the rate of growth. Therefore the needs of an individual boy require evaluation of his growth and sexual maturity.[34] The RDA for the male fifteen to twenty-two years of age is 3,000 kcal. Assuming a ratio of 6 mg of iron per 1,000 kcal, the RDA of 18 mg of iron could be met if the diet were not excessive in carbohydrate or fat. To meet iron needs and prevent anemia, the adolescent boy should choose foods of high nutrient density.

Peak growth velocity during adolescence in the girl occurs before the onset of menses. The girl needs less iron for increase in muscle mass and blood volume than the boy, and at an earlier age, followed by the need to compensate for iron lost in menstrual blood. Because of wide individual variations in the amount of menstrual blood lost, some girls have a greater risk of anemia than others. In a review of studies on women between menarche and menopause, Hallberg et al.[35] found a range of 1.6 to 199.7 ml of blood lost per period in most women, and loss as high as 970 ml in women with menorrhagia. Bowering et al.[32] summarized balance studies showing average losses of 8 to 18 mg of iron per period and a variety of studies reporting average losses of 8 to 38 mg. Individual women ranged from 0.3 to 110 mg of iron lost per period. It is not surprising that hypochromic anemia is more often found in women with high blood losses. Although some variation from one menstrual period to another has been recorded for individual women, much greater variation occurs between women. It is obvious that the menstrual history of a teenage girl must be evaluated to determine her risk of iron deficiency. Age at menarche, regularity of periods, frequency of the cycle, length of periods, and amount of blood lost are major determinants of the need for iron replacement. The use of contraceptives must also be considered, since blood loss may be reduced with the use of oral contraceptives but increased by intrauterine devices.[15]

The average monthly iron loss from menses may be assumed to be the equivalent of 0.4 to 0.5 mg of iron daily, with wide variations. The girl with infrequent or short periods and small blood loss per period may be able to maintain satisfactory hemoglobin levels on a generally good diet. The girl with excessive losses will probably need therapeutic iron, but emphasis should still be placed on providing a high dietary iron intake because of the uncertainty that iron supplements will be taken regularly. Higher absorption of iron from meat than from eggs or plant sources makes the inclusion of generous amounts of meat in the diet of the adolescent girl important. The diet should also contain adequate ascorbic acid, which enhances iron absorption. After fourteen years the RDA decreases from 2,400 to 2,100 kcal, while the iron allowance remains at 18 mg, placing stress on the need for foods high in iron but lower in calories.

### Growth Retardation

More complex in its etiology, growth retardation is therefore more difficult to evaluate and treat. Not all short children are retarded in growth. As discussed in previous chapters, size is determined by a combination of factors. By considering parental size, genetic potential has been taken into account in some of the growth standards which have been developed. However, increase in height in some population groups once considered genetically small has shown that improvement of the environment may modify heredity as a predictor of size. Growth may also be altered by congenital abnormalities, metabolic defects, and illness. However, our concern in this text is with growth retardation which may be caused, at least in part, by nutritional inadequacy.

The definition of growth retardation has depended on the comparison of the height of the child with an accepted standard. The problems of deciding on a meaningful standard were discussed in chapter 4.

Shortness of stature has been found more often in the United States in children of families with low income than with high income. The TNSN,[36] with its intentional concentration on the poor, found that 18% to 46% of children in various age groups were below the fifteenth percentile of the Stuart-Meredith height standards. Shortness for age was more common in children under eight years, especially in low income ratio states. The PNS[1] found that smaller size for age, lower dietary intakes of some nutrients, and lower biochemical indexes all tended to be clustered in children in the lowest of four income groups. There was little consistent sex or ethnic difference in frequency of short stature, but the relationship between shortness and economic level led to the conclusion in both surveys that insufficiency of food as a result of poverty was a major factor in growth retardation. These findings are consistent with observations that low birth weight is more frequently found in infants born to mothers in low socioeconomic groups.

Vulnerability to insufficient nutrient intake is greatest when the growth rate is fast, demanding a large and constant supply of growth materials. Rates of growth are most rapid during the fetal period, in the first postnatal year, and during adolescence. Although these specific age groups have usually been selected for special attention in nutrition programs, the need for adequate diets at all ages of childhood must not be overlooked.

A deficiency of protein or of any of the minerals or vitamins essential to the formation of body tissues may interfere with normal anabolism. If caloric intake is inadequate, deamination of protein to meet the body's primary need for energy decreases the availability of amino acids for formation of cells, enzymes, hormones, and other body compounds necessary for growth. When nutrient intake is low, physiological adaptation activates a variety of mechanisms to increase absorption and conservation of nutrients. If intake continues to be deficient, metabolic adaptation becomes inadequate. The body becomes more susceptible to infection, both in frequency and severity of illness, which may cause anorexia and alteration of function of gastrointestinal cells so that absorption becomes less efficient. Normal cell metabolism is altered and the synthesis of protein and other compounds is diminished. Thus the cycle of inadequate intake and progressive failure of metabolic adaptation results in growth retardation and other symptoms of deficiency.

The cycle of poverty, inadequate food, and limitation of physical and mental well-being has been repeatedly demonstrated. The infant born to a malnourished mother may be small at birth, with immature function which interferes with feeding. In a poor home environment, with a diet low in quantity or imbalanced with respect to his physiological needs, he has limited opportunity for catch-up growth. It is all too clear that the prevention or treatment of growth retardation necessitates attention to the total socioeconomic environment. Nutrition education to improve the diet must be combined with programs of income maintenance to make purchase of adequate food possible.

Failure to thrive is another syndrome of growth retardation which is being increasingly recognized. The failure to maintain a satisfactory rate of increment in height or weight may be due to organic problems, but careful investigation and differential diagnoses of some cases have led to identification of maternal deprivation when there is no demonstrable organic reason for the interference with expected growth. Study of the behavioral patterns of these mothers has shown both underfeeding and understimulation. This may not be willful neglect but may be unawareness of the mother of her child's needs and how she is providing for them. Emotional and psychological problems are often involved, and there may be stress due to marital discord, unwanted pregnancies, or too many children. This syndrome is not limited to low income families. The mother tends to become hostile toward the child or to withdraw from adequate care of him.[37] Although some cases have included physical abuse, the most difficult to identify are those which have only signs of neglect. Nutritional deprivation is usually associated with sensory deprivation, and growth retardation results.[38] The mother may bring her child to medical attention with a complaint about his growth, concerned primarily with weight in the first two years and with height at older ages. Treatment with adequate diet and increased attention in the hospital usually result in rapid weight gain. Long-term therapy must include psychological support and treatment of the mother to modify the underlying causes of her behavior.

Dietary improvement to ensure a balance of protein, minerals, and vitamins required for growth with calories to satisfy energy needs must be an essential component of any program for the prevention and treatment of growth retardation, but the underlying cause is usually economic or psychological and requires multidisciplinary teamwork. Only when the basic problem is the ignorance of the mother about nutrient needs and food values can nutrition education alone be expected to have a major effect. Programs of food supplementation by direct provision, by food stamps or certificates, or by school feeding programs may ameliorate the situation during those periods of the life cycle for which they are intended, but the ultimate solutions must be economic and political.

## Impairment of Brain Development

The effects of undernutrition on intellect and behavior have been intensively investigated in recent years.[39] The obvious difficulties of human studies and the lack of long-term follow-up after dietary improvement have made conclusions sometimes premature and tenuous. Retardation in physical growth has long been recognized as a result of undernutrition. Development of techniques for cell studies have permitted brain analyses and measurement of brain growth under certain conditions. Infants who died of severe malnutrition showed deficits in brain size, especially in the cerebrum and cerebellum, and abnormalities of morphology, biochemistry, and physiology.[40] Laboratory experiments established alteration in behavior as well as brain growth retardation in animals as a result of undernutrition at critical stages of brain growth.

The most critical period of human brain development probably extends from the twelfth week of pregnancy, when neuronal multiplication has been reported to increase, to the third or fourth postnatal year, when rapid myelination may have passed its peak.[41] Growth rates of various parts of the brain are not uniform. Comparative degrees of vulnerability of the brain and long-term effects of malnutrition in interruption of brain growth are not yet clear. Experimental animals are poor models of human brain growth because of species variation in timing.[40] Cell studies in humans must of necessity be postmortem, and the measurements of intelligence and behavior have not always been applicable to various cultures. However, recent studies suggest that at least some of the early effects of malnutrition on cognitive function may be reversible and that the synergism between undernutrition and environmental stimulation must be considered.[42–44]

Malnutrition is a biological result of complex social, cultural, and economic factors, especially in its effect on intellect and behavior. Children so poorly nourished prenatally or postnatally that they are physically or mentally retarded usually come from deprived environments. The interaction of poor nutrition and poor environment makes it difficult to sort out the effects of either cause. The undernourished child is often apathetic, lethargic, poorly motivated to perform, easily fatigued, and unable to concentrate for extended periods of time. Greater susceptibility to infection may result in further deterioration of health and nurture and increase social isolation. Parental neglect may be one of the causes of malnutrition, whether due to poverty, ignorance, or lack of time or energy. The child's inactivity and unresponsiveness further limit interaction with parents and environment, decreasing external stimulation and opportunities to learn and develop skills.[45] Behavior patterns are disrupted and the child may be indifferent, irritable, or excessively active. Therefore it is difficult to determine whether delays in cognitive development are due primarily to malnutrition or to environmental factors.

Most early studies on the aftereffects of malnutrition were done on children in developing countries who survived and remained in their impoverished environments or on nutritionally rehabilitated children who were returned to environments which caused the original mal-nutrition. Recent studies have shown that if both the nutritional state and the environment are improved, reversibility of deficits in physical growth, head circumference, and psychological function are pos-sible.[43-46] Therapeutic programs are increasingly combining medical, nutritional, and educational components.

In contrast to the studies of severe malnutrition in developing coun-tries, the effects of short-lived or moderate degrees of malnutrition on mental performance have been less intensively investigated. In a follow-up of children whose mothers had been well-nourished before and after a period of wartime food shortage during their pregnancies, Stein et al.[47] found no significant effects on adult performance. Since only moderate degrees of malnutrition are observed in the United States, behavioral changes of children are more likely to be due to decreased ability to concentrate for learning than to structural dam-age to the brain or central nervous system.[48] Programs to improve the nutritional status of young children should also stress intellectual and experiential stimulation, both at home and in day-care centers.

## Dental Caries

In both the TSNS[36] and the National Health Survey (NHS)[49] dental caries were found to be a major problem with children of all ages. In the NHS the average number of decayed, missing, and filled teeth (DMF ratio) increased from 1 at six years to 4 at twelve years and to 8.7 at seventeen years. Girls had slightly higher ratios than boys. White children had slightly higher ratios than black children, despite the earlier eruption of teeth in the black children. By seventeen years only 6% of all subjects examined had teeth without decay or fillings. The number of affected teeth was not related to income or to parents' education. However, as income rose the amount of dental treatment increased so that the number of decayed teeth was less and of filled teeth more. In the lowest income group 25% of the teenage group had at least three decayed teeth needing treatment.

In the TSNS, Spanish-American children had the least dental care. Up to the age of six years, the DMF ratio in deciduous teeth rose more rapidly in Spanish-American and white children than in black children and there were slightly fewer DMF teeth in the high income ratio states than in the low income ratio states. The DMF ratio increased in all groups after six years, rising from an average of six affected teeth at six years to eleven at seventeen years. Again a higher degree of dental care was found in white children. The level of carbohydrate from foods that were primarily sugar eaten between meals was related to the DMF ratio, but there was no correlation between dental state and similar carbohydrates consumed at meals.

The normal formation and mineralization of teeth depend on genetic, nutritional, and hormonal factors. Deciduous teeth begin to form about the sixth week of fetal life. The incisors, which are the first to calcify, begin to have mineral deposition about the fifth fetal month, and calcification of the deciduous teeth is completed in the second molars about three years of age. At the time of eruption, starting at about five months and terminating at three years, enamel is completely developed but dentin continues to form until the roots are completed. In the permanent teeth, calcification begins in the first molars at about the time of birth and may not be complete in the third molars until eighteen to twenty-five years. Therefore the period of deposition of minerals in teeth spans from the fifth fetal month to young adulthood.[50]

A number of nutrients are required for normal tooth development. Protein forms the matrix, and calcium and phosphorus are the major minerals in hydroxyapatite crystals. Vitamin D is essential for calcium and phosphorus absorption and deposition, vitamin A for formation of the enamel layer and ascorbic acid for the dentin layer. A deficiency of any of these nutrients may result in structural weakness and lead to caries susceptibility. The incorporation of fluoroapatite crystals into tooth structure increases resistance to decay.

After eruption, caries-susceptibility of the tooth, presence of a fermentable carbohydrate, and organisms capable of fermenting the carbohydrate in the mouth contribute to caries. Acid formation facilitates solution of the tooth enamel and exposes the tooth to decay. Sucrose is the carbohydrate most likely to be fermented in the mouth, and the hazard is greater with sweet foods which cling to the teeth and allow a longer time for bacterial action. Fluorine in drinking water or by topical administration has been shown in some studies to reduce caries incidence by 50% to 60% (see chapter 7).

A diet adequate in the formative nutrients is important throughout the period from conception to young adulthood for healthy tooth formation as it is for healthy bone growth. Protein should form the nucleus of the diet, with milk the major source of calcium. To supply other essential nutrients, emphasis should be placed on citrus fruits as a source of ascorbic acid, liver or yellow and green leafy vegetables for their vitamin A content, irradiation of milk, and fluoridation of water. After eruption of teeth, fluorine continues its protective influence, and sugar intake should be restricted, particularly between meals. If sweet and sticky foods are eaten, they should be followed by brushing the teeth, rinsing the mouth with water, or eating an apple or other crisp food which helps to clean the surfaces of the teeth.

## Obesity

In the United States and other technologically advanced countries, obesity has become a health problem of major concern. Although it is not limited to affluent populations, the greater availability of food, financial resources to purchase food, and the use of equipment and transportation which decrease physical activity contribute to an imbalance between caloric intake and energy output. Increase in life expectancy and elimination or treatment of infectious diseases which used to shorten life have focused attention on the relationship between excessive weight and the development of degenerative diseases. Programs for weight loss in adults, although they may be temporarily successful, have rarely resulted in long-term weight reduction. Obesity which begins in childhood seems to be more refractory to treatment than when it begins after linear growth has ceased. Therefore attention has turned toward prevention of excessive fat deposition in children.

The prevalence of obesity at various ages in childhood has not been well established, but estimates vary from 3% to 20%.[51] There has been little agreement on a definition of obesity during the growth years. The normal amount of fat varies with age and sex, as shown in chapter 3, so the diagnosis of excessive adiposity is different for the nine-month-old child and for the six-year-old or the adolescent. Standards used in various published reports have been weight 20% or 30% or more above "ideal" weight for age and sex, or above the eighty-fifth, ninetieth, or ninety-fifth percentile of weight for age in the Stuart-Meredith or other acceptable table. Some studies have used ponderal index (height in inches divided by the cube root of weight in pounds) less than 12.4 or skinfold thickness measurement contrasted with the standards of Seltzer and Mayer[52] (see appendix 2). Some attempts have been made to distinguish between the child who is heavy because of large muscle and skeletal mass and the child who is obese because of excessive adipose tissue. Unfortunately, methods of evaluating body composition, such as body density, isotope dilution, and potassium-40 determinations, are not adaptable to most examining situations.

The basic cause of obesity is intake of calories in excess of the body's need. That statement is deceptively simple, and the etiology of obesity is frustratingly complex. There are many different reasons for either high consumption or low output of calories, and the reasons vary from one individual to another. Little concern is elicited about excessive body fat until it has already developed, so the study of obesity is usually retrospective and subject to errors of interpretation of retrospective data. Among the etiological factors are genetics, metabolic derangement, endocrine disorders, physiological alterations in senses of smell and taste, and emotional and psychological disturbances.[53,54] Caution should be used in the interpretation of findings in obese individuals in contrast to those of normal weight since physiological and psychological differences may be the result of increased adiposity rather than causes.

Parental obesity increases the likelihood of a child's becoming obese. It has been estimated that if neither parent is obese the child has a 7% chance of obesity, and the odds increase to 80% if both parents are obese.[55] However, since the child shares the food patterns and life style of the parents, it is difficult to sort genetic from environmental influences.[56] Studies of children reared in foster homes have produced inconsistent results. Inadequate thyroxine production is relatively rare as a cause of obesity, but some studies have been done on other hormones, including growth hormone, corticosteroids, and insulin, to elucidate their effect on lipid metabolism both before and after the development of obesity. Hypothalamic control of appetite and satiety and variations in blood levels of glucose, lipids, and amino acids may play a role in the regulation of food consumption.[57]

Lower levels of physical activity have been demonstrated in obese individuals than in those of normal weight,[54,55,58,59] but this may be a result of excesssive weight as well as a cause. Children who spend a large proportion of their free time watching television expend less energy than if they were engaged in sports or other active play and may become obese if caloric intake is too high. On the other hand, a decrease in physical activity may follow the development of obesity as the body becomes larger and more unwieldy and the child more reluctant to expose himself to taunts of his playmates.

Recent studies of the number and size of adipocytes show promise of increasing our understanding of body changes. Since measurement of DNA is not reliable for identifying the number of adipose cells, current counting methods depend on the presence of a minimum of

0.01 $\mu$g of lipid within the cell. As a result, a falsely low count may be obtained in the nonobese individual when small adipocytes escape count.[60] As obesity develops, previously noncounted cells accumulate lipid and contribute to a higher count.[61] However, it has been postulated that obesity occurring during childhood is accompanied by hyperplasia of fat cells and that obesity which develops during adulthood is associated with increase in size but not in number of fat cells.

It is logical that adipocytes, like other body cells, can be replicated at any age during the years of growth, but increase in fat depots is not linear (see chapter 3). Periods of acceleration of fat deposition occur during healthy growth, especially during the last half of fetal development, the first nine months of postnatal growth, and the prepubertal or early pubertal period in both sexes. Females tend to increase subcutaneous fat tissue throughout adolescence while the average male has a greater deposition of muscle than of fat.[62] Whether these are "critical" periods in hyperplasia and the development of obesity is not yet clear. Cell studies may be expected to determine the rate of cell replication, the age when the adult number and size of cells are achieved, and whether there is a relationship between adipose cellularity and feeding behavior. If cell number is a predictor of obesity and can be limited by dietary means, and if some ages are particularly susceptible to dietary manipulation, the implications in prevention of obesity are obvious.

Prevention of obesity must begin with the feeding of the neonate. Hunger awareness of the newborn and how the mother responds to the cues of her infant may establish the pattern of the infant's learning to discriminate between physiological need and the use of food for nonphysiological reasons.[53] The mother who responds to the baby's hunger by feeding him promptly but allows his appetite to control both the time of feedings and the amount of intake helps the infant to identify hunger and satiety as meaningful bodily sensations. On the other hand, overfeeding by urging the infant to finish a bottle may lead to confusion of hunger discrimination. Overweight is more common among bottle-fed than among breast-fed infants.

At later ages the use of food as a pacifier, as a reward for compliant behavior, or as punishment for disapproved behavior may further distort the child's normal concept of hunger and satiety as indicators of inner needs by imposing social and psychological components which may be inappropriate to his learning about the meaning of food. In addition, overfeeding of formula or solids and the prolonged use of high-carbohydrate formulas may provide more calories than physiologically needed and result in excessive weight gain.

The concept that a plump baby is a healthy baby and that rapid weight gain is desirable should be revised. The weight of the infant should be monitored and excessive gain identified as soon as possible. However, the use of skim milk for weight control is inappropriate for the young infant,[63] as discussed in chapter 5. A better program is the restriction of carbohydrate, both in formulas and in supplementary foods. The introduction of solid foods is not essential until four to six months, and earlier feeding of solids may contribute to high caloric intake.

During the preschool period, when appetite is often reduced, efforts should be made to avoid foods high in carbohydrate, especially as between-meal snacks. Fruit, raw vegetables, bits of meat, or a glass of juice or milk will supply essential nutrients with fewer calories than sweets. Obesity is less often a problem during the preschool years than slow weight gain, but the establishment of good eating patterns should be encouraged.

Throughout childhood it is important to distinguish between normal increases in weight and adipose tissue and the undesirable high increase in adiposity. Interpretation of weight gain in children is different from the interpretation of gain in adults for whom growth and maturation are complete. Garn et al.[64] observed that fatter children of both sexes are taller, have larger skeletal mass and higher hemoglobin and hematocrit levels, and mature earlier than children of lesser weights. Weight as a sole criterion of the need for treatment is insufficient, and evaluation of maturational stage should be undertaken before a program of weight control is considered.

Methods of weight control which may be effective with adults are usually not applicable to children. It is most important to realize that weight *reduction* in children should be undertaken only in unusual cases and under strict medical supervision. Weight loss includes loss of lean body mass as well as of fat.[62] Reducing caloric intake sufficiently to cause loss of weight interferes with protein anabolism. A loss of more than 1% of body mass results in marked depression of growth.[65] The long-term result may be lower final height attainment and therefore increased risk of adult obesity because of a shorter stature. Better results are obtained if caloric restriction is designed only to limit further weight gain while height is allowed to increase; this requires careful monitoring. Adherence to a special diet is often poor. Children are rarely motivated before adolescence to follow dietary restrictions, and parental control is difficult when the child has access to foods outside the home. Therefore parents often find that their role in diet modification is to decrease the availability in the home of foods high in carbohydrate and fat and to increase the availability of snacks and desserts lower in calories but high in essential nutrients.

The exaggerated interest of the teenage girl in weight reduction may lead to poor nutritional state. The number of adolescent girls who wish to lose weight is higher than the number who are overweight.[66] They often resort to vigorous reducing programs with unbalanced diets. As discussed in chapter 5, the RDA for calories decreases at fifteen years while the RDA for other nutrients remains elevated. This necessitates selection of foods with high nutrient density. Unless the diet provides adequate iron replacement of menstrual losses, the risk of iron-deficiency anemia is high. It is also important at this age to maintain high body content of nutrients in preparation for successful pregnancy. Nutrition counseling for the teenage girl should encourage limitation of foods high in carbohydrate or fat but low in essential nutrients. A wide variety of foods is more likely to meet her requirements than a reducing diet which is limited to a few foods.

The use of hormones and other drugs as aids to weight restriction should be avoided in childhood. At best, such medications have had little long-range value in the treatment of obesity; at worst their effects on the growing organism may be harmful due to interference with normal metabolic processes.[67]

The level of physical activity and energy expenditure are important components of weight control. The relative inactivity of many children in our present society[66] affects caloric balance, muscle tonus, and general health. Passivity is often accompanied by increased exposure to food, and boredom may lead to higher food consumption. Since dietary restriction is often difficult, especially with young children, they should be encouraged to participate in active sports and outdoor activities.

The familiar advice to eat less and exercise more is basically sound and is effective in some cases of overweight. However, it does not attack the underlying disturbances which may have initiated the weight increase. Treatment should deal with existing obesity as a complex syndrome, not as a simple entity. Similarly, prevention of obesity can be effective only if the major etiological factors are better understood and appropriate educational programs initiated. Longitudinal studies are needed of the metabolic, morphological, and psychological states before and during the active phase of development of excessive adiposity as well as after obesity has occurred. Only if we learn why and how individuals become obese can we develop effective programs of prevention.

# References

1  Owen, G. M.; Kram, K. M.; Garry, P. J.; Lowe, J. E.; and Lubin, A. H. "A Study of Nutritional Status of Preschool Children in the United States, 1968–1970." *Pediatrics* 53(1974[suppl., pt. 2]):597–646.

2  Moore, W. M.; Silverberg, M. M.; and Read, M. S., eds. *Nutrition, Growth and Development of North American Indian Children.* DHEW publication no. (NIH) 72–26. Washington, D.C.: Superintendent of Documents, 1972.

3  Bruhn, C. M., and Pangborn, R. M. "Food Habits of Migrant Farm Workers in California." *Journal of the American Dietetic Association* 59(1971):347–55.

4  Larson, M. B.; Dodds, J. M.; Massoth, D. M.; and Chase, H. P. "Nutritional Status of Children in Mexican-American Migrant Families." *Journal of the American Dietetic Association* 64(1974):29–35.

5  Segal, J. A. *Food for the Hungry: The Reluctant Society.* Policy Studies in Employment and Welfare, no. 4. Baltimore: Johns Hopkins Press, 1970.

6  Lewin, K. "Forces behind Food Habits and Methods of Change." In *The Problem of Changing Food Habits.* National Research Council bulletin 108. Washington, D.C.: National Academy of Sciences–National Research Council, 1948.

7  Mead, M. "Culture Change in Relation to Nutrition." In *Malnutrition and Food Habits*, edited by A. Burgess and R. F. A. Dean. London: Tavistock Publications, Ltd., 1962.

8  Council on Foods and Nutrition, American Medical Association. "Malnutrition and Hunger in the United States." *JAMA* 213(1970):272–75.

9  Carter, J. P.; Vander Zwagg, R.; Darby, W. J.; Leose, E. J.; Lauter, F. H.; Dudley, B. W.; High, E. G.; Wright, D. J.; and Murphree, T. "Nutrition and Parasitism among Rural Pre-school Children in South Carolina." *Journal of the National Medical Association* 62(1970):181–91.

10  Van Duzen, J.; Carter, J. P.; Secondi, J.; and Federspiel, C. "Protein and Calorie Malnutrition among Preschool Navajo Indian Children." *American Journal of Clinical Nutrition* 22(1969):1362–70.

11  Van Duzen, J.; Carter, J. P.; and Vander Zwagg, R. "Protein and Calorie Malnutrition among Preschool Navajo Indian Children: A Follow-up." *American Journal of Clinical Nutrition* 29(1976):657–62.

12  Birch, H. G., and Gussow, J. D. *Disadvantaged Children: Health, Nutrition, and School Failure.* New York: Harcourt, Brace and World, Inc., and Grune & Stratton, 1970.

13  Committee on Maternal Nutrition, Food and Nutrition Board. *Maternal Nutrition and the Course of Pregnancy.* Washington, D.C.: National Academy of Sciences–National Research Council, 1970.

14  Rath, C. E.; Caton, W.; Reid, D. E.; Finch, C. A.; and Conroy, L. "Hematological Changes and Iron Metabolism of Normal Pregnancy." *Surgery, Gynecology, and Obstetrics* 90(1950):320–26.

15   Pritchard, J. "Prevalence of Iron Deficiency in the United States with and without Anemia in Adult Women." In *Extent and Meanings of Iron Deficiency in the U.S.: Summary Proceedings of a Workshop, March 8–9, 1971.* Washington, D.C.: Food and Nutrition Board, National Academy of Sciences.

16   De Leeuw, N. K. M.; Lowenstein, L.; and Hsieh, Y. "Iron Deficiency and Hydremia in Normal Pregnancy." *Medicine* 45(1966):291–315.

17   Svanberg, B; Ardivson, B.; Norrby, A.; Rybo, G.; and Solvell, L. "Absorption of Supplemental Iron during Pregnancy: A Longitudinal Study with Repeated Bone Marrow and Absorption Measurements." *Acta Obstetricia et Gynecologica Scandinavica* 48(1975[suppl.]):87–108.

18   Food and Nutrition Board. *Recommended Dietary Allowances,* 8th ed. Washington, D.C.: National Academy of Sciences–National Research Council, 1974.

19   Committee on Iron Nutritional Deficiencies. *Extent and Meanings of Iron Deficiency in the U.S.: Summary Proceedings of a Workshop March 8–9, 1971.* Washington, D.C.: Food and Nutrition Board, National Academy of Sciences.

20   Gutelius, M. F. "The Problem of Iron Deficiency Anemia in Preschool Negro Children." *American Journal of Public Health* 59(1969):290–95.

21   U.S. Department of Health, Education, and Welfare. *Ten-State Nutrition Survey, 1968–1970: IV. Biochemical.* DHEW publication no. (HSM) 72–8132. Washington, D.C.: Superintendent of Documents, Government Printing Office, 1972.

22   Garn, S. M., and Clark, D. C. "Nutrition, Growth, Development and Maturation: Findings from the Ten-State Nutrition Survey of 1968–1970." *Pediatrics* 56(1975):306–19.

23   American Academy of Pediatrics Committee on Nutrition. "Trace Elements in Infant Nutrition." *Pediatrics* 26(1960):715–21.

24   American Academy of Pediatrics Committee on Nutrition. "Iron Balance and Requirements in Infancy." *Pediatrics* 43(1969):134–42.

25   Fomon, S. J. *Infant Nutrition,* 2d ed. Philadelphia: W. B. Saunders Co., 1974.

26   Bing, F. C. "Assaying the Bioavailability of Iron." *Journal of the American Dietetic Association* 60(1972):114–22.

27   Waddell, J. "The Bioavailability of Iron Sources and Their Utilization in Food Enrichment." *Federation Proceedings* 33(1974):1779–83.

28   Rios, E.; Hunter, R. E.; Cook, J. D.; Smith, N. J.; and Finch, C. A. "The Absorption of Iron as Supplements in Infant Cereals and Infant Formulas." *Pediatrics* 55(1975):686–93.

29   Rivera, J. "The Frequency of Use of Various Kinds of Milk during Infancy in Middle and Lower Income Families." *American Journal of Public Health* 61(1971):277–80.

30   Purvis, G. A. "What Nutrients Do Our Infants Really Get?" *Nutrition Today* 8(1973):28–34.

31   Cook, J. D., and Monsen, E. R. "Food Absorption in Human Subjects: III. Comparison of the Effect of Animal Proteins on Nonheme Iron Absorption." *American Journal of Clinical Nutrition* 29(1976):859–67.

32   Bowering, J.; Sanchez, A. M.; and Irwin, M. I. "A Conspectus of Research on Iron Requirements of Man." *Journal of Nutrition* 106(1976): 985–1074.

33   Hepner, R. Discussion. In *Nutrient Requirements in Adolescence*, edited by J. I. McKigney and H. N. Munro. Cambridge, Mass.: M.I.T. Press, 1976.

34   Gaines, E. G., and Daniel, W. A., Jr. "Dietary Iron Intakes of Adolescents: Relation of Sex, Race and Sex Maturity Ratings." *Journal of the American Dietetic Association* 65(1974):275–80.

35   Hallberg, L.; Högdahl, A.; Nilsson, L.; and Rybo, G. "Menstrual Blood Loss: A Population Study." *Acta Obstetricia et Gynecologica Scandinavica* 45(1966):320–51.

36   U.S. Department of Health, Education, and Welfare. *Ten-State Nutrition Survey, 1968–1970: III. Clinical, Anthropometry, Dental.* DHEW publication no. (HSM) 72–8131. Washington, D.C.: Superintendent of Documents, Government Printing Office, 1972.

37   Whitten, C. F. "T. L. C. and the Hungry Child." *Nutrition Today* 7 (1972):10–14.

38   Pollitt, E. "Failure to Thrive: Socioeconomic, Dietary Intake and Mother-Child Interaction Data." *Federation Proceedings* 34(1975):1593–97.

39   Subcommittee on Nutrition, Brain Development, and Behavior of the Committee on International Nutrition Programs. *The Relationship of Nutrition to Brain Development and Behavior.* Washington, D.C.: National Academy of Sciences–National Research Council, 1973.

40   Winick, M. *Malnutrition and Brain Development.* London: Oxford University Press, 1976.

41   Dobbing, J. "Cellular Growth of the Brain: Infant Vulnerability." *Pediatrics* 55(1975):2–6.

42   Frisch, R. "Present Status of the Supposition that Malnutrition Causes Permanent Mental Retardation." *American Journal of Clinical Nutrition* 23(1970):189–95.

43   Graham, G. G. "Environmental Factors Affecting the Growth of Children." *American Journal of Clinical Nutrition* 25(1972):1184–88.

44   Barnes, R. H. "Dual Role of Environmental Deprivation and Malnutrition in Retarding Intellectual Development." *American Journal of Clinical Nutrition* 29(1976):912–17.

45   Latham, M. C., and Cobos, F. "The Effects of Malnutrition on Intellectual Development and Learning." *American Journal of Public Health* 61(1971):1307–24.

46   McKay, H. E.; McKay, A.; and Sinisterre, L. "Behavioral Intervention Studies with Malnourished Children: A Review of Experiences." In *Nu-

*trition, Development and Social Behavior,* edited by D. J. Kallen. DHEW publication no. (NIH) 73–242. Washington, D.C.: Superintendent of Documents, Government Printing Office, 1973.

47 Stein, Z.; Susser, M.; Saenger, G.; and Marolla, F. *Famine and Human Development: The Dutch Hunger Winter of 1944–1945.* London: Oxford University Press, 1975.

48 Read, M. S. "Malnutrition, Hunger and Behavior: II. Hunger, School Feeding Programs and Behavior." *Journal of the American Dietetic Association* 63(1973):386–91.

49 Kelly, J. E., and Harvey, C. R. *Decayed, Missing, and Filled Teeth among Youths 12–17 Years, United States.* Vital and Health Statistics series 11, no. 144. DHEW publication no. (HRA) 75–1626. Washington, D.C.: Superintendent of Documents, Government Printing Office, 1974.

50 Timiras, P. S. *Developmental Physiology and Aging.* New York: MacMillan Co., 1972.

51 Knittle, J. L. "Obesity in Childhood: A Problem in Adipose Tissue Cellular Development." *Journal of Pediatrics* 81(1972):1048–59.

52 Seltzer, C. C., and Mayer, J. "A Simple Criterion of Obesity." *Postgraduate Medicine* 38(1965):A101–7.

53 Bruch, H. *Eating Disorders: Obesity, Anorexia Nervosa and the Person Within.* New York: Basic Books, 1973.

54 Dwyer, J. T., and Mayer, J. "Overfeeding and Obesity in Infants and Children." *Bibliotheca Nutritio et Dieta* 18(1973):123–52.

55 Mayer, J. "Obesity during Childhood." In *Childhood Obesity,* edited by M. Winick. New York: John Wiley & Sons, 1975.

56 Garn, S. M., and Clark, D. C. "Trends in Fatness and the Origins of Obesity." *Pediatrics* 57(1976):443–56.

57 Garrow, J. S. *Energy Balance and Obesity in Man.* Amsterdam/London: North Holland Publishing Co., 1974.

58 Johnson, M. L.; Burke, B. S.; and Mayer, J. "Relative Importance of Inactivity and Overeating in the Energy Balance of Obese High School Girls." *American Journal of Clinical Nutrition* 4(1956):37–44.

59 Spargo, J. A.; Heald, F.; and Peckos, P. S. "Adolescent Obesity." *Nutrition Today* 1(1966):2–9.

60 Hirsch, J. "Cell Number and Size as a Determinant of Subsequent Obesity." In *Childhood Obesity,* edited by M. Winick. New York: John Wiley & Sons, 1975.

61 Widdowson, E. M., and Shaw, W. T. "Full and Empty Fat Cells." *Lancet* 2(1973):905.

62 Heald, F. "Juvenile Obesity." In *Childhood Obesity,* edited by M. Winick. New York: John Wiley & Sons, 1975.

63 Schubert, W. K. "Fat Nutrition and Diet in Childhood." *American Journal of Cardiology* 31(1973):581–87.

64   Garn, S. M.; Clark, D. C.; and Guire, K. E. "Growth, Body Composition, and Development of Obese and Lean Children." In *Childhood Obesity*, edited by M. Winick. New York: John Wiley & Sons, 1975.

65   Wolff, O. H. "Obesity in Childhood." *Quarterly Journal of Medicine* 24 (1955):109–23.

66   Huenemann, R. L.; Hampton, M. C.; Behnke, A. R.; Shapiro, L. R.; and Mitchell, B. W. *Teenage Nutrition and Physique.* Springfield, Ill.: Charles C Thomas Co., 1974.

67   Rivlin, R. S. "The Use of Hormones in the Treatment of Obesity." In *Childhood Obesity*, edited by M. Winick. New York: John Wiley & Sons, 1975.

# Chapter Seven

## Basic Methods of Improving the Nutriture of Children

Important among the methods of improving the nutritional status of children are certain overall dietary measures that operate on a mass scale without knowledge or effort on the part of the children concerned. Notable among these measures are (1) raising the nutrient level of the diet automatically by enriching certain common foods and combinations eaten regularly by most people, and (2) feeding adequately children who are in group care in the many types of institutions, schools, and other situations where meals are served.

In any consideration of improved nutriture, standards are paramount—standards of nutritive content, quality, and safety in foods and standards for dietary adequacy which serve as goals for improvement. In the United States various government agencies are charged with responsibilities involved in establishing and maintaining food standards. For example, the U.S. Public Health Service, under the Public Health Service Act, formulates safety standards for certain foods. The most familiar PHS standard is for "grade A" milk. The

U.S. Department of Agriculture (USDA) issues regulatory standards for meats and poultry and voluntary grade standards for quality in some 300 food and farm products. The USDA also establishes guidelines for meals served in schools and at other sites and to preschool children in day care. The federal Food and Drug Administration (FDA) of the U.S. Department of Health, Education, and Welfare establishes food standards of identity under the authority of the Federal Food, Drug, and Cosmetic Act. These standards are *regulatory*: they set certain ingredient requirements that many food products must meet to be legally manufactured, shipped, or sold in interstate commerce.

In addition, the FDA has instituted a program of nutrition labeling for packaged and canned products based on nutrient standards. Nutrition labeling is voluntary on the part of the manufacturer, unless he adds a nutrient or makes a nutritional claim, either on his packaged product or in his advertising. If a claim is made, or a nutrient added, nutrition labeling becomes mandatory. In itself the concept of labeling, properly applied, assumes improved nutrition. A label describes the nutrient content of a given product in relation to established nutrient standards, called U.S. RDAs (U.S. Recommended Daily Allowances). They are a modification of the RDAs (Recommended Dietary Allowances) which have been alluded to throughout the text, and they replace the MDRs (Minimum Daily Requirements) formerly used as standards by FDA. For practical purposes in labeling, the many RDA categories of dietary allowances for males and females of different ages have been condensed to four groups: adults and children four or more years of age; children under four years of age; infants; and pregnant and lactating women. The highest values from RDA, for the combined ages, form the U.S. RDAs. Nutrition labels thus provide the public with a tool which may stimulate interest in upgrading the diet and furnish high dietary standards in line with improved nutritional status.[1,2]

Professional agencies and organizations in the United States have consistently given support and provided counsel to movements designed to raise the nutrient level of diets.[3,4] They were, for example, the first to call for the nutrient enrichment of single conventional foods, with prescribed nutrients, to be added at specified levels. Such measures have resulted in the release of greater amounts of certain nutrients into the national food supply and thus the greater likelihood that most individuals will benefit nutritionally.

## Improving Nutritional Values of
## Conventional Foods

The food enrichment movement began in the 1930s when there was accumulated evidence that nutritional deficiency conditions of a subacute type were fairly widespread. Also, dietary surveys showed that more than one-third of family diets could be classified as "poor." On the basis of these findings, consideration was given by various professional bodies to the possibility of making good the more glaring dietary deficiencies by adding certain nutrients to everyday foods. The American Medical Association, through its Council on Foods and Nutrition, took the initiative in endorsing the procedure of enriching and fortifying foods.* In a resolution, passed by the Council in 1939, it (1) encouraged the addition of vitamins, minerals, and other dietary essentials to conventional foods in amounts to restore them to high natural levels, when in the interest of the public, and (2) opposed the indiscriminate fortification of conventional foods. Conventional foods were interpreted to be the traditional, primarily single-entity foods identified as dietary staples. The Council specifically endorsed the addition of vitamin D to milk, vitamin A to margarine, iodine to table salt, calcium, iron, thiamin, riboflavin, and niacin (later) to cereal products. This early action was to have a far-reaching influence on enrichment and fortification programs during the ensuing years.

### Enriched Bread and Flour

It was logical that flour and bread be the foods chosen for enrichment because they are consumed daily in significant amounts by practically everyone, and they are used in larger than average quantities by low income groups whose diets are most in need of nutritional improvement. Furthermore, thiamin, riboflavin, niacin, and iron, reduced considerably by the milling process, could be restored to flour without changing the appearance, taste, or any physical characteristic of the original product.

In 1940, the Food and Nutrition Board of the National Academy of Sciences–National Research Council recommended levels of en-

---

*The Council on Foods and Nutrition was officially terminated by the American Medical Association in December 1975.

richment for white flour and baker's bread. In May 1941, the enrichment program was inaugurated when the National Nutrition Conference for Defense endorsed the recommended levels. Following the
issuance of a federal standard of identity, by FDA, for enriched flour,
the flour and bread began to appear on the market. There have been
minor changes over the years in levels required for individual nutrients. Table 7.1 shows nutrient levels for enriched flour as they
appear in the Code of Federal Regulations for 1976.

In 1943, War Food Order no. 1, requiring nationwide enrichment
of white bread and rolls, was issued, and by the end of the war, when
this order was revoked (1946), nineteen states had made enrichment
compulsory. By 1953, bread and flour enrichment was required by
law in twenty-seven states and Puerto Rico. In other states it was
widely practiced on a voluntary basis. Today, changes in procedures
alter the situation. Most enrichment of flour now takes place at the
mill, suggesting that flour enrichment is fairly universal without the
need for state action.

Teamwork has been responsible for this progress in food enrichment. The Food and Nutrition Board has taken a series of actions
favorable to enrichment and has issued several publications on flour
and bread enrichment which have given support to educational programs in its behalf. The American Medical Association has supported
the movement consistently. In 1953, 1961, 1968, and 1973 these two
groups issued statements reaffirming, in principle, policies proclaimed
earlier.

It is estimated that a considerable proportion of all the white flour
milled now reaches the consumer enriched, either as flour or as bread
products. One measure of progress lies in the increased amounts of
enrichment nutrients which have entered the U.S. food supply (the
quantity of foods from all sources that are moved into channels for
civilian consumption) annually since 1940. In 1940, the year before
enrichment, these nutrients in milligrams per capita per day in the
U.S. food supply were as follows: thiamin, 1.5; riboflavin, 1.92;
niacin, 18.1; and iron, 14.2. In 1974 corresponding amounts were
1.9, 2.3, 23.4, and 18.2 for thiamin, riboflavin, niacin, and iron, respectively. Thus, there has been a significant increase of certain nutrients which are known to be low in many diets. On a percentage
basis, the average person would theoretically have increased his intake
of thiamin by 27%, his riboflavin by 20%, his niacin by 29%, and
his iron by 28%.[5]

**Table 7.1** Enrichment Standards for Certain Conventional Foods (mg/lb Unless Otherwise Indicated)

| | Enriched Flour | Enriched Bread, Rolls, Buns | Enriched Corn Meal | | Enriched Rice | | Enriched Macaroni Products | | Enriched Noodle Products | |
|---|---|---|---|---|---|---|---|---|---|---|
| | | | Mini-mum | Maxi-mum | Mini-mum | Maxi-mum | Mini-mum | Maxi-mum | Mini-mum | Maxi-mum |
| Thiamin | 2.9 | 1.8 | 2.0 | 3.0 | 2.0 | 4.0 | 4.0 | 5.0 | 4.0 | 5.0 |
| Riboflavin | 1.8 | 1.1 | 1.2 | 1.8 | 1.2 | 2.4 | 1.7 | 2.2 | 1.7 | 2.2 |
| Niacin* | 24.0 | 15.0* | 16.0* | 24.0* | 16.0 | 32.0 | 27.0 | 34.0 | 27.0 | 34.0 |
| Iron | ≤16.5 | ≥8.0≤12.5 | 13.0 | 26.0 | 13.0 | 26.0 | 13.0 | 16.5 | 13.0 | 16.5 |
| *Optional Additions* | | | | | | | | | | |
| Calcium | 960.0† | 600.0† | 500.0 | 750.0 | 500.0 | 750.0 | 500.0 | 625.0 | 500.0 | 625.0 |
| Vitamin D USP units | | | 250.0 | 1000.0 | 250.0 | 1000.0 | 250.0 | 1000.0 | 250.0 | 1000.0 |
| wheat germ or partly defatted wheat germ | Not more than 5% by weight | Not more than 5% by weight of flour ingredient | | | | | Not more than 5% by weight of finished food (partly defatted wheat germ) | | Not more than 5% by weight of finished food (partly defatted wheat germ) | |

SOURCE: Data from Code of Federal Regulations, Food and Drug Administration (FDA), 1976.

*Tryptophan not to be considered as source of niacin.

†Enriched flour and bread may contain added calcium in such quantity that total calcium content, respectively, is 960 and 600 mg/lb.

## Bread Standards

Official enrichment standards for bread were delayed in coming. Extended hearings on bread were held in 1941, and in July 1943 an order was proposed embodying a definition. However, this order was never issued. Instead, War Food Order no. 1, mentioned above, requiring the enrichment of bread (not flour), had taken effect in January 1943. It was not until after this war order was rescinded in 1946 that the then Federal Security Agency resumed consideration of the matter.

Hearings were held again in 1948–49. The proposed standards for enriched bread and rolls did not deviate from those proposed in 1943. They were consistent with those for enriched flour and the two were interrelated in that bread made from enriched flour would meet the enriched bread standard. Standards of identity for five types of bread and rolls were published by the Food and Drug Administration in the *Federal Register* for 15 May 1952. These became effective ninety days later (see table 7.1 for 1976 standards for enriched bread).

There was concern that the addition of enrichment ingredients would decrease the use of milk in bread. At first this fear seemed unfounded. Bakers were using milk solids in pan breads at the same level in 1948 as in 1939, that is, 4.1 lb on the average per 100 lb of flour. However, a gradual decline in this practice ensued and by the mid-1970s the amount of milk used had dropped dramatically. Whereas in 1951 the major use of nonfat dry milk was for baking purposes—44% of all that produced for domestic use—by 1975 the figure had dropped to 7%. As will be shown presently, the nonfat dry milk solids were merely diverted to other foods.

---

### Enriched Corn Meal

The high consumption of corn meal and grits in southern sections of the United States soon made evident the desirability of enriching corn products. The Food and Nutrition Board urged enrichment of corn in a series of resolutions between 1941 and 1949. In 1946, the Board recommended nutrient levels for enriched corn products corresponding substantially to those in effect for enriched white flour. Whereas emphasis was originally placed on enriching degerminated products, by 1947 the Board urged that "universal enrichment of *all corn products* should be achieved as promptly as possible, especially in areas of the United States where the average per capita consumption of corn products equals or exceeds fifty pounds."

On 13 May 1947, definitions and standards for enriched corn products were issued under the Federal Food, Drug, and Cosmetic Act. Table 7.1 shows the minimum and maximum levels of nutrients for enriched corn meal, as of 1976.

## Enriched Rice

It was soon evident that rice, as an important dietary component of some populations of the United States, should also be enriched. The Food and Nutrition Board urged the step in 1949, and in May 1952 advocated hearings for the determination of standards for enriched rice. Table 7.1 presents the minimum and maximum nutrient levels of enrichment for rice, in effect in 1976.

## Enriched Macaroni Products and Enriched Noodle Products

As pastas came to be used by the general population in this country, as alternates for breads and potatoes, or combined with other foods in mixed dishes, there was a need for standards of enrichment. The Code of Federal Regulations of 1976 sets standards of identity for enriched macaroni products and for enriched noodle products. The former include not only enriched macaroni itself, but enriched spaghetti and enriched vermicelli; the latter include enriched noodles, enriched egg noodles, enriched egg spaghetti, and enriched egg vermicelli. Table 7.1 presents the standards from the Code of Federal Regulations of 1976.

## Other Cereal Foods

Most cereal breakfast foods are voluntarily enriched if nutrients are lost in processing, and many are fortified with additional nutrients. These cereals all must carry nutrient labeling. Cereals fortified with 50% or more of U.S. RDA per serving must be labeled as dietary supplements. Cereal breakfast foods undoubtedly add significant amounts of standard enrichment nutrients to the diets of this country. Infant cereals are subject to the same regulations as other cereals.

It is apparent from this section that the use of enriched cereal products can result in diets improved with respect to the specific nutrients added. Essentially the same improvement could be accomplished by the use of these cereals in whole grain form. It is often argued that this is the preferred way and the educational efforts to that end should supplant legislation for enrichment. It is more realistic, however, to face the fact that highly milled, white cereals are preferred by the majority of the people and that educational programs to convince them of the value of whole-grain products have made little headway.

## Fortified Margarine

All margarine manufactured for use in the United States today is fortified with vitamin A. In 1941, the Food and Nutrition Board endorsed the addition of vitamin A to oleomargarine as follows:

> Resolved that the addition of vitamin A to oleomargarine as permitted by paragraph 6 of the Food and Drug Administration, promulgated in the *Federal Register* June 7, 1941, is in the interest of better nutrition, particularly of low income groups, and therefore, is fully approved by this Committee; that such additions of vitamin A should be made to all margarine intended for table use.

Fortification was optional at first, but if vitamin A was added, federal standards set up in May 1952 required at least 15,000 IU per pound, an amount close to the year-round average for butter. Vitamin D was also an optional ingredient. The 1976 Code of Federal Regulations makes *mandatory* that the finished margarine must contain not less than 15,000 IU of vitamin A per pound, and that vitamin D, still an optional ingredient, should, when used, be added in quantity not less than 1,500 IU per pound. However, because of concern for excessive intake of vitamin D, it is usually omitted.

## Iodized Salt

Simple goiter is endemic in areas where the salt, water, and vegetation are poor in iodine. The Ten-State Survey has reported finding goiter in nongoiter areas, indicating that it may not always be due to a deficiency of iodine, but, in some cases perhaps to an excess. Iodine deficiency is easily corrected through the daily use of table salt to which small amounts of iodine have been added by the manufacturer. This salt tastes no different from noniodized salt. The effectiveness of iodized salt, when it has been added to or withdrawn from populations in goiter belts, has been proved repeatedly.

Iodization of all table salt has been advocated consistently by such organizations as the American Public Health Assosciation, the American Medical Association, and the Food and Nutrition Board. The RDAs for 1974 indicate a range of daily allowances of iodine from 35 to 45 $\mu$ in infancy to 100 $\mu$ or more in adult life and approximately 150 $\mu$ in late adolescence, pregnancy, and during lactation.[6] The current fortification provides 76 $\mu$ iodine per gram of salt. Unfortunately, only slightly more than half of the table salt consumed in the United States is iodized, and use of salt, iodized and plain, has declined significantly in recent years. Salt added to preprocessed foods is usually not iodized, nor is bulk salt that is bought for restaurant use.

---

### Fortified Milks

Milk was early considered a logical and desirable carrier of additional vitamin D because of the favorable action of vitamin D in utilization of calcium and phosphorus in the milk. In 1933, in its advisory service to industry, the American Medical Association considered for its acceptance seal, fresh milk fortified with vitamin D. It later included for acceptance, whole powdered milk and evaporated milk, the amount of fortification of any form of milk not to exceed 400 IU per quart.

The Food and Nutrition Board has made a series of recommendations favorable to the use of vitamin D milk. In the 1941, 1943, and 1945 editions of the *Recommended Dietary Allowances*, the Board proposed a range of 400 to 800 IU of vitamin D per day for all ages of children and for women during pregnancy and lactation. Beginning with the 1948 edition, the single value of 400 IU has been proposed for those same ages and conditions. The lower figure was adopted in order to avoid the danger of excess intake of vitamin D. At present, much of the pasteurized whole milk on the market is fortified with 400 IU of vitamin D to the quart.

In recent years the fortification of skim and low-fat milks with vitamin A has become mandatory. See table 7.2 for fortification standards.

As mentioned earlier, nonfat dry milk solids are now added to many foods, notably skim and low-fat milks and other dairy foods. However, it is not considered an enrichment factor and it is not regulated as such. Table 7.3 shows how nonfat milk solids, manufactured in this country in 1975, were used to raise the nutritive level of human

**Table 7.2** Fortification Standards for Milks of Different Fat Content

| | Milks of Specified Percent Fat | Vitamin D (IU) | Vitamin A (IU) | Nonfat Milk Solids |
|---|---|---|---|---|
| Fluid whole milk* | ≥3.25 | 400/qt (optional) | Not less than 2,000 per qt (optional) | No provision |
| Fluid low-fat milk* | 0.5, 1.0, 1.5, or 2 | 400/qt (optional) | Not less than 2,000 per qt (mandatory) | Optional |
| Fluid skim milk* | <0.5 | 400/qt (optional) | Not less than 2,000 per qt (mandatory) | Optional |
| Evaporated milk | ≥7.5 | 25/oz (mandatory) | 125 per fluid oz (optional) | No provision |
| Nonfat dry milk fortified with vitamins A & D† | ≤1.5 by weight of milk fat | 400 per reconstituted quart (mandatory) | 2,000 per reconstituted quart (mandatory) | No provision |

SOURCE: Data from Code of Federal Regulations, Food and Drug Administration (FDA), 1976.
*Must be pasteurized or sterilized.
†There are also standards for a nonfortified dry milk, identified as nonfat dry milk.

diets that year. More than one-third went into dairy foods such as ice cream, yogurt, cottage cheese, and low-fat and skim milk. A similar amount was packaged and sold as instant nonfat dry milk for household use.

Table 7.3          Disposition of Nonfat Dry Milk Solids for Domestic Use in 1975

|  | % of Total |
|---|---|
| Domestic Nongovernment Use | 100.0 |
| Added to dairy foods | 36.4 |
| Packaged for home use | 32.6 |
| Prepared mixes | 12.4 |
| Bakery | 7.0 |
| Meat processing | 3.5 |
| All other (confectionary, soups, chemicals) | 8.1 |

SOURCE: Data from American Dry Milk Institute, Chicago.

## Fluoridated Drinking Water

Fluorine is an essential trace element. Its judicious use in drinking water serves as a deterrent to dental caries, thus qualifying it as a factor in improving the nutriture of children. In 1916, it was postulated that mottled enamel of teeth resulted from something in drinking water. In 1931, there was published evidence that high levels of fluorine in the water caused the mottled enamel but, somehow, contributed to low incidence of dental caries. It was found that fluorine is incorporated in the structure of teeth and is required for resistance to dental caries. It was also found that local water supplies vary greatly in fluorine content, from almost none to 10 ppm or more. This finding led to consideration of the desirability of adding fluorine to those waters of low fluorine level.

Dental, public health, and medical authorities and national professional organizations endorsed the practice of fluoridating local public water supplies as practical and safe, when found to be deficient in fluorine. And, because dental decay is a critical health problem, local health officers soon advised fortifying drinking water with specified, limited amounts of fluorine. Local communities endorsed the plan in many cases and implemented the process in their own areas. Studies were instituted in various sections of the country to compare the results, in terms of dental caries, using different levels of fluorine in the drinking water.

In general it was found that water supplies naturally containing 0.8 to 1.5 ppm of fluorides, or fortified to that approximate level, were beneficial in reducing the incidence of dental caries. Currently the Federal Environmental Protection Agency advises that concentration of fluorides in public water supplies be adjusted slightly to allow for variations in water consumption—greater consumption of water occurs when ambient temperatures are higher. For example, if the annual average maximum daily air temperature is 53.7° F and below, the maximum amount of fluorine present in the water should be 2.4 mg per liter of water. As the air temperature increases to 79.3° to 90.5° F, the maximum amount of fluorine present in the water should be 1.4 mg per liter.

## Overview

Undoubtedly the total nutritional impact of the basic measures just described, on the diets of children, is considerable although the precise benefits are unknown. These fundamental, across-the-board efforts should be continued and, in some cases, expanded judiciously but it cannot be inferred that they alone are sufficient to insure dietary adequacy. Still essential are aggressive, well-planned educational programs directed toward the formation of good food practices, based on the selection of varied, nutritionally sound diets.

## Other Influences on Dietary Content

There are many less comprehensive influences on the nutrient quality of the diet which deserve consideration. Not to be overlooked is the matter of variation in nutrient values within the same classes of foods, due to differences in their genetic constitution. For example, different kinds of corn vary considerably in niacin content, sweet potatoes in vitamin A value, cabbage and apples in ascorbic acid content, and cereal grains in thiamin. Plant varieties may be selected and propagated, therefore, for their high nutrient content, with a view to improving the quality of the diet. Genetic manipulation of corn to raise the level of certain amino acids is an example. Also, methods of growing and harvesting a food may further affect its nutritive content. The amount of ascorbic acid in a tomato, for instance, is influenced by the amount of exposure to sunlight shortly before it is harvested. Such differences in nutrient values may seem relatively minor in the overall process of obtaining adequate amounts of given nutrients. However, they assume importance if the increase in a nutrient is significant, if the food is normally eaten in large quantities, or if the nutrient is not readily available from other sources.

## Formulated and Fabricated Foods

A relatively new influence on food selection and dietary adequacy are formulated and fabricated foods. They are discussed here briefly, not as basic influences on child nutriture at present, but as factors whose potential is not fully foreseen. The Food and Nutrition Board and the American Medical Association have followed the movement closely. In their joint policy statement of 1968, they devoted considerable space to "new and formulated foods." Additional information and recommendations in 1973, in the separate policy statements of the two organizations, suggest the strides made in the manufacture, identification, and labeling of these new foods.[3,4]

No official definitions for formulated and fabricated foods have been agreed upon. The 1973 policy statement of the American Medical Association proposes that *formulated foods* are mixtures of two or more food stuffs or ingredients, other than seasonings, processed or blended together, and that *fabricated foods* are prepared principally from ingredients specifically designed to achieve a particular function not possible with common food ingredients.

Rapid developments in food technology hastened the introduction of formulated and fabricated foods. The very magnitude of the operation makes it impossible for the public to fully comprehend it. Applying standards of identity and nutrition labeling regulations is a monumental task in itself. A complicating factor is the rapidity with which standards and regulations must be altered to meet changing situations. Any attempt to give here more than a glimpse of the types of solutions sought would be impractical.

### Formulated Foods

Formulated foods are of many types that serve multiple purposes: convenience food, snacks, meal replacers, and complete meals. Such food combinations are subject to nutrition labeling if the manufacturer chooses to make nutritional claims for his product or if nutrients are added. The principles of nutritional improvement of formulated foods are similar to those for conventional foods. The American Medical Association policy statements suggest that meal replacers, such as liquid meals, "should provide 25 to 50% of the daily allotment of nutrients, except calories, established for all nutrients included in the RDA."[4]

*Nutritional Quality Guidelines.* The Food and Drug Administration is in the process of establishing nutritional quality guidelines for certain classes of processed foods. Frozen "heat-and-serve" dinners constitute the first class of products for which nutritional quality guidelines have been established. If a grouping of frozen foods in a meal is labeled a "heat-and-serve" dinner, it must meet specific nutritional requirements. FDA has decreed that such dinners shall contain at least the following components:

1. One or more sources of protein derived from meat, poultry, fish, cheese, or eggs.
2. One or more vegetables or vegetable mixtures, other than potatoes, rice, or cereal-based products.
3. Potatoes, rice, or cereal-based products (other than bread or rolls) or another vegetable or vegetable mixture.

The guidelines also include a detailed statement of mandatory and optional nutrient levels for the dinners.

### Fabricated Foods

Fabricated foods are mixtures structured or engineered into finished food products from various ingredients. Many fabricated food mixtures contain textured vegetable proteins which are combined with other ingredients to produce products similar in appearance and flavor to conventional foods, for example, bacon. If a fabricated food contains certain levels of specified nutrients present in a food it seeks to imitate or substitute for, it need not be labeled an imitation. It can be called by a special name, such as breakfast strips, as in the case of fabricated bacon.

Fabricated foods are a subject for discussion among nutritionists. Concerns lie in the possibilities that the new foods are not investigated thoroughly enough before being put on the market; that they may not contain nutrients in concentrations similar to those of their traditional counterparts; that they may lack, particularly, certain micronutrients; or that there may be an imbalance of the nutrients present.

Constant and thorough monitoring of fabricated foods is urged in behalf of sound nutrition practice in planning the meals of families and children.

## Improving the Nutriture of Children through Group Feeding

The history of group feeding of children throughout the world has been that of a continuing effort to improve their nutritional status.[7] In the United States there were scattered examples of supplementary feeding in the early 1900s. The primary purpose was always to upgrade the basic diet of the children served. The need for programs of a more comprehensive nature was indicated as women joined the work force and were required to seek outside arrangements for providing their children with lunch, and sometimes other meals, on a regular basis. The trend toward more group feeding, particularly in schools, continues to date.

In most cases, group feeding of children in the United States is considered more than a mere feeding operation. Often it is regarded as an indirect type of nutrition education whereby children learn to know and enjoy foods which contribute significantly to their nutritional well-being. Also, planned educational experiences often accompany the feeding operations in the belief that they will encourage better eating practices as a permanent outcome. Some of the major agencies and organizations which are responsible for such programs are considered below in light of their purposes and activities in relation to improved child nutrition.

### Child Nutrition Programs

The federal government of the United States authorizes child nutrition programs under P.L. 94–105, enacted October 1975. It is cited as the National School Lunch Act and Child Nutrition Act of 1966, amendments of 1975.[8,9] The programs offer food service to children in various types of group situations. P.L. 94–105 authorizes changes in previous legislation which affect present food programs: school lunches and breakfasts; child-care and summer food programs for the community. The general trend is toward liberalization of the concept of serving children, that is, making school breakfasts more available, extending school-type meals to child-care institutions, and broadening the types of agencies eligible to join. The law also addresses itself to the problem of plate waste in the school lunch and it authorizes changes in the special food program for women, infants, and children (WIC).[8] If schools and child-care institutions agree to participate in the programs described, they must comply with the following regulations: (1) conduct the food program on a nonprofit basis for all children regardless of race, color, or national origin; (2) furnish free or reduced-price meals to children unable to pay full price, without discrimination against or identification of these children; (3) provide meals that meet established nutritional criteria.[10]

## The National School Lunch Program

The National School Lunch Program (NSLP) is a joint responsibility of the federal government, state governments (with a few exceptions), and local communities. The ultimate contribution of the program rests with the local community and its schools.[9] The program is administered by the Food and Nutrition Service (FNS) of the U.S. Department of Agriculture. The purpose of NSLP is to furnish nutritionally adequate lunches for schoolchildren and, simultaneously, to provide them with educational experiences which encourage good food practices (see appendix 5, which traces important legislative steps in the development of the school lunch program in the United States).

The USDA offers a Type A lunch pattern as the basis for planning adequate school lunches for children. It has served as a guide for some forty years and throughout that period has undergone minor changes which have kept it in line with modern knowledge of nutrition and accepted practices in food service. In general, the Type A pattern has, through the years, moved toward a more explicit statement of meal content and more definitive application to age groups as designated by the RDA. It is expected that one-third or more of the nutrients proposed by the RDA, for different age levels, will be supplied by the school lunch. The Type A lunch pattern calls for a suitable assortment of common foods in designated quantities. The pattern itself has come to symbolize adequacy in the school lunch. Its reliability as a standard is tested regularly for nutrient content by analyzing actual meals served in schools. In the recent past there has been some disposition to displace the Type A food pattern with nutrient standards. However, independent studies, sponsored by USDA, report that significant nutritional differences have not been found between meals planned using the Type A food pattern and those planned directly by the nutrient standard approach.[11]

Concern for excessive plate waste in school lunchrooms has led to analyses of the reasons for rejection of the foods and study of ways to deal with the problem. Findings suggest there may be several causes for rejection, including the lack of nutrition education, the selection of menus served, preparation of the food, size of food portions served, seating arrangements, and the atmosphere of the lunchroom. One attempt to reduce plate waste has been to allow senior high school students to choose less than the Type A lunch. The students may now select as few as three of the Type A items. (The present items of the lunch pattern are meat or meat alternate, milk, two or more fruits and/or vegetables, and grain.) This plan to lessen plate waste will undoubtedly result in more clean plates, but at the same time it avoids, rather than meets, a fundamental challenge of the school lunch, that of improving food practices. Rejection of foods in the Type A pattern emphasizes the need for greater efforts to provide well-planned meals that children enjoy: well-cooked, good-tasting foods, attractively served in friendly surroundings, free from hurry and pressures. Active student participation in all phases of the lunch program and combined efforts of interested, involved teachers, parents, and food service personnel have been features of programs where plate waste is kept to a minimum. Vigorous, practical nutrition education at all grade levels is essential in such a plan. In-service education programs are currently under way to train teachers and lunchroom managers to act as a team, in attacking problems of food acceptance (chapters 9 and 10).

It is difficult to determine the full nutritional impact of the school lunch, as a single factor, on the nutritional status of the children of the United States, although there are many indications of benefits attained. In most cases, especially among needy children, it may be supposed that a school lunch usually contributes more of the assortment of nutrients needed—more consistently every school day—than does lunch from other sources. This was borne out in a survey of 54,000 children in grades 4 through 12 in Massachusetts schools; 72% of the children who ate the Type A lunch at school consumed a meal rated adequate, in contrast to 42% of those who brought their lunch from home, 28% who went home for lunch, 23% who bought à la carte in school, and 21% who ate in the neighborhood store.[12]

It is known also that the school lunch contributes significantly to the daily nutrient intake of children. In the Ten-State Survey the

lunch was found to supply 30% to 50% of daily nutrient intakes in
low-income-ratio states and 20% to 40% in high-income-ratio states.
Black children, presumably in greater need, received higher propor-
tionate nutrient contributions from the school lunch than did white
children.[13]

Certainly the increasing numbers of schools, lunch programs, and
children, alone, offer practical measures of progress. In 1944 it was
estimated that approximately one million Type A lunches were served
daily. In 1976, more than twenty-six million children participated in
the National School Lunch Program—an impressive record of growth.
These figures are more significant in light of the fact that the proportion of free and reduced-price lunches advanced steadily throughout
that period.

Several provisions of P.L.94–105 are notable. One is the new interpretation of the word *school* as "any public or licensed nonprofit
private child-care institution."[9] It includes, but is not limited to,
orphanages and homes for the mentally retarded and it represents a
considerable extension of the benefits of the school lunch program.
To join the program, institutions no longer need to be conducting
educational programs. A second new provision relates to the problem
of student acceptance of the served lunch. The secretary of agriculture is authorized, as one phase of a larger study, to examine the
degree and cause of plate waste in the school lunch program as it
may be related to lack of adequate menu development, the service of
competitive foods, and the nature of the Type A lunch pattern. The
secretary of agriculture is also authorized to make cash grants to state
educational agencies for the purpose of conducting experimental or
demonstration projects to teach schoolchildren the nutritional values
of foods and the relationship of nutrition to human health.

### Food Programs for Children

*Summer Food Service Program.* The Summer Food
Service Program (SFSPC) is directed to school-age children, usually
from May to September, in districts in economic need. Sponsors may
serve breakfasts, lunches, suppers, and snacks. All meals are served
free to the children. Federal assistance consists of cash reimburse-
ments and commodity foods to public and nonprofit private institutions serving school-age children. These include settlement houses,
recreation centers, residential camps, and summer day camps. Individual children may receive breakfast and/or lunch and/or dinner
and/or between-meal supplements, depending on how long they spend

at the meal site. The objective of the programs is to raise the nutrient intake level of children in nonschool, largely nonresidential situations, particularly of those from low income areas where a large proportion of the mothers work outside their homes. To support this objective, the USDA has established certain minimum guidelines for the meals and snacks. This program has the potential of providing a child with 100% of his daily dietary allowances if he consumes all or nearly all of his food at a specified location.

The concept of the summer food program is to continue, for school-age children, the benefits of school feeding in a structured vacation schedule of recreation, crafts, and study. Many communities see this as a way of extending the health benefits of the school nutrition program throughout the year.

*Child-Care Food Program.* The concept of the year-round day-care program, largely for preschool children, is to meet the health, nutrition, and social needs of young children in group care. The program is no longer confined to very needy children. All public and private day-care centers can join if they are nonprofit. Day-care facilities must be licensed to operate by a designated state agency. Staff members must meet qualifications for training and experience required for working with preschool children. Nutrition counseling is often provided by outside agencies. Institutions, including family day-care homes, Head Start centers, settlement houses, recreation centers, and institutions providing day care for handicapped children, approved for participation, are expected to implement essentially the same meal guidelines as those for the school lunch and breakfast programs. Money and food are provided for breakfasts, lunches, suppers, and snacks. The meals are served free to needy children. Meals include specific types of foods in minimum amounts in accordance with the ages of the children.[9]

Often the most conspicuous nutrition measure of the day is the noon lunch, but the entire day's routine contributes to the success or failure of that meal. Rested, contented children, who play actively are usually ready to eat at meal time. Tasty, attractive, nutritionally adequate meals, served in a relaxed environment, with the children seated comfortably, adds to the enjoyment of the meal and to its educational potential. Participation by children in preparing or serving the meal, and some opportunity to make choices for their lunch often help to create interest in food and eating. Many day-care facilities provide for parental participation in the program as a means of relating group activities of the children to life in their own homes.[14,15]

Thus group care, at its best, does far more than provide physical care for children. Within its particular purpose and means, it furnishes an environment which contributes to the total nutritional well-being of the children under care.

### School Breakfast Program

The original purpose of the School Breakfast Program (SBP) was to provide breakfast at school for children from needy homes and/or for those children traveling long distances to school. The program originated in 1966 with the passage of the Child Nutrition Act. The legislation provided for a program on a two-year pilot basis. The SBP has been continued from time-to-time by a series of legislative extensions. P.L.94–105(1975) reaffirmed congressional support of SBP. Since 1973 the funding ceiling has been removed and the program has spread to all schools that indicate need. Growth of the program has been phenomenal. It is administered by the Food and Nutrition Service of the USDA, much as is the National School Lunch Program.

Breakfasts served must meet guidelines set by the USDA. Each meal must include at least a specified amount of milk, fruit or full-strength fruit juice or vegetable juice, and enriched bread or cereal. Schools are encouraged to serve a meat, or meat-alternate, as often as possible. (For exceptions to this pattern see below, "Trends in Group Feeding"). It is generally assumed that a school breakfast should furnish at least one-fourth of the RDA for the different age groups of children who are served. If breakfast is served in their schools, students from needy families are eligible for free and reduced-price breakfasts under the same guidelines which serve for the school lunch program. Other pupils in those schools can buy the breakfast at a reasonable price. Some USDA-donated commodities are provided the participating schools. Breakfast assistance payments are made to the states on a formula involving the number of paid, reduced-price, and free breakfasts served.[10]

The importance of breakfast as a nutritional measure is generally recognized, particularly for children. Unfortunately it is a meal often poorly selected, inadequate in amounts of food, or skipped entirely. Studies show that children who miss breakfast stand a poor chance of having an adequate day's diet.[16] It is difficult to make up in the other meals of the day for the nutrients not obtained in breakfast. Early studies showed that, as the quality of children's breakfasts declined from excellent to poor, the quality of the total day's diet declined in direct proportion.[17]

The data available on breakfast habits of children come largely
from surveys of segments of the school population in designated areas.
A twenty-four-hour dietary recall on a sample of 80,000 schoolchildren in Massachusetts, for example, revealed that only 5% of the
children ate a good morning meal on that day; 13% ate *no* breakfast;
and 24% (or a projected 257,000 children) came to school with an
inadequate breakfast.[12]

What are the implications of such findings in terms of nutriture
and behavior in children? The answers are limited and mixed but
generally point to advantages of a good breakfast. A recent reviewer
has emphasized the scarcity of published data on the subject, but
cites one well-known study which provides measurable evidence fa-
voring an adequate morning meal.[18,19] The study, conducted at the
University of Iowa over a period of ten years, devoted one segment
to schoolboys twelve to fourteen years of age. Maximum work rate
and maximum work output in the late morning hours were significantly better when the boys had eaten a basic breakfast than when
they had eaten no breakfast. Also, according to careful records kept
by the teacher, a majority of the boys had a better attitude and ex-
hibited better scholastic achievement during the experimental period
when they ate breakfast than when it was omitted. On the other hand,
reactions to certain tests were negative. For example, there was no
effect from omitting breakfast on the magnitude of neuromuscular
tremor, or on simple and choice reaction times, maximum grip
strength, and grip strength endurance. In other studies in the series,
no differences in results were observed when the boys ate a basic
cereal breakfast and when they had a bacon-and-egg breakfast.

There are many reports of a subjective nature which point to improved behavior and better scholastic performance following breakfast and other school feeding programs. Many such reports come from
anecdotal records of teachers and comments of parents. However, the
cumulative indication of these observations is that feeding programs
decrease the apathy of children, which in turn leads to improved attitudes, awareness, and greater school accomplishments. Apparently,
the hungry child is disinterested and irritable when confronted with
difficult tasks. It seems likely that "hunger may influence learning and
behavior primarily in terms of the ability to concentrate, rather than
of structural change in the brain and central nervous system."[18]

## Special Milk Program

There is a long history of milk service to children in schools. Under
the Special Milk Program (SMP), milk is available to children

whether or not the school also has a lunch or a breakfast program. There is a specified scale of reimbursement. All public and private schools, and child-care institutions, including summer camps, are eligible to participate. Full endowment for the cost of the milk may be allowed if it is served free of charge to needy children. The purpose of SMP is to encourage milk drinking among children, particularly for those who do not receive adequate amounts at home. Children who carry their lunch to school are thus provided with milk to accompany their packed lunch.

## Trends in Group Feeding

With technological advances, followed by the advent of new foods, there are departures in group feeding practices in government child-feeding programs. For example, USDA has authorized the service of certain alternate foods, such as textured vegetable protein products and formulated grain-fruit products. The former may now be used in combination with meat and other animal products to meet 30% of the minimum requirement of the 2 oz of cooked meat required in one of the choices offered by the Type A school lunch pattern. Various questions have been raised by nutritionists with respect to the use of such foods in child nutrition programs. As indicated earlier in the chapter, major concern lies in the posssibility that nutrients may not be present in concentrations similar to those of their traditional counterparts, that certain micronutrients may be lacking, or that the nutrients present may be in imbalance.

The formulated grain-fruit products, advised by USDA chiefly for programs where there are limited kitchen facilities, are of several types. All are designed to meet the USDA standard for a School Breakfast or SFSPC meal when served with ½ pt of milk. These formulated products are questioned on the same grounds of possible nutrient inadequacy as expressed for the textured vegetable proteins. A further criticism is for the high sugar content of some of these products. In addition, nutrition educators have pointed out that children who have become accustomed to eating a fortified sweet cake at the school breakfast may be confused and come to regard all cakes as equally nutritious.

An increase in the variety of milks available in the child nutrition programs has also been inaugurated. On 13 August 1973, the USDA issued a regulation which authorized "fluid types of unflavored whole milk or low-fat milk or skim milk or cultured buttermilk which meet

State or local standards for such types of milk and flavored milk made from such types of milk which meet such standards." This order represents a change from the original stipulation of unflavored whole milk only.

New food serving methods have also been introduced in the child-feeding programs, chiefly to meet problems of limited kitchen facilities. These methods include delivering meals to individual schools from satellite kitchens; providing an individual lunch to each child in a cup-can, which calls for combining the components of Type A lunches in stews and other mixtures; using canned and frozen convenience foods when the situation dictates. Such methods may introduce factors that reduce appetite appeal of the meals. Also, when meals must be transported, held, and reheated, obviously there must be concern not only for the bacteriological safety of the foods, but also for the retention of nutrients.

Competitive foods, chiefly available from vending machines, continue to be a nutritional problem in schools. The responsibility for regulating the sale of such foods in child nutrition programs has been transferred from USDA to state and local school officials. Often competitive foods are available to children at the same hours and in essentially the same setting as the school meals. Nutritionists have urged that all foods served in the school should be under the supervision of persons knowledgeable in child nutrition. If competitive foods are to be allowed in the school, the choice of items and the conditions under which they are sold should be rigidly controlled in the interest of conforming to the basic nutritional purpose of child nutrition programs.

## National Advisory Council on Child Nutrition

The National Advisory Council on Child Nutrition is composed of thirteen members—four from the USDA and nine from outside the department—representing specific fields such as school administration, nutrition, food service, and education. It is the responsibility of the Council to make a continuing study of official child nutrition programs for the purpose of determining how they may be improved.[10] The first two annual reports of the Council in 1972 and 1973 singled out for top priority the following problems: strengthening nutrition education, reaching schools currently without meal programs, increasing student participation in child nutrition programs, using school facilities and experience for summer feeding programs, and making sure that the use of new food products is properly monitored and accompanied by nutrition education. Later the Council addressed itself to such topics as preservice nutrition education of teachers, nutritional bases for child nutrition meal patterns, and plate waste and ways to deal with it. The Council is a practical, working group. It is dedicated to finding answers to important questions facing the child nutrition programs.

## Special Supplemental Food Program for Women, Infants, and Children

The Women, Infants, and Children Program (WIC) supplies food supplements to pregnant and lactating women and to infants and young children, who are declared to be at "nutritional risk" by competent medical, nutrition, or health officials. Applicants must also qualify for free or low-cost medical care, thus encouraging better total health care. While the WIC program does not provide for serving children in groups, as do those programs just described, it represents a fundamental concept for protecting the nutritional welfare of children, largely through preventive measures.[8,9]

A two-year pilot program, begun in 1974, was authorized by the Child Nutrition Act of 1966, amended. P.L.94–105, enacted in 1975, extended WIC through the fiscal year ending 30 September 1978, and stated as its purpose: "to provide supplemental nutritious food as an adjunct to good health care during such critical times as growth and development, in order to prevent the occurrence of health problems."[9] The level of support was raised by the new law and eligibility was broadened to include women from the time of pregnancy through six months postpartum and children to the fifth birthday. The Food and Nutrition Service of USDA administers WIC and funds are made available to participating state health departments or comparable state agencies; to Indian tribes recognized by the Department of Interior; or to Indian Health Services of DHEW. These agencies distribute funds in needy areas to local public health or welfare agencies or private nonprofit groups, largely through health clinics. Such funds are used to carry out health and nutrition programs under which specified food supplements are provided and to pay administrative costs, including those for nutrition education.

The supplemental foods are those containing nutrients known to be lacking in the diets of populations at nutritional risk and, in particular, "those foods and food products containing high quality protein, iron, calcium, vitamin A, and vitamin C."[9] Concessions may be made for including formulated foods designed specifically for women and infants, and flexibility is provided to take into account medical problems and cultural eating patterns. The WIC food "package" contains iron-fortified infant formula, fortified milk, cheeses, eggs, high-iron breakfast cereal, and high-vitamin fruit and vegetable juices. The food is available at specified time intervals and the amounts are determined by the ratio of woman-child participants served in a given household. Three food delivery systems are the ones used most frequently: vouchers for recipients to purchase the foods in market; home delivery; and direct distribution to recipients at dispersal centers. Emphasis is placed on the fact that these foods are issued as *supplements* to their home meals and are not intended as their sole diet. Also it is urged that the foods are for specified vulnerable members of the family and not for general family consumption.

Poor nutritional status and inadequate income are considered critical risk factors in determining eligibility for WIC. The women may demonstrate one or more of the following characteristics: known inadequate nutritional patterns, unacceptably high incidence of anemia, high prematurity rates, or inadequate patterns of growth (underweight, obesity, or stunting). Infants and children under five years of age are at risk if they show a deficient pattern of growth, by minimal standards, as reflected by an excess number of children in the lower percentiles of height and weight. Also included in this category may be those who are in the parameter of nutritional anemia or who are from low income populations where nutritional studies have shown inadequate infant diets. State or local participating agencies are required to maintain adequate medical records on all participants in WIC.

The new law specifies that nutrition education shall accompany the WIC food assistance program, but there is need for greater emphasis on this component.[9] Different methods of nutrition education have been applied—formal and informal—with the latter largely the favored approach. Only a small percentage of participants reported they had learned from the educational program, but those who did so attributed it to simple advice given mainly on a one-to-one basis, advice that related to their own specific food problems, offered by persons who were acquainted with their home situations. In general, recipients felt more was gained from suggestions which involved small changes, undertaken one at a time, than from formal educational procedures which involved sweeping dietary reforms.

Two advisory committees were named by P.L.94–105 to guide and direct WIC: one committee, composed of representatives of government agencies and professional organizations dealing with child nutrition, to study the operation of the WIC Program in depth and to recommend to the Secretary of Agriculture the best methods of evaluating and assessing health benefits of the program, and a second committee, a National Advisory Council on Maternal, Infant, and Fetal Nutrition, which was appointed to make a continuing study of WIC. It is composed largely of professionally trained persons, inside and outside the government, particularly those concerned with or active in the supplementary feeding program, at different levels of responsibility. The Council is directed to report annually to the president and Congress on recommended administrative or legislative changes.

A medical evaluation of the WIC program has been made by the Department of Nutrition, School of Public Health, the University of North Carolina. The evaluation covered the period from 28 November 1973 to 1 June 1976, and involved nineteen projects in fourteen states. The report offers the following evidence of improvement resulting from participation in the WIC program: improved nutrient intakes among mothers; desirable weight gains among pregnant women; marked increase in birth weights, especially of those infants belonging to minority groups; reduced incidence of anemia in mothers, infants, and children; increased head circumference in infants; increased rate of growth in height and weight for infants and children.[20-22]

## Other Types of Group Feeding for Children

Traditional group feeding in child-care institutions has decreased over the years. Many children once placed in orphanages which accommodated large groups are now living in foster homes where there may be one child or, at most, only a few children. All foster homes are licensed, under different procedures, in the various states. Nutritional guidelines for feeding the children also vary. In general, local agencies which place the children require foster parents to provide meals which meet certain standards of nutritional adequacy.

Group feeding of children has come to offer special educational opportunities for dealing with certain health conditions in children. The ultimate purpose is to provide a daily diet, therapeutic or other, which meets accepted dietary standards as one step toward achieving and maintaining satisfactory nutritional status. Two examples are discussed below—one explores the group approach to weight reduction in a summer camp for girls. The other examines approaches made with small groups in a nutrition clinic and with larger groups in a summer camp. Both of the latter involve diabetic children.

## Camps for Overweight Children

How obese children can lose weight and improve their nutriture at the same time is a real challenge. One-third or more of the U.S. population is said to be overweight, with 5% to 10% of schoolchildren obese. A large proportion of obese children will probably remain that way unless well-planned programs are instituted to treat the condition. Prolonged obesity in childhood is the most difficult type to cope with and gives the least promise of success in weight reduction and maintenance in adulthood. Approaching weight loss in the teenage population has many perplexing aspects.

Obese children, especially teenagers, often attempt weight reduction on their own initiative. Their concept of the process is to seize upon a current popular fad reducing diet in the expectation it will result in prompt weight loss that will be sustained. This fails to take place when motivation is no longer sustained, when perseverance with the diet ends, and when family and friends no longer support the undertaking. Unsuccessful efforts of this type are due basically to lack of comprehension of the child obesity problem, failure to understand nutritional needs of the obese person, and the absence of a structured plan which takes into account the many factors involved in safe, steady weight loss. The seriousness of the problem has resulted in efforts to render professional aid to such children, in groups. One method has been to teach them through organized summer camps. There are several such camps, for girls and for boys. One long-established camp for obese girls (eleven to eighteen years of age) which operates successfully on principles of sound nutrition, is described here.

The camp is owned and managed by a physician and a nutritionist.[23] It was their purpose to create a setting in which they could study teenage obesity in depth while at the same time helping the girls to meet their frustrating problem of overweight.

The camp operates on several well-defined nutrition principles calculated to meet its objectives. Important among them is the service of three nourishing well-balanced meals daily, accompanied by periodic instruction in nutrition to provide the girls with bases for understanding their own condition. The owners believe that few things are as important as regularity in meals and an adequate break-fast. Accordingly, calories are so distributed throughout the day that all three meals are in demand. Total energy intake in the meals for the day ranges from about 1,000 to 1,400 calories. Meals are served attractively, but they consist of ordinary foods readily available in regular food markets and of sufficient variety to satisfy most appe-tites. Desserts, such as fresh fruit, served at meals, may be reserved by the girls for snacks between meals. The overall purpose is to main-tain good nutrition on an adequate diet low enough in calories to lose weight gradually.

For their instruction in nutrition, the nutritionist meets the campers as a group twice a week. Individual counseling is provided as needed. The girls learn about nutrients, the different functions they perform in the body, and the consequences of deficiencies. They also learn about body build, the differences in bone structure, fat padding, and musculature among individuals. The influence of heredity is consid-ered, as well as individual variations in rate of growth. Actual weight is deemphasized; there is no calorie counting and the girls are weighed only three times during the seven weeks of camp life. At the close of camp each summer, parents are brought together for a symposium on childhood obesity. This provides them with background information and prepares them to be supportive of the girls in their efforts to con-tinue their weight loss program.

The girls learn that special dietetic foods are not needed, that ordi-nary foods have the same functions, and that neither possesses any magic in losing weight. So-called forbidden foods, such as cake, pie, and candy, are not excluded entirely from camp fare nor proposed for total exclusion outside. The nutritionist teaches the doctrine of "por-tion control," that is, that frequency and quantity of food are the key concepts. Moderation, rather than abstinence, is set as the reasonable goal, thus avoiding the psychological trauma of depriving the girls of favorite foods. The thrust is toward a knowledgeable, confident, motivated girl who will acquire a new attitude and approach toward food selection.

It goes without saying that the camp organization has important features, other than food itself, which contribute to the total program for reducing body weight. One is physical activity. The girls are en-couraged to increase their physical exercise. However, this measure is not urged unduly because of the extreme effort required (as in tennis, swimming, volleyball) on the part of those girls greatly over-weight, and because of the comparative scarcity of facilities outside the camp to continue regular exercise of this type. More important, the girls are under constant stimulation to broaden their range of interests (music, painting, writing). This creates a more positive outlook on their weight situation and tends to direct their attention toward new permanent interests and away from the constant obsession with food and eating and the introspection and depression which usually accompany it. This combination of approaches has gratifying results. "Each year," the nutritionist reports, "we have ascertained that 40% of our campers achieve and maintain their desired weight."[24]

Many other advantages accrue which add to the probabilities that weight losses will be sustained. For example the girls, separated from their parents at the camp, learn self-reliance and independence with respect to meal selection—they learn, through nutrition counseling, how to cope in the real world with food choices in restaurants, the school lunch, home meals, and snacks. They discover that the matter of weight loss is up to them. A whole new life opens; they learn new ways to enjoy food. Many overweight girls enter camp with a poor image of themselves. Families are embarrassed by their fatness and there are few social affairs. Efforts are made to reverse this image. At camp, much emphasis is placed on body carriage and build, on clothes, fashion, style, dress sizes. Periodic postcamp counseling sessions with the nutritionist provide stimulation for continued interest in diet and other routines which contribute to weight loss.

## Group Approach to Diabetic Counseling

Educational programs to deal with feeding diabetic children are not new. They are part of a continuing effort to help young people understand and carry out the management of their disease and at the same time lead a normal life and maintain good nutrition. Child patients are expected to "comprehend, integrate, perform and assume responsibilities for a multiplicity of areas for survival."[25] Understanding of diabetes, as related to food, is fundamental. This background is usually acquired by the child through individual instruction, using his own situation as the focus. But there has been increasing recognition of the importance of making dietary management more effective and more palatable through the use of modern educational techniques. One aspect of these techniques is the innovative nutrition-related group-learning activities.

Many such activities have originated with the children themselves, based on a felt need for the aid and reassurance which can follow informal exchange of experiences. Group approaches of many types have been tried. Those described here arose with outpatient diabetic children in a nutrition clinic in a hospital.[26] In all cases the focus was on group meal situations which gave rise to pertinent dieting discussions. One such type took the form of brown-bag lunch sessions of a few preadolescents and teenagers with the clinical nutritionist. It offered opportunity for peer group learning through interchange of personal experiences with diabetic-related food problems based largely on school-social pressures. The lunch itself was the departure point for discussion. From time to time it extended from brown bags to eating facilities in the hospital, such as the cafeteria or snack bar.

A breakfast "workshop," initiated by teenage boys, represented another type of small group session during which self-selected topics concerned with diet and nutrition were discussed. The problems of dietary excesses at parties, the effects of pregnancy on diabetes, and information on current diabetes research, relevant to the children, were among those included. Appropriate staff joined the group as needed to give guidance.

Patients and their families were also involved in planning and preparing a picnic-type barbeque. This occasion gave opportunity for sharing ideas with other families and members of the medical team. It was another device to inform and reassure both parents and child patients as they pursued their task of managing the diabetic diet.

One project arose in response to a critical need—that of how to cope with the matter of sweets at holiday season. Both parents and child patients requested help to solve the problem of holiday dietary indiscretions. It was called a holiday food teach-in workshop in which parents and patients worked together to produce traditional holiday foods. They were taught "how to modify the free sugar content of recipes, to evaluate the finished product for approximate glucose load potential, and portion the whole approximately to meet the diet-insulin structure." To add interest and provide effective learning, a sample of each family's product was displayed with a label giving its approximate glucose load potential, lettered in grams of carbohydrate and its equivalence in 5-gm sugar cubes. At the appointed time each child patient was given a specified amount of glucose load "money" designated in 5-, 10-, and 15-gm denominations to "spend" for the holiday food items and show proof of its appropriateness.[26] Activities of the type described are judged by participants to have resulted in a better understanding of the processes involved in helping child diabetics to face the realities of their disease and to help them assume responsibility for the medical-diet therapy.

Diabetic camps for children provide a setting for community living where child patients may benefit from shared experiences with their peers as well as acquire new professional direction. There are some sixty diabetic camps in the United States, located in practically every state. Many of them are sponsored by the American Diabetes Association, usually in cooperation with local diabetes organizations and/or various civic groups. In an atmosphere of informal exchange, a child discovers early that his fellow campers are experiencing the same emotional problems and facing the same questions of dietary management as he is.[26] This realization helps to create conditions for maximum learning and tends to normalize attitudes toward a shared problem.

## References

1   National Nutrition Consortium, Inc., with Ronald M. Deutsch. *Nutrition Labeling: How It Can Work for You.* Bethesda, Md.: National Nutrition Consortium, Inc., 1975.

2   Peterkin, B.; Nichols, J.; and Cromwell, C. *Nutrition Labeling: Tools for Its Use.* Washington, D.C.: U.S. Department of Agriculture, 1975.

3   Food and Nutrition Board, National Academy of Sciences–National Research Council. "How Far Shall We Go in the Enrichment, Fortification and Formulation of New Foods?" *Journal of the American Dietetic Association* 64(1974):255–56.

4   Council on Foods and Nutrition, American Medical Association. "Improvement of the Nutritive Quality of Foods: General Policies." *JAMA* 225(1973):1116–18.

5   *Food Consumption, Prices, and Expenditures.* Supplement for 1974 to Agricultural Economic report no. 138. Washington, D.C.: U.S. Department of Agriculture, 1976.

6   Food and Nutrition Board. *Recommended Dietary Allowances,* 8th ed. Washington, D.C.: National Academy of Sciences–National Research Council, 1974.

7   Martin, E. A. *Roberts' Nutrition Work with Children.* Chicago: University of Chicago Press, 1954.

8   Jenkins, D. D. "New Legislation for Child Nutrition Programs." *Food and Nutrition* 6(1976):2–5.

9   U.S. Congress. House. *National School Lunch and Child Nutrition Programs.* Pub. L. 94–105. 94th Cong., 1975, H.R. 4222.

10  Pearson, J. "Child Nutrition Programs of the Food and Nutrition Service, U.S. Dept. of Agriculture." In *Nutrition Program News.* Washington, D.C.: U.S. Department of Agriculture, 1973.

11  Jansen, R. J.; Harper, J. M.; Frey, A. L.; Crews, R. H.; Shigetomi, C. T.; and Lough, J. B. "Comparison of Type A and Nutrient Standard Menus for School Lunch: III. Nutritive Content of Menus and Acceptability." *Journal of the American Dietetic Association* 66(1975):254–61.

12  *Focus on Nutrition: You Cannot Teach a Hungry Child.* Boston: Bureau of Nutrition Education and School Food Service, Massachusetts Department of Education, 1970.

13  U.S. Department of Health, Education, and Welfare. *Ten-State Nutrition Survey, 1968–1970: V. Dietary.* DHEW publication no. (HSM) 72–8133. Washington, D.C.: Superintendent of Documents, Government Printing Office, 1972.

14  Juhas, L. "Nutrition Education in Day Care Programs: A New Challenge to Our Profession." *Journal of the American Dietetic Association* 63 (1973):134–37.

15  Chenoweth, A. D. "Standards and Progress in Day Care Programs." *Journal of the American Dietetic Asssociation* 60(1972):197–200.

16  Myers, M. L.; O'Brien, S. C.; Mabel, J. A.; and Stare, F. J. "A Nutrition Study of School Children in a Depressed Urban District." *Journal of the American Dietetic Association* 53(1968):226–33.

17  Sidwell, V., and Eppright, E. "Food Habits of Iowa Children: Breakfast." *Journal of Home Economics* 45(1953):401–5.

18  Read, M. S. "Malnutrition, Hunger and Behavior: II. Hunger, School Feeding Programs and Behavior." *Journal of the American Dietetic Association* 63(1973):386–91.

19  *A Complete Summary of Iowa Breakfast Studies.* Chicago: Cereal Institute, 1962.

20  Edozien, J. C.; Switzer, B. R.; and Bryan, R. B. *Medical Evaluation of the Supplemental Food Program for Women.* Vol. 1. *Study Design, Methods and Performance Data.* Vol. 2. *Results.* Vol. 3. *Summary and Conclusions.* Chapel Hill, N.C.: Department of Nutrition, School of Public Health, University of North Carolina, 1976.

21  Bendick, M., Jr.; Campbell, T. H.; Blawden, D. L.; and Jones, M. *Efficiency and Effectiveness in the W.I.C. Program Delivery System.* Miscellaneous publication no. 1338. Washington, D.C.: U.S. Department of Agriculture, Food and Nutrition Service, 1976.

22  "Four Views of W.I.C.: A Unique Environment for Nutrition Education." A commentary by four participants. *Journal of Nutrition Education* 8 (1976):156–59.

23  Peckos, P. S.; Spargo, J. A.; and Heald, F. P. "Adolescent Obesity: Nutrition Guidelines for Teenagers." *Nutrition Today* 2(1966–67):22–27.

24  Peckos, P. S. "The Teenage Obesity Problem: Why?" *Food and Nutrition News* 42(1970–71):1–4.

25  Lum, B. L. "Nutrition Education for the Child with Diabetes." *Diabetes Educator* 1(1975):6–10.

26 Lum, B. L. "Preventing Ketoacidosis in the Child with Juvenile-Onset Diabetes Mellitus: II. The Learning Environment." *Journal of the American Dietetic Association* 69(1976):161–64.

# Chapter Eight

## Nutritionists and Nutrition Programs

This chapter and those which follow are devoted to constructive programs designed to help children become and remain well nourished. The present chapter introduces the chief agencies, organizations, and institutions concerned with nutritional health—the mechanisms through which nutrition education and service programs operate. Inseparable from the programs are the nutrition-trained personnel who plan and implement them. Qualifications of nutritionists as gauged by scientific training and experience are therefore essential in the total program perspective.

Nutrition services in this country had their beginning in health agencies. The first agency to develop a formalized nutrition program (1906) was the Community Service Society of New York City. The American Red Cross initiated its nutrition program two years later, and by 1911 the first nutrition service for a visiting nurse association was established in Boston. Nutrition services were introduced into other organizations one by one in the ensuing years.

In the meantime, nutrition services were being incorporated into official agencies dealing with health and food. Such work has been carried on by state health departments since 1915 to 1920, when the Massachusetts and New York health departments employed their first nutritionists. The Shepard-Towner Act, passed by Congress in 1921, was administered by the then Children's Bureau until the expiration of the act in 1929. This act gave grants-in-aid to states, "for the promotion of the welfare and hygiene of maternity and infancy." During that period, several additional state health departments inaugurated nutrition services.

With the passage of the Social Security Act in 1935, federal funds were again made available for extension of health services to mothers and children and for strengthening public health services in general. State health departments were enabled to employ nutritionists from the funds administered by the Children's Bureau and the Public Health Service. As a result, the number of nutritionists serving with state health departments increased rapidly. Between 1940 and 1950 the number rose from 85 to 170. These state programs were then the major ones employing nutritionists. At the same time other health agencies were adding nutrition services or expanding current facilities.

The exact number of nutritionists serving various agencies in the United States at a given time is impossible to determine. It was estimated in the mid-1950s that the total number employed by federal, state, and local agencies, both governmental and nongovernmental, fell within the range of 350 to 400. Of this number, approximately 200 were employed by state health departments and another 75 by local health departments. There are no reliable data on comparable positions at the present time. Informed guesses from several sources suggest that the previous total may have increased several-fold. Approximately one-half of the current number is estimated to be involved in direct counseling, with the remainder in administrative positions.[1] Growth in numbers of personnel has paralleled the broadening of nutrition services and efforts to upgrade professional education and training of nutritionists preparing to conduct the programs.

## Qualifications of Nutritionists

During nearly fifty years the requirements for training and experience of personnel in public health nutrition positions have gradually been evolved, mainly through the joint efforts of allied professional groups. In the mid-1930s a joint committee of the American Home Economics Association and the American Dietetic Association acted to consider "problems of qualification, functions and preparation of nutritionists for the field of public health." The first report of this committee was made in 1938; it was revised in 1941 and again in 1945. Each report was accepted by the sponsoring organizations. The 1941 and 1945 editions were also approved by the Governing Council of the American Public Health Association.[2]

The 1945 edition of the report outlined educational qualifications for three grades of nutrition positions: (1) the *director* of a nutrition service in a health agency, with responsibility for a staff of workers; (2) the *nutritionist* who acts primarily as a consultant and neither has responsibility for supervision of a staff of workers nor receives close technical supervision; and (3) the *staff nutritionist* working under close technical supervision of a director of nutrition service. The basic educational qualifications at each of the three levels was, in brief, a bachelor's degree in home economics with a food and nutrition major and, for the first two levels, at least one year of full-time graduate credit, which provided training in the nutrition-public health field.

Since 1945, additions and revisions have been made from time to time.[3,4] In 1976 a new compilation was issued titled *Personnel in Public Health Nutrition*. This report was the work of a committee chosen by the Faculties for Graduate Training in Public Health Nutrition and the Association of State and Territorial Public Health Nutrition Directors.[5] Task force subcommittees were composed of members of these two organizations, of other concerned groups, and of federal, state, and local agencies. The report describes the roles, responsibilities, qualifications, education, and training of nutrition personnel in public health. Major consideration is given here to sections of the report dealing with nutrition in maternal and child health. A recommended general pattern for training in public health nutrition is outlined first. (See chapter 9 for qualifications of nutrition educators.)

Guidelines have been developed for a master's degree program in public health nutrition.[5] They call for courses in the area of study conforming in general to those in "Suggested Objectives for the Graduate Preparation of Nutritionists for the Public Health Field."[3] The program would be under the direction of a full-time faculty member who has had advanced preparation in the science of nutrition and broad experience in the field of applied nutrition. This preparation would also include knowledge of public health administration and public health practice. The faculty would include other members specifically educated in human nutrition at advanced levels. The courses would be apportioned to the curriculum in a manner approved by the institution and in accordance with its policies. It is recommended that course content may well fall into three categories, approximately as follows: one-third in advanced nutrition, including the science of nutrition, nutritive needs of the life cycle, and special needs in disease and under varying conditions; one-third in public health areas, such as organization and administration of community health services, including program planning; and one-third in related courses in social and behavioral sciences and education.

Field work is required and would be under the supervision of a public health nutritionist. It would be practical, wide-ranging, and appropriate to the function of a public health nutrition program: to give a broad understanding of the role of the public health nutritionist in public health; to provide opportunity to integrate theory with professional practice; and to help students learn how to assess nutritional needs and how to plan, evaluate, and implement programs to meet those needs.

Master's degree programs in public health nutrition are currently available in eighteen universities in the United States. To assure a supply of well-trained public health nutritonist personnel, some funds are available, from public and private sources, to students studying for advanced degrees. One source is public health special purpose traineeship grants from the U.S. Public Health Service.

Undergraduate educational training leading to a bachelor's degree lays the foundation for master's degree programs. The former would include appropriate courses in chemistry, physiology, and microbiology; in basic, normal nutrition, advanced human nutrition, and nutrition in disease; in principles of learning; in behavioral sciences; in principles of food selection and preparation; and in food service systems management. Highly desirable is undergraduate work in human growth and development and mathematics. Summer experience in the field of public health nutrition and orientation in community and community organization is recommended.

## Training for Maternal and Child Health Service

Continuing concern for the nature of health problems of the mother-infant-child population, plus increases in the numbers of persons to be served, demand more and better trained nutritionists for maternal and child health programs. Specialized needs of mentally retarded and crippled children make added demands. "Increased awareness that the mentally retarded and multihandicapped require specialized comprehensive care has resulted in an increase in the number of clinical mental retardation programs, expansion of state and local maternal and child health and crippled children's services for the mentally retarded, and development of University Affiliated Training Programs to prepare persons in the multidisciplines in the area of mental retardation."[5]

The responsibilities of a nutritionist in maternal and child nutrition are outlined briefly:[5]

Plans and coordinates nutrition components of the comprehensive health and medical care for mothers and children

Provides consultation in maternal and child nutrition to nutrition workers with varying levels of training and to other health professional personnel

Promotes nutrition services in multidisciplinary team work

Participates in multidisciplinary research as needed

The basic requirement for preparation in the area of nutrition in maternal and child health is a master's degree in public health nutrition, as outlined above, with certain specified emphases. Specific and in-depth education in maternal and child health, with particular stress on nutrition during the life span, is essential; clinical training and experience in the health care of mothers and children is desirable. Course work and the experiences related thereto should include the following:

1. Nutrition as it is related to preconception, pregnancy, interconception, infancy, early childhood, and adolescence, including the physical, psychological, and socioeconomic implications throughout the consecutive periods of life

2. The meaning of adequacy and inadequacy of growth and development from conception to maturity in terms of physical, mental, and social progress

3. Special needs of handicapped mothers and children, including their nutritional care as an integral part of diagnosis, prevention, treatment, and rehabilitative measures

4. Public health programs and services for mothers and children, including current concepts of medical care and delivery of health services affecting them, their families, and the communities[5]

The public health nutritionist of today must indeed be a well-qualified person with strong academic training and practical experience. The importance of such a background has long been appreciated, even though the opportunity for its attainment has been possible only in recent years. A half century ago, Lydia J. Roberts pointed out the unique and varied background essential to what was then known as a "social dietitian":

In outlining the training and the personal qualities required to make a successful social dietitian, we have been obliged to draw from the knowledge and technique required for numerous special fields. Directions for producing such a worker might indeed be summed up as follows: Take (a) all the knowledge of nutrition, (b) the special knowledge and experience of the hospital dietitian with diet therapy, (c) the sympathy, understanding and teaching ability of both the primary and high school teacher, (d) the knowledge of human problems, and some of the technique of the social worker, and (e) the knowledge of factors influencing human behavior possessed by the psychologist.[6]

### Priorities in Nutrition Services

Public health nutritionists play multiple roles. It has been suggested that the very variety of their activities tends to diffuse the impact of their contributions. A recent survey of nutrition programs in state health agencies has confirmed this diversity of roles and has brought to focus the need for examining and evaluating the projects involved with a view to establishing priorities. As a result of this analysis of programs, the following four major areas of involvement emerge as the "matrix" within which optimum nutrition programs can evolve at state level.[7] They are offered here in condensed form as functional guidelines:

*Nutritional Surveillance*: To obtain information on nutrition problems unique to the state, which will become the foundation for well-founded nutrition programs based on identified current nutritional needs. Surveillance, as opposed to single surveys, provides continuing or planned periodic study. It may be concerned with such subject areas as dietary patterns of the community, nutritional status of selected population groups, or availability of health and nutrition services. Data collected for other purposes, by different departments of the agency, may supplement, effectively, nutritional surveillance data.

*Nutritional Standards*: To set nutritional standards should be a primary responsibility of the state health agency, including standards of meal content in group facilities under its jurisdiction; professional standards for personnel involved in such facilities; guidelines for nutrition education programs; and standards for evaluating the nutritional status of individuals involved in surveillance. It is doubly important that standards be set and provisions be made to assure their implementation when nonnutritionists are used to extend nutritional care.

*Nutritional Consultation*: To provide assistance in the identification of problems, at the local level, and interpretation of these problems in terms of program needs and assistance in setting up operational programs. (It is conceded that direct patient counseling and usually institution counseling should be performed at the local level.) Consultation should be provided by state units to appropriate state agencies and to government branches with regard to long-range and immediate nutrition needs and program plans for people of the state.

*Applied Nutrition Research*: To design, implement, and evaluate model programs, which, if successful, can be instituted at the local level.

(Chapter 10 of the previous edition of this text [1954] presents a detailed overview of the scope, organization, and procedure patterns of nutrition programs in the 1950s in state and local health departments and in other agencies engaged in nutrition activities at that period.)

## Nutrition Programs Worldwide

At present there is throughout the world a network of agencies, organizations, and activities which deal with phases of nutrition and nutrition education. Each has its own objectives and its own procedures for attaining them. In an effort to furnish a brief overview of the extent and scope of such programs, as they relate to nutrition, certain essential facts have been reduced to capsule form in tables 8.1 through 8.4. Table 8.1 covers domestic programs in the United States which involve nutrition; table 8.2 includes organizations in the United States which largely address themselves to nutrition policy; table 8.3 lists federal agencies which direct nutrition services to needs of developing nations; and table 8.4 describes nutrition activities of United Nations agencies.

The purpose of the tables is merely to give a bird's-eye view of the many nutrition activities carried on here and abroad. Continuous changes in agencies, organizations, and programs make it impossible to assure accuracy of information from day to day and the multiplicity of programs involved makes it impractical to include more than a fraction of them. Nevertheless, the information has served its purpose if it leaves the reader with the concept of a worldwide framework of nutrition planning and performance. Research, as it relates to program planning and implementation, is included, that is, in the collection of nutrient data on foods, in acquiring knowledge of diet practices, and in applying procedures for nutritional surveillance of populations.[8] Practically all of the agencies mentioned have functions beyond the range of nutrition and few confine their nutritional efforts to any one age group. It is assumed that nutrition programs concerned with maternal and family nutrition, as well as those directed primarily to children, are pertinent for consideration here. Emphasis has been placed largely on programs to improve normal nutrition, rather than on those for disease control. Organizational relationships of nutrition programs within agencies have been a secondary consideration.

## Domestic Programs in the United States: Federal, Regional, State, and Local-Level Activities

It is apparent from table 8.1 that several well-known nutrition services originate from two official departments of the federal government: the Department of Health, Education, and Welfare (DHEW) and the U.S. Department of Agriculture (USDA). Within DHEW, most of the agencies listed operate under the U.S. Public Health Service. Within USDA, a variety of nutrition programs function under Food and Nutrition Service; Agricultural Research Service; Economic Research Service; and Extension Service. Other programs at the national level are those supported by food industries, some of which carry on educational activities in nutrition of a general nature rather than focusing on product or brand name promotion. Finally, there are several national service agencies which play a cooperative and supportive role with respect to nutrition. Many agencies function at regional, state, or local levels—in some cases all three. This is true of the Extension Service. Local service organizations, with nutrition components, may be independent or may be connected with a state and/or federal program. The state and local nutrition committees and associations, composed largely of professionals who unite to encourage local nutrition activities and to improve nutritional conditions in the community, are distinctive.

## Agencies, Organizations, and Groups in the United States Concerned with Nutrition Policy

There are many movements in this country which serve in behalf of good nutrition but which do not perform traditional program functions. These include national group movements such as White House Conferences, periodic national nutrition education conferences, and emergency nutrition programs such as the National Nutrition Pro-

**Table 8.1**  Domestic Programs with Nutrition Components—Federal, Regional, State, Local

| Sources | Major Nutrition Program Areas | Characteristic Nutrition Activities |
|---|---|---|
| U.S. Department of Health, Education, and Welfare (DHEW) | **U.S. Public Health Service**<br><br>Maternal and Child Health Service (MCHS)<br><br>Its nutrition program is directed to improvement in nutritional status of mothers and children, including the disadvantaged, mentally retarded, and physically handicapped<br><br>Program direction is toward prevention | MCHS counsels departmental staff and outside agencies, at the planning level, on nutrition programs for mothers and children; emphasis is on preventive measures<br><br>Sponsors studies, symposia, and workshops to increase nutrition knowledge of infancy, childhood, adolescence, pregnancy, and lactation and of effective methods to provide required nutrition services<br><br>Prepares and/or sponsors publications on nutritional care of mothers and children for use by professionals and the lay public<br><br>Strengthens maternal and child health programs nationally by sharing findings of research in subject areas and in educational method with nutritionists in state and local health departments |
| | National Institutes of Health (NIH)<br><br>Areas involving child nutrition are served by various of the institutes, more specifically, through its National Institute of Child Health and Human Development (NICHD) | NICHD conducts and supports biomedical and behavioral research in areas that include maternal and child nutrition, and research on problems of human development with special reference to mental retardation<br><br>Findings are disseminated to professionals and the public to improve the health of children and their families |
| | Food and Drug Administration (FDA)<br><br>Activities are directed toward protecting the health of the nation against impure and unsafe products | The Bureau of Foods of FDA conducts research and develops standards for composition, quality, nutritive content, and safety of foods, food additives, and colors |

| | |
|---|---|
| In the Bureau of Foods are concentrated programs related to foods and nutrition | It coordinates and evaluates FDA's surveillance and compliance programs relating to foods |
| | FDA has instituted a program for nutrition labeling of packaged and canned foods to inform consumers of the nutrient content of items purchased |
| National Center for Health Statistics (NCHS) | Collects clinical, biochemical, and dietary data on a probability sample of U.S. population, 6 to 74 years of age, of varied incomes |
| Health and Nutrition Examination Survey (HANES) | Data collected in time cycles to provide a national surveillance system for measuring nutritional status and monitoring change, over time |
| *Purpose:* to measure periodically the prevalence of certain health and nutrition conditions | Growth charts, with reference percentiles for boys and girls, 2 to 18 years of age, prepared by NCHS and CDC |
| Center for Disease Control (CDC) | Assists certain states to gather, compile, and analyze growth and biochemical data on children from low income homes |
| Survey activities carried on through CDC's *Nutrition Activities* as a phase of *Preventable Disease* | Analyzes data provided by several other states on growth, obesity, and anemia of children |
| *Purpose:* to identify specific high-risk population groups | Does laboratory work of HANES |
| Indian Health Services (IHS) | Provides educational programs, conducted by professionals, in nutrition/dietetics, to improve the food patterns and nutriture of adults and children on the reservations |
| Nutrition service is an important aspect of total health services on Indian reservations | Offers consultation for mothers of infants and young children; distributes foods under the WIC program (see USDA below) |

**Table 8.1** (*Cont.*)

| Sources | Major Nutrition Program Areas | Characteristic Nutrition Activities |
|---|---|---|
| | Education Division U.S. Office of Education (OE) | Counsels state and local nutrition educators through divisions of health education at the state level |
| | In respect to nutrition and related subjects, OE largely functions through state departments of education | Provides guidance for home economics educators of the states through vocational home economics supervisors |
| U.S. Department of Agriculture (USDA) | Food and Nutrition Service (FNS) Nutrition and technical services | Reviews the technical and nutritional aspects of USDA food and nutrition programs; makes recommendations to the secretary of agriculture |
| | Special meal programs for school and preschool children | Administers child nutrition programs with state and local cooperation: National School Lunch and School Breakfast programs; child care and summer food service programs; and the Special Milk program |
| | Commodity allocation | Makes available supplemental foods to pregnant and lactating women, infants, and children up to age 5 (WIC Program); provides foods through cooperating state and local agencies to Child Nutrition Programs |
| | Food stamp program | Provides needy persons and families, through state and local welfare agencies, with food coupons to increase their food-purchasing power |
| | Nutrition education | Aids school nutrition education programs: develops plans and teaching tools; provides for in-service nutrition education of classroom teachers and school lunch personnel |

## Extension Service (ES)

ES is an educational arm of USDA. Nutrition programs were originally directed primarily to rural families; now they are extended to cities, towns, and suburbs as well

Federal nutrition specialists in ES explore, plan, and develop educational programs and create nutrition education tools

Assist professional ES staffs at state and county levels to adapt nutrition research findings and implement program plans

Utilize ES's *Expanded Food and Nutrition Education Program* (EFNEP) to teach low income homemakers how to feed their families more nutritious meals—instruction by paid aides, trained for the job but not professionally educated in nutrition

## Agricultural Research Service (ARS)

Human nutrition research in ARS is concerned with optimum nutritive requirements for healthy individuals, nutrient composition of foods, nutrient intake and food habits of the U.S. population

Certain activities are carried on by regional staffs with different specialties

*Nutrition Institute:* Covers a broad spectrum of basic research on nutrient values and human requirements; disseminates findings to other federal agencies and educators and interprets them to consumers

*Consumer and Food Economics Institute:* Maintains the Nutrient Data Research Center (NDRC); studies family food intakes; appraises food practices; publishes materials, including *Nutritive Value of American Foods, in Common Units,* handbook 456; *Household Food Consumption Data;* food guides, food cost plans for households at different economic levels; and *Nutrition Program News*

*Human Nutrition Laboratory* (N. Cent. Region): Conducts basic research on nutrients (for example, trace minerals) to establish incidence, functions, requirements, and boundaries for use

*Experiment Stations:* State Experiment Stations at land grant colleges conduct applied human nutrition research, frequently related to local problems; studies include nutritive intakes and food patterns of different age groups of children

**Table 8.1** (*Cont.*)

| Sources | Major Nutrition Program Areas | Characteristic Nutrition Activities |
|---|---|---|
| | Economic Research Service (ERS) | Publishes such periodicals as *Food Situation* and *Food-Consumption, Prices, Expenditures* which provide basic data for program planning |
| | As one aspect of a broad economic research program on use of agricultural resources, ERS investigates trends and relationships between food prices and family income and food consumption practices | |
| National industry-supported organizations representing basic foods | American Butter Institute<br>American Dry Milk Institute<br>American Egg Board<br>American Institute of Baking<br>Cereal Institute<br>Evaporated Milk Association<br>National Cheese Institute<br>National Dairy Council<br>National Live Stock and Meat Board<br>Nutrition Foundation<br>Potato Board<br>Wheat Flour Institute | Provide information on processing, distribution patterns, and nutritive values of foods represented (some organizations confine their activities to these services)<br><br>Offer program plans and consultation services, by professional staff, in nutrition education<br><br>Provide instructional materials for nutrition education programs<br><br>Sponsor nutrition research, symposia, and conferences to further nutrition knowledge and its application |

| | |
|---|---|
| National Health Service Organizations which include certain nutrition services | |
| American Heart Association | Offers printed dietary recommendations and nutrition advice for prevention of heart disease |
| American Red Cross | Maintains nutrition consultant at national headquarters; provides disaster feeding services |
| The National Foundation—March of Dimes | Cooperates with medical organizations in urging the need for nutritionists in the management of pregnancy and the newborn |
| American Lung Association | Integrates nutrition education in its programs for improved general health |

(These organizations also function at local levels)

| | |
|---|---|
| State and local agencies with nutrition components | |
| State departments of education | Provide consultation in nutrition education and consumer and home economics education for the state's school systems |
| Health education divisions of state agencies provide nutrition advisory services for school personnel of the state | State education agency manages the distribution of money and commodities to schools of the state participating in the National School Lunch program |
| Some states have nutrition educators who perform this service | |
| State departments of health | Conduct surveys to identify the state's nutrition problems, as bases for program planning |
| Programs conducted by nutrition-trained personnel vary widely depending on organization of the department, emphasis placed on nutrition, size of staff | Establish standards for group nutritional care and food service guidelines, for the state |
| Types of activities often carried on are listed | Consult with local health agencies on cooperative nutrition activities |
| | Advise administrators and other agencies of the state of the nutrition needs of the people |

**Table 8.1** (*Cont.*)

| Sources | Major Nutrition Program Areas | Characteristic Nutrition Activities |
|---|---|---|
| | Local health agencies | |
| | City, county health departments; neighborhood health centers | |
| | Maternal, child clinics | Provide direct consultation on nutrition problems of mothers, infants, children; prenatal classes, group consultation; dietary counseling on meal-planning problems, considering ethnic food patterns, ages, and income |
| | Neighborhood health centers | |
| | Institution services | Child day care: Uphold nutritional standards and meal guidelines established by licensing organization or other designated group |
| | Staff consultation | Furnish nutrition information and counsel to health educators, social workers, staff nurses, others |
| | Visiting Nurse Association | Provide indirect nutrition counseling for staff nurses who advise mothers. |
| | Infant Welfare Society | |
| | Hospital, maternal-child clinics | Provide direct and/or indirect nutrition counseling for mothers |
| | State and local nutrition committees—professional nutritionist organizations | Dispense accurate, pertinent nutrition information to the community; take leadership role in behalf of sound dietary practices in area |

gram, World War II. There are also organizations (table 8.2) largely composed of professionals trained in the science of nutrition, whose overall purpose is to work toward sound nutrition policy for the United States. These organizations have different origins and they function differently, but they have certain common objectives: they seek to obtain coordinated action on the part of responsible nutrition science authorities and guide the application of food and nutrition knowledge for the public good.

Such organizations include the Food and Nutrition Board of the National Academy of Sciences–National Research Council, the U.S. Senate Select Committee on Nutrition and Human Needs, the National Nutrition Consortium, and the private scientific organizations which are represented in the Consortium and/or support its program. Also, the universities, colleges, teacher-education institutions, teaching hospitals, and professional schools might well be added. In their position of educational leadership they are potentially the largest single influence for nutritional improvement. Private foundations, with their encouragement of research and support of higher education in health, nutrition, and medicine, contribute substantially to a closer understanding and enunciation of nutrition policy.

## U.S. Agencies Functioning Internationally

The United States has cooperated with other nations in helping to raise the level of nutrition and health throughout the world. It seems suitable to review, briefly, some of the major organized efforts directed to that end. While programs have usually been aimed toward total populations, children, as vulnerable members of those populations, have received major consideration. Agencies serving international nutrition needs are essentially of four types: those official agencies of the U.S. government which have certain overseas commitments; the specialized United Nations agencies devoted entirely to international programs; foundations and other privately supported organizations largely engaged in research to further the aims of the planned programs; and the variety of service organizations which include improved nutrition among their objectives.

## International Nutrition Programs Developed by the Agencies of the U.S. Federal Government

Three departments of the federal government of the United States are the chief contributors to nutrition phases of international programs:

**Table 8.2**  Agencies, Organizations, and Groups in the United States which Function in Making Nutrition Policy

| Agencies, Organizations, Groups | Representative Groups and Functions | Characteristic Nutrition Contributions |
|---|---|---|
| General objectives: | | |
| Policy-making Advisory | Food and Nutrition Board, National Academy of Sciences–National Research Council | Develops and publishes at five-year intervals the *Recommended Dietary Allowances* (**RDA**) for U.S. citizens |
| | The Board serves as a national advisory body in the field of food and nutrition. It recommends nutrition research and helps interpret nutritional science in the interest of public welfare. | Proposes policies for the development of new foods and the nutrient fortification of conventional foods |
| | | Establishes principles and procedures for the evaluation of safety of foods. |
| | | Outlines specifications of identity and purity of food chemicals |
| Legislative | Select Committee on Nutrition and Human Needs, U.S. Senate* | Proposed legislation to coordinate and concentrate responsibilities for government nutrition activities (chapter 9) |
| | A committee of the U.S. Senate which seeks to upgrade nutrition in the United States, largely through improvement of governmental processes which relate thereto | Endorsed and promoted the guidelines for a National Nutrition Policy developed by the National Nutrition Consortium |
| | | Collected and made available to health and nutrition professionals pertinent printed information on nutrition research and nutrition programs |
| | | Formulated and issued dietary goals for the United States |

| | | |
|---|---|---|
| | National Nutrition Consortium | Prepared guidelines for the development of a National Nutrition Policy |
| | A committee of representatives of professional organizations whose major purpose is to help develop and implement national nutrition policy in the United States | Sponsored the development of guidelines for nutrition labeling |
| | | Urged that paid nutritional services be included in regulations for health maintenance organizations |
| | | Assisted in the review and revision of the proposed rule-making of the Federal Trade Commission, as related to nutrition advertising |
| Private professional organizations | Scientific groups supportive of sound nutrition policy in areas of their special concern | |
| | American Institute of Nutrition | Professional society of experimental nutrition scientists: members encourage, engage in, and coordinate nutrition research |
| | American Society for Clinical Nutrition | Physicians and research scientists engage in teaching, research, and information exchange, in human nutrition |
| | American Dietetic Association | Professional organization of nutritionists and dietitians; advances the science of dietetics and nutrition; promotes education in these fields |
| | Institute of Food Technologists (functions in nutrition through its Expert Panel on Food Safety and Nutrition) | Professional society of technical personnel, promotes application of science and engineering in the production, processing, packaging, distribution, preparation, and utilization of foods |
| | Society for Nutrition Education | Society of nutrition educators which promotes better nutrition with programs to improve nutrition education through research, education, and communication |

**Table 8.2** (*Cont.*)

| Agencies, Organizations, Groups | Representative Groups and Functions | Characteristic Nutrition Contributions |
|---|---|---|
| | American School Food Service Association | Organization of persons engaged in food service to schools and colleges; dedicated to improving the nutritional background of personnel and the serving of nutritionally adequate and acceptable school meals |
| | American Academy of Pediatrics (functions through its Committee on Nutrition) | Society of physicians, for treatment of children; issues policy statements for members and other professionals on nutrition issues |
| | American Public Health Association | Association of professional workers from many fields brought together by a common interest in public health |
| | American Home Economics Association | Professional organization seeks to improve the quality and standards of individual and family life, including nutrition, through research, education, and cooperative programs |
| | American Nurses Association | Nationwide association of nurses concerned with the professional advancement of its members; orientation in nutrition is a phase of their program both in training and in-service, through convention programs and periodicals |

*Reorganization of the U.S. Senate committee structure calls for the transfer of Select Committee duties to a standing subcommittee on agriculture, nutrition, and forestry and to other specified senate committees. The U.S. House of Representatives' agriculture subcommittee on domestic marketing, consumer relations, and nutrition conducts similar programs with respect to nutrition.

the Departments of State; of Health, Education, and Welfare; and of Agriculture. Table 8.3 provides a brief overview of the types of services rendered by each department. The text and table 8.3 also point out the many ways in which each agency cooperates with others in the U.S. government and with the international agencies serving the same populations abroad.

*Department of State:*
*Agency for International Development*

The Agency for International Development (AID) had an unusual beginning in 1949. In Point 4 of his inaugural address that year, the president of the United States appealed to the American people to "embark on a bold new program to make benefits of scientific advances and industrial progress available for the improvement and growth of underdeveloped areas." He outlined the need as falling roughly into two categories: "Technical, to improve food production, health, education and productive skills; and financial, to develop transportation, water control and power, and productive industries."

Eighteen months later the Congress passed the Act for International Development which established what came to be known as the Point 4 Program, as a new phase of U.S. foreign policy. Soon thereafter the program took the name of the act and eventually became known as AID. The basic act, with amendments, was continued in the Mutual Security Act of 10 October 1951. These acts declared it to be the policy of the United States to aid the peoples of underprivileged areas to help their economies and themselves by the exchange of technical knowledge and skills, as a means of raising the standards of productivity and living.

The implications for good nutrition of utilizing technical assistance in agriculture alone are obvious. Most of the people in the world are farmers and more food is the first need in many countries. Much of AID's work, therefore, has been in agriculture. The overall objective of the agricultural program has been to achieve a better-nourished people and thus to build stamina and health toward stronger nations. The program has simply offered a means of self-help. It has made skills available, but the transfer, adaptation, and practical application of those skills has rested largely with the people themselves. Training has been provided in two ways: (1) "on-the-job" training, whereby trainees have been hired in their own countries and assigned to work with technicians sent there from the United States, and (2) advanced training, given to technicians who could benefit by studying in the United States.

**Table 8.3** International Nutrition Programs Conducted by Agencies of the U.S. Federal Government

| U.S. Agencies | Program Areas | Representative Nutrition Services for Developing Countries |
|---|---|---|
| Agency for International Development (AID) | Nutrition programs of the State Department originate in the Office of Nutrition of AID | Develops patterns of procedure for planning nutrition education programs where needed |
| U.S. Department of State | Act for International Development, 1951, declared it to be the policy of the United States to aid peoples of the developing areas by the exchange of technical knowledge and skills as a means of raising their standards of productivity and living | Evaluates nutrition programs and has developed a field guide to measure the effectiveness of nutrition education techniques[9] |
| | | Conducts investigations, conferences, workshops, tests, and assembles data to determine directions for programs in such areas as breast feeding, nutrient fortification of staple cereals, and vitamin A deficiency problems[10] |
| | Foreign Assistance Act of 1961 laid the ground work for establishing AID as an agency in the Department of State | Urges use of growth charts, as part of a parent-involved program, to detect early signs of malnutrition in children |
| U.S. Department of Health, Education, and Welfare (DHEW) | International nutrition programs of DHEW arise largely in National Institutes of Health (NIH) and Maternal and Child Health Service (MCHS) | NIH sponsors, through INCAP, a major long-term research study in Guatemala. Purpose: to clarify relationships between malnutrition and intellectual development. Subjects: pregnant mothers and their offspring |
| | NIH engages in nutrition research abroad chiefly through other agencies, such as the Institute of Central America and Panama (INCAP) | NIH also sponsors research elsewhere abroad in such areas as anemia, vitamin A deficiency, and calcium metabolism in certain bone diseases |
| | MCHS acts in the capacity of nutrition consultant to AID, a service implemented | MCHS cooperates with AID to sponsor program-planning conferences to implement nutrition activities, including the growth charts, and to publish nutrition education materials[11] |

through a cooperative arrangement by sharing staff

| | | |
|---|---|---|
| U.S. Department of Agriculture (USDA) | International services for human nutrition arise in various areas of USDA, among them: Agricultural Research Service (ARS) through regional and state experiment stations | ARS provides research data and practical procedures for increasing crop yields and breeds certain cereal grains for higher protein content. Findings can contribute to a food supply higher in quantity and quality in developing countries. |
| | Economic Research Service (ERA) | ERS focuses on worldwide food supply and demand conditions; provides direct assistance and coordinates USDA's overall program to aid agricultural development in low income countries; furnishes AID with such technical services as evaluating its nutrition programs; directs field tests for acceptance of newly developed foods |

Nutrition education activities go hand in hand with the agricultural programs. Representative areas of nutrition education and services provided by AID are outlined briefly in table 8.3. Strengths of AID programs are enhanced by effective cooperation with agencies in their own government, with the UN specialized agencies, and with a host of agricultural and other agencies of international origin or emanating from individual developing nations.

### Department of Health, Education, and Welfare

DHEW participates in international nutrition programs largely through its Institutes of Health (NIH) and its Maternal and Child Health Services (MCHS) (table 8.3). NIH activities are chiefly of a research nature. MCHS activities are consultative and advisory in character. The major service of MCHS is to AID, but it also consults on nutrition problems with other overseas agencies when mothers and children are involved.

### Department of Agriculture

USDA functions in international nutrition programs through many avenues, chiefly under two main divisions: Agricultural Research Service (ARS) and Economic Research Service (ERS). ARS supplies basic information and data from its research laboratories and ERS renders technical assistance in the field of agriculture to AID and other agencies in practically all phases of their programs which relate to food production (table 8.3).

### Agencies of the United Nations (UN)

The specialized agencies concerned with nutrition are shown in table 8.4. While each agency has its own goals, together the agencies join in planning for better use of resources in an effort to bring about higher standards of living.

### United Nations International Children's Fund (UNICEF)

UNICEF was created by the General Assembly of the United Nations in December 1946. It was established primarily to meet the emergency needs of children particularly in war-devastated countries. By vote of the General Assembly in 1950 it was continued for a

**Table 8.4**    Agencies of the United Nations: International Programs Involving Nutrition*

| UN Agencies | Origin and Development | Nutritional Objectives | Nature of Nutrition Programs |
|---|---|---|---|
| United Nations International Children's Fund (UNICEF) | 1946, UNICEF was created by the General Assembly of the UN, to meet emergency health needs of children | To improve the quality of life for needy mothers and children throughout the world (80% of the budget now assigned to permanent programs) | Works with other agencies and with local governments to monitor the nutriture of populations, especially the children |
| | 1953, it was accorded permanent status as a UN agency | To provide food as well as nutritional services when disaster strikes | Aids local nutrition programs with UNICEF personnel, administrative direction, and equipment and supplies needed for child-care centers and health clinics |
| | It is the only agency concerned solely with the welfare of mothers and children | To pursue objectives of the country assisted, not of UNICEF; local governments must request aid and suggest projects *they* think are important | Trains local personnel to work with mothers, children, and families; fosters community gardens and school feeding programs |
| | UNICEF is supported by voluntary contributions of governments, groups, and individuals; local governments served provide matching funds | To prepare governments to take over and continue programs when UNICEF withdraws | |
| United Nations Educational, Scientific, and Cultural Organization (UNESCO) | 1946, UNESCO was launched when twenty countries had signed its constitution | Overall: to wipe out illiteracy as a first step in raising the standard of living throughout the world | Establishes educational centers: trainees at centers are school teachers from countries served by UNESCO; teachers are taught how to apply improved methods in their own countries |
| | It is an independent body with its own membership and budget; it receives from the UN appropriations for technical assistance activities | To help people everywhere acquire an understanding about the world's food and ways they can help make it available to all | Teaches reading; reading is taught in connection with food, |

**Table 8.4** (*Cont.*)

| UN Agencies | Origin and Development | Nutritional Objectives | Nature of Nutrition Programs |
|---|---|---|---|
| | | | homemaking, and agriculture to provide knowledge for improved community life |
| | | | UNESCO programs are conducted in cooperation with other UN agencies and with various organizations; there is an international exchange of personnel |
| United Nations Food and Agriculture Organization (FAO) | 1945, first session convened in Quebec<br><br>Secretariat includes five technical divisions: agriculture, economics, fisheries, forestry, and nutrition<br><br>Three organizations which are outgrowths of FAO: 1963—Freedom From Hunger Campaign (FFHC); 1964—Young World Appeal (YWA); 1968—Young World Development (YWD) | Overall: to raise the nutritional level of the people in developing countries; infants, children, adolescents, and expectant and nursing mothers receive special consideration<br><br>To deal with nutrition in relation to production, distribution, and consumption of food<br><br>To work with health, nutrition, agricultural specialists in the countries being served, to bring to each country specific needed help<br><br>To strive for increased food | Nutrition programs with local governments<br><br>Technical assistance to establish projects: materials, supplies, equipment, experts to aid<br><br>Research to develop and exploit high nutrient, high-yield grains<br><br>Educational activities to improve nutrient intakes: supplementary feeding programs for mothers and young children; school feeding; home food management<br><br>Training and educational programs for local personnel: on-the-job |

| | | | |
|---|---|---|---|
| | | production, better management, improved training of leaders | training, travel-study grants, regional institutes |
| World Health Organization (WHO) | 1948, WHO launched at International Health Conference in New York<br><br>WHO recognizes nutrition as an essential element in concept of health; a nutrition section was established early<br><br>1949, a Joint Committee on Nutrition with FAO was organized<br><br>Pan American Health Organization (PAHO) is the regional office of WHO for governments of the Western Hemisphere | Overall: to achieve positive health, not merely combat disease<br><br>To assist member nations to assess their own health and nutrition needs, to plan nutrition services, to implement programs to meet needs<br><br>To direct programs toward improved general health and the prevention and elimination of dietary deficiency diseases | Conduct surveys in member countries to determine levels of health, extent of nutritional deficiencies<br><br>Provide educational training in nutrition for medical, public health and paraprofessional personnel serving mothers and children<br><br>Sponsor and conduct research to assess the nature of nutritional deficiencies<br><br>Center program efforts on nutritional anemias, endemic goiter, protein-calorie malnutrition, xerophthalmia |

*Publications from agencies described in table 8.4 are available as follows: UNICEF: 331 East 38th St., New York, N.Y. 10016; UNESCO and FAO: UNIPUB Inc., Box 443, New York, N.Y. 10016; WHO: Geneva, Switzerland.

three-year period, with a view to making it a permanent organization. The General Assembly provided for the support of UNICEF by voluntary contributions of governments and individuals. In 1953 it voted to continue UNICEF indefinitely.

UNICEF has been referred to as an "international cooperative" on behalf of children. It has received contributions from those countries able to help with money and goods, and has distributed that aid to countries whose needs could not be met from their own resources. The UNICEF executive board acts upon requests from governments for international aid.

Although emergencies arise constantly which call for special feeding projects, most of the fund's aid today goes to help countries deal with long-standing maternal and child welfare programs. All aid is given in close collaboration with other UN agencies, notably FAO and WHO. Aid is of the following types: (1) Assistance for the building and expansion of basic child welfare services, including supplies for clinics. It also helps to train local child-care personnel by equipping training centers and furnishing the services of experts. (2) Provision of milk and other needed foods to assist supplementary child-feeding programs and in many cases, equipment and basic supplies for making the food available on a continuing basis. The governments of the assisted countries agree to participate and carry on as UNICEF withdraws its support. The more specific objectives and activities of UNICEF are outlined in table 8.4.

### United Nations Educational, Scientific, and Cultural Organization (UNESCO)

UNESCO, another of the specialized United Nations agencies concerned in some measure with nutrition, came into existence officially on 4 November 1946, when twenty countries signed its constitution. The purpose of UNESCO, as stated in Article 1 of its constitution, is to contribute to peace and security by promoting collaboration among the nations of the world through education, science, and culture. A primary goal of this agency is to wipe out illiteracy as a first step in raising the standard of living throughout the world. UNESCO's function, with respect to nutrition, is to help people everywhere acquire an understanding and philosophy about the world's foods and ways in which they can help to make it available to all (table 8.4).

UNESCO has headquarters in Paris. It operates through a conference, an executive board, a director general, and its secretariat.

To carry out its world program, UNESCO works with other specialized agencies of UN and with international, nongovernmental organizations. A national cooperating body is set up in each member country. It serves as a link between UNESCO and the other bodies or individuals concerned with education, science, and culture in each country.

### Food and Agriculture Organization (FAO)

Of the specialized agencies concerned with nutrition, the Food and Agriculture Organization (FAO) was the first of the permanent UN agencies to come into existence after World War II. Its broad purpose was to improve the nutritional status of the disadvantaged people of the world.

The first steps in the formation of FAO were taken when the United Nations' Conference on Food and Agriculture was convened at Hot Springs, Virginia, in May 1943. Forty-four nations were invited to send representatives to the conference, which recommended the formation of the United Nations Interim Commission on Food and Agriculture. The commission was set up in Washington, D.C., in July 1943, to make plans for a permanent international organization. It drafted a constitution and a report on suggested structure and functions of FAO. When more than twenty governments had indicated acceptance of the proposed constitution, the first session of FAO was convened in Quebec in October 1945. Forty-two nations became charter members. By 1975 there were 136 member countries.

The history of FAO is rooted in two international organizations no longer existent: the League of Nations and the International Institute of Agriculture. Nutrition was added to the small Health Section of the League of Nations in 1930. As the economic depression of the 1930s was felt around the world, the League Assembly sought to find in nutrition the solution to a situation which created food surpluses in one part of the world and hunger in others. It was at an assembly of the League that Lord Bruce of Australia coined the now famous phrase that called for "the marriage of health and agriculture."

Various nutrition commissions were established by the League. One of these examined human requirements for calories and nutrients and issued a report which was a landmark on the subject. National nutrition committees were set up in a number of countries, with the responsibility of advising governments on the steps needed to improve the nutrition of their peoples. World War II halted these activities but the work of the League helped to make governments aware of the importance of good nutrition safeguarding the health of their populations. And it is not unlikely that the League experience helped the nations to grasp the importance of FAO when it was proposed shortly thereafter.

FAO has been called "a child of the science of nutrition."[12] Nutrition functions through the Food Policy and Nutrition Division, which is part of the Economic and Social Policy Department of FAO. A major role of the Division is to integrate nutritional objectives into the more general activities of FAO, with respect to production and trade in foods. The work of the Division is carried out by three services: Food Standards and Food Sciences, Food and Nutrition Development Strategy, and Nutrition Policy and Programs. The Director General of FAO said recently: "Insofar as the problem of world hunger is basically an economic problem, nutrition must be regarded as an integral part of the framework of economic planning . . . production plans must increasingly be geared to nutritional requirements."[13]

The nutrition activities of FAO are described fully in publications available from FAO headquarters in Rome, and from regional offices located on the different continents. The overall objectives and general nature of nutrition programs are outlined briefly in table 8.4. Information on its auxiliary organizations is also available from FAO. The auxiliary organizations include *The Freedom from Hunger Campaign*, which seeks to create a better understanding of world hunger and ways to approach solutions; *Young World Development*, a youth organization of the American Freedom-from-Hunger Foundation; and *Young World Appeal*, whose purpose is to involve young people throughout the world in supporting programs to eliminate hunger.

### World Health Organization (WHO)

Of the specialized agencies concerned with nutrition, WHO was the last of the permanent UN agencies to come into existence (1948). Its objectives with respect to nutrition are broad. It has functioned particularly in helping health departments in member countries to develop nutritional services and in showing practical ways to conquer widespread dietary deficiency diseases.

WHO was empowered by its constitution to act as the directing and coordinating authority on international health work. It had its origin in an International Health Conference which was called in

New York in June 1946. WHO come into being officially on 7 April 1948, when twenty-six members of the UN had accepted the constitution drafted at the 1946 meeting. By 1975, WHO had a total membership of 131 countries in all parts of the world.

While WHO has cooperated closely with sister agencies of the UN, it has its own constitution—referred to as the "Magna Carta of Health"—and its own governing bodies, the latter being the World Health Assembly and the executive board. The overall program of WHO's operational services covers three broad fronts: (1) organization of public health services; (2) campaigns against communicable and nutritional deficiency diseases; and (3) general promotion of health. The emphasis in all WHO's work has been, as its constitution specifies, on achieving positive health and not merely on combating disease.

The nature of WHO's nutrition activities and their objectives are summarized briefly in table 8.4. Comprehensive accounts of such activities are available in printed literature from WHO headquarters in Geneva or its regional offices. (The regional office of WHO in the Western Hemisphere is the Pan American Health Organization [PAHO] located in Washington, D.C. It serves the governments of Latin America particularly.) WHO, alone, makes a unique contribution to the improvement of nutrition and health in developing countries and, in cooperation with other UN agencies, helps to create conditions which make nutritional progress possible.

### Cooperation between United Nations Agencies

Cooperative nutrition programs and activities between UN agencies have been emphasized here as essential to the total international efforts. A prime example of such cooperation is the long-established FAO-WHO Expert Committee on Nutrition. A major product has been the adoption of realistic dietary standards for populations of the developing countries of the world. Other projects have dealt with the identification and treatment of nutritional deficiency diseases in those countries. Such joint programs have served to strengthen the programs of each organization and to avoid duplication of effort. In general, FAO programs have dealt with nutrition in relation to the production, distribution, and consumption of food, while WHO has considered nutrition in relation to the maintenance of health and prevention of disease. The Joint Committee on Nutrition reviews the programs of both agencies at its periodic meetings and studies new problems of joint concern.

Foundations and Other Cooperating Organizations

"If human nutrition is meaningful, it can only be so when based solely on an efficient agricultural industry." This statement was made in 1975 by President Emeritus Harrar of the Rockefeller Foundation.[14] He added that conventional agriculture "is still the principal hope for an improving world economy and universally improved human nutrition." These statements might be regarded as principles upon which the far-flung research projects of the privately supported research programs of the Rockefeller and Ford foundations are based, as they relate to world food and nutrition problems. These foundations early recognized that greater quantities of food were required, as well as a food supply higher in nutritive content if people of developing nations were to survive.

The records of the agricultural-nutrition research programs of the Ford and Rockefeller foundations are impressive ones. Their findings, which have resulted in dramatically increased yields of wheat and rice from hybrid strains, are known around the world.[15] But their greatest gains were made when they acted jointly with other agencies and local governments. Together, the two foundations took responsibility for establishing the International Rice Research Institute in the Philippines. They have also contributed to the development of hybrid varieties of corn with increased amounts of certain amino acids; to the crossing of grains such as wheat and rye to increase protein and provide a rugged strain; to improving varieties of sorghum grains and various legumes which can be grown under adverse weather conditions. These are token evidences of the contributions toward better-fed nations.

In 1971 a Consultative Group on International Agricultural Research (CGIAR) took responsibility for long-term basic plans for improved agriculture designed to bring continuing benefits to many parts of the world. Eight international centers for tropical agriculture are now functioning in Colombia, Nigeria, the Philippines, Mexico, India, Peru, Kenya, and Ethiopia.[16] The CGIAR is a group of donor countries, development banks, foundations, and agencies which have agreed to provide funds for international agricultural research. The centers and institutes are autonomous but they work together closely, sharing plans, procedures, and results. Each has a program largely dealing with tropical agriculture, emphasizing the nutritional needs of areas served. Scientists from developing countries advise, teach, and assist. A major objective is to involve and train local or visiting students, with arrangements made for advanced education outside the country, when indicated.

Characteristic of the overall plan is its cooperative nature, its concept of continuity in education and service, and its recognition and application to current agricultural and nutritional problems. Cooperation is exemplified in one of the eight centers—the International Institute of Tropical Agriculture (IITA), in Ibodan, Nigeria. Its research is performed by a team of agricultural scientists; its support is provided by AID along with the Ford and Rockefeller foundations, the Canadian International Development Agency, the Overseas Development Ministry of the United Kingdom, the International Bank for Reconstruction and Development, the UN Environment Program, and the governments of Nigeria, West Germany, Belgium, the Netherlands, and Iran. Nigeria contributed the 2,500 acres of land for the facility.[17]

## Voluntary Service Organizations

Privately supported organizations which render types of nutrition services in developing countries are chiefly of two origins: (1) denominational church organizations, such as Catholic Charities, American Friends' Service Committee, and Lutheran World Relief, which have foreign service commitments and (2) community-supported groups such as CARE, World Education, Save the Children Foundation, International Red Cross, and Salvation Army.

Traditional U.S. voluntary organizations in foreign service have participated in nutrition programs chiefly by helping distribute government-donated foods, by aiding refugees, and by dispensing disaster relief. Such cooperation continues as needed but gradually voluntary agencies have enlarged their scope. U.S. legislative action has extended the ways in which food relief may be utilized and has made it possible to expand voluntary services.[18]

AID has an active cooperative program with voluntary agencies. Its formal contacts with the agencies are through the Office of Private and Voluntary Cooperation of the Bureau of Population and Humanitarian Assistance. There has been a new and increasing emphasis among voluntary agencies on development assistance, which includes practical programs, such as organizing child-care centers at community level and conducting research and training activities. To encourage such development programs, AID establishes two new types of grants which may be used by voluntary agencies to sustain long-term programs and expand staff.

## References

1   Select Committee on Nutrition and Human Needs of the U.S. Senate. *Nutrition and Health II: Nutrition and Health Revised with a Study of the Impact of Nutritional Health Considerations on Food Policy.* Washington, D.C.: U.S. Government Printing Office, 1976.

2   "Educational Qualifications of Nutritionists in Health Agencies." *American Journal of Public Health* 36(1946):45–50.

3   Robb, E. "Suggested Objectives for the Graduate Preparation of Nutritionists for the Public Health Field." *Journal of the American Dietetic Association* 26(1950):269–74.

4   "Educational Qualifications of Nutritionists in Health Agencies." *American Journal of Public Health* 52(1962):116–21.

5   Steering Committee on Roles, Qualifications, and Training of Nutrition Workers in Health Agencies. *Personnel in Public Health Nutrition.* Chicago: American Dietetic Association, 1976.

6   Roberts, L. J. "The Dietitian in Social Service." *Journal of the American Dietetic Association* 5(1930):286–94.

7   Nichaman, M. Z. "Nutrition Programs in State Health Agencies." *Nutrition Reviews* 32(1974):65–67.

8   Select Committee on Nutrition and Human Needs of the U.S. Senate. *The Role of the Federal Government in Human Nutrition Research.* Washington, D.C.: U.S. Government Printing Office, 1976.

9   *A Field Guide for Evaluation of Nutrition Education.* Washington, D.C.: Office of Nutrition, Technical Assistance Bureau, Agency for International Development, U.S. Department of State, 1975.

10  *Vitamin A Xerophthalmia and Blindness*, vols. 1–3. Washington, D.C.: Office of Nutrition, Technical Assistance Bureau, Agency for International Development, U.S. Department of State, 1973.

11  *Nutrition Education in Child Feeding Programs in Developing Countries.* Washington, D.C.: Office of Nutrition, Technical Assistance Bureau, Agency for International Development, U.S. Department of State, 1974.

12  Aykroyd, W. R. "FAO." *Nutrition Abstracts and Reviews* 23(1953): 229–43.

13  Boerma, A. H. "The Thirty Years War against Hunger." *Food and Nutrition (FAO)* 1(1975):3–7.

14  Harrar, J. G. *Nutrition and Numbers in the Third World.* Washington, D.C.: Agricultural Research Service, U.S. Department of Agriculture, 1975.

15   Annual and special reports of the Ford and Rockefeller foundations.

16   Rhoad, D. L. "Of Seed and Man: I." *War on Hunger* 10(1976):1–5.

17   Shuler, A. "Of Seed and Man: II." *War on Hunger* 10(1976):1–4, 11–13.

18   Snead, B. "The Voluntary Role of Foreign Aid." *War on Hunger* 10 (1976):5–9.

# Chapter Nine

## School Nutrition Programs

### Needs, Procedures, Personnel

Thus far the text has largely considered the science of nutrition as it relates to child development. The importance of nutrition education in this process has been implied throughout. The two ensuing chapters will deal more specifically with basic understandings of nutrition education and explore ways of applying them, primarily to structured situations as found in schools. The responsibilities of nutritionists in this area vary greatly with circumstances. They may initiate programs, assume leadership for them, or merely cooperate actively with others as the occasion demands. The special province of nutritionists in all cases is to provide sound nutrition information and to guide and consult in the interpretation of such information, within the context of the educational activity.

The meaning of the term *nutrition education* has in the main been taken for granted. Recently individuals and organizations have sought to analyze and define it in terms of its objectives. One definition describes nutrition education succinctly as the development of an understanding capable of producing intelligent decisions and actions. Thus, it is the meaningful interpretation of knowledge, not merely the acquisition of information. Bosley offers a more comprehensive definition which embraces several elements proposed also by others:

Education in nutrition is founded on the philosophy that nutrition is a major component in the quality of well-being of man and his environment. It is conceived as having its roots in the physical and social sciences and of having specific aims and goals. Nutrition education is not incidental or accidental. Good nutrition education is planned. True education takes time. Further, it requires a sufficient knowledge of the science to be able to identify the needs of those to be educated, a knowledge of the learning process and a good understanding of appropriate techniques to be employed in various types of educational programs.[1]

Reduced to a simple analogy, the educational process is sometimes characterized as a bridge between findings of nutrition research and the acceptance and application, by recipients and users, of the information. The desired outcome of such a transfer is obviously good nutritional status and sound health. The content and methods of education in nutrition cover a wide span depending on the age, background, and needs of those to be educated. Both content and method are presently under fire, as proving inadequate in application. Poor food practices of children and varying degrees of failure in human nutrition, discussed earlier in the text, tend to support this allegation. National, state, and local agencies and individuals are currently motivated to increase the amount and improve the quality of nutrition education. A series of events and actions kindled this effort.

## Movements to Stimulate Nutrition Education

### White House Conference

In 1969, the White House Conference on Food, Nutrition, and Health proclaimed the need for a strong nationwide nutrition education program.[2] Such a program should encompass the broad area of nutrition and would cover all segments of the population, but children would receive major consideration. Nutrition education of schoolchildren at all grade levels was emphasized as essential to nutritional health throughout life. Three of the many recommendations made by panels of the conference suggest their sweeping nature:

> That a unified, sequential nutrition education curriculum, designed for pre-kindergarten through adults, to teach the basic concepts of food and nutrition, be distributed to every school in the United States.

That . . . every school or school district employ a professional person responsible for coordinating nutrition education and nutrition services.

That state departments of education be urged to require that all elementary school teachers and secondary teachers of health education, biology, chemistry, home economics, and physical education complete a course in food use and principles of nutrition . . . that all currently employed teachers complete a similar course for maintenance and certification.

These and other recommendations served as rallying points for professional groups across the United States. Following the conference, panel members sought state and local support for the recommendations and tried to implement them. Response was difficult to measure but, clearly, there was no significant nationwide progress attributable to the basic recommendations listed here. However, seeds had been sown for a national nutrition policy which would recognize nutrition education as a basic tenet of the total policy and would lend broad support to the initial recommendations.

One stated purpose of the White House Conference had been to lay the groundwork for a national nutrition policy which would assure concerted, purposeful effort in nutrition programs and education—at home and in international commitments. Realization of the need had been accentuated by the growing number of separate agencies and organizations dealing with nutrition problems and by increased recognition of the significant role other food-related fields play in nutrition programs and services. Involved are individuals and groups concerned not only with the status of national health but with guiding agricultural, economic, social, and educational policies as they are inseparably associated with production, distribution, and use of food supplies. Together they represent broad, significant dimensions of nutrition today. There is at present no overall federal policy designed to unify and coordinate these forces toward achieving the maximum in nutritional health for the population. A start has been made.

## National Nutrition Consortium

Gradually the framework of a national nutrition policy for the United States has emerged.[3] Guidelines and goals were developed and programs suggested by a group of professionals called the National Nutrition Consortium, a policy-making group representing major scientific societies (table 8.2). The policy guidelines cover the gamut of food and nutrition considerations of national and international importance. A first goal is to assure an adequate wholesome food supply at reasonable cost to meet the needs of all segments of the population. In order that an individual utilize food to his greatest benefit, he should have some basic understanding of food and nutrition in relation to requirements for health. Among the many programs proposed to meet goals set forth by policy guidelines is nutrition education at all childhood levels. "In schools: nutrition should be a basic curriculum requirement in all elementary schools and high schools. The school lunch program should be used to assist in nutrition education through correlation with teaching in the classroom. All teachers should receive training in nutrition."[3]

### Legislation

A national nutrition policy moved nearer to reality when the National Nutrition Education Bill of 1974 was introduced in Congress.[4] It was sponsored by seven members of the Senate Select Committee on Nutrition and Human Needs, at the behest of and with the assistance of concerned professional groups. The Consortium's guidelines provided substance for the bill. While this bill (S–3864) was not successful, it was the forerunner of other efforts which will undoubtedly continue until there is some measure of accomplishment. Similar new legislation is already under consideration in both the U.S. Senate and the House of Representatives. The 1974 bill called for a three-year pilot program that would introduce a comprehensive nutrition education curriculum into the nation's schools. In the absence of a national mandate, several state legislatures have acted to support various aspects of nutrition education programs, in their states.

### Official Endorsements

The National Advisory Council on Child Nutrition (established by P.L. 91–248) in its first annual report to the president of the United States in 1972, placed nutrition education as a high priority. In this and later reports the Council stressed the importance of classroom instruction in nutrition and the inclusion of nutrition education as a curriculum component in all grades and in secondary schools. The Council has urged also that some preparation in nutrition be required of all teachers (chapter 7).

Meantime, sentiment for more meaningful nutrition education has spread as a result of endorsements by such professional organizations as the Society for Nutrition Education,[5] the American Dietetic Association,[6] and the American Home Economics Association,[7] and with the advocacy and encouragement of various professional symposia and conferences. Such backing has largely taken the form of position papers and resolutions or testimony before government bodies to urge legislative action for increased financial support of nutrition education.

## Program Procedures

There appears to be wide acceptance of the concepts that nutrition education is a factor in achieving physical health and that effective nutrition education is dependent on properly conceived program planning and implementation. Despite this awareness, there is scant evidence that the nation's schools have made significant progress in nutrition education. Professional leadership at the national level is essential and should be accelerated but, alone, it is insufficient to generate sustained program growth. If there is to be permanent progress, there must also be participation, at the grass roots, by qualified persons knowledgeable and concerned with local conditions and needs. A primary step in such cooperation is in the development, jointly, of effective nutrition education curricula.

## The School Curriculum

A curriculum, in its broadest sense, is said to consist of everything that happens to learners while they are in the school setting. A curriculum *guide* is the framework for an organized plan for learning. Such a guide in a specified field, such as nutrition education, is ideally developed as one segment of the total school curriculum. Its basic objective is an instrument, relevant at different school levels, through a sequential progressive program, growing suitably in depth and sophistication from preschool through grade 12.

*Guidelines for Curriculum Development*

One reason ascribed to failure of school nutrition education is that curriculum guides are often developed and imposed on schools by persons apart from the local scene. Teachers avoid the use of such guides because they are unrealistic and inapplicable. The result is little systematic nutrition education. The purpose in this chapter is to offer a cooperative approach to curriculum building which would avoid that error. The plan proposes minimum guidelines, not precise steps to be taken. The suggestions are intended primarily for nutritionists who are in a position to advise, guide, and/or participate in the development and implementation of sound viable nutrition education curricula, which are acceptable in school classrooms.

Many blueprints for curriculum planning have been offered. Those of recent design usually propose a combined effort of personnel having expertise in method and subject matter, with potential users at the classroom level. Griffin conceives of curriculum development as a three-step process carried on at different stages by appropriate groups.[8] He considers his plan particularly appropriate for nutrition education. It is predicated on cooperation between principal participants at each of three levels, as well as between the levels. The three levels of Griffin's plan are summarized here briefly with suggested adaptations to nutrition education.

*Societal Level.*   The principal purpose of this level is to blend the knowledge, skills, and experience of the science of nutrition with the power of official policy-making bodies, to define the broad goals of the curriculum in terms of what is expected: in learner behaviors, in learning experiences, and in problem-solving opportunities. The persons involved are principally discipline and policy experts. The former might be nutrition scientists at national or state levels. The latter might be nutrition educators with national or state agencies or organizations. The outcome sought at the societal level is to establish certain patterns for the nutrition education curriculum which will serve as guidelines and background for the second and third planning levels.

*Institutional Level.*   At this level school personnel, working together, make decisions about what the curriculum should be in a given school or school system, with local nutrition and education experts and in cooperation with representatives of the community, including parents. The objective is a community-based project developed within the boundaries established at the societal level. A dialogue is conducted between the first two levels, with modifications being made at both levels. At the institutional level, organizing principles are considered as well as evolution techniques, procedures, and strategies, all on a broad base. They do not pertain to what happens to an individual child in a particular school setting. Thus, at the institutional level alternatives are provided from which, at the instructional level, an individual teacher can arrive at a personalized curriculum. Griffin cautions of the consequences if the institutional level is bypassed. He says, "Until you get support and the necessary expertise of the people who are holding power in institutional settings . . . you are creating a dysfunctional situation. . . . It [a program] must be surrounded with an institutional commitment in order to really make a difference."[8]

*Instructional Level.*   This level is the one closest to the learner. It involves teachers, children, parents, and others concerned with decision making in the classroom or other school setting. Again, decisions are made within the parameters of preceding levels. However, at the instructional level, teachers and learners are expected to make adaptations to their own particular setting. Children with their teachers establish their own objectives, decide the learning activities most suitable in their own situations, and what problems they propose to solve.

## Curriculum Planning, U.S. Schools

Apparently no specific pattern is followed in developing nutrition curriculum guides for schools in this country. A 1976 survey suggests that guides in current use followed a variety of procedures. As one aspect of a comprehensive study of kindergarten through grade 12 curriculum guides, for nutrition and related subject areas, Cooper and Go examined seventy-eight of them for sources.[9] They found that one guide originated with a federal government agency, thirty-three with state education agencies, eleven with local school districts, twelve with state universities/extension, and the remainder with association/ commercial groups.

Efforts have also been made to discover how school personnel *think* nutrition education curricula should be developed and function. Judgments were obtained from nearly 300 experienced staff members serving at institutional and instructional levels.[10] Approximately half the group were classroom teachers, one-fourth were curriculum specialists, and one-fourth were school principals. Each was personally questioned by a trained interviewer soliciting attitudes toward and suggestions for a proposed new nutrition education curriculum.

The administrators expressed need, generally, for effective nutrition education in their schools and for better organized, coordinated, and sequentially planned programs. The curriculum, they said, should be made more interesting, creative, and relevant. Four out of five administrators and teachers thought nutrition should be taught at all grade levels. Both groups mentioned frequently that teaching nutrition should start in kindergarten and progress in scope and complexity throughout the grades. Both also listed a number of possible ways to organize a new nutrition curriculum but more in each group leaned toward separate grade or grade-grouping packages than toward curriculum guides alone. Most teachers and administrators (60% and 77%, respectively) expressed the belief that nutrition should be integrated with other subjects.

### Curricula and School Organization

Some educators believe that the very structure of the school tends to inhibit the development and implementation of nutrition curricula. Experts in the field, especially those from the outside, find that the school is a closed system difficult to penetrate. Components of the organization are conventional and inflexible in function; there is lack of goal clarity and the roles of school personnel are often not specific; teachers work in isolation from each other; and the school frequently lacks meaningful relations with other community agencies.[8] In initiating a nutrition education program from the outside, goals must coincide with those of the school if the program is to succeed. Support systems, such as teacher training programs, materials, and equipment, must often be provided. Endorsement of the program at the administrative level is essential.

Normal variations in the internal organization of schools are also a factor in curriculum planning. Schools are classified as ungraded, open education, highly individualized, and traditional. Most classify as traditional. The nutrition education segment of the school curriculum usually applies to the elementary school and to certain subject areas in the upper grades and high school. The term *elementary school* commonly refers to kindergarten or grades 1 to 6 or 8; *junior* or *middle school* refers to grades 6 to 8 or 7 to 9; and *secondary* or *high school* refers to grades 9 or 10 to 12. In the elementary grades nutrition is taught as a separate subject or is integrated with other subject areas such as health, home economics, social studies, social science, physical education, language arts.[10] At junior and secondary school levels, where subject matter is departmentalized, nutrition lends itself to integration with courses such as biology, home economics, science, consumer education, and health education.

Cutting across all levels are school feeding programs available in almost all schools: breakfast, lunch, snacks. The school lunchroom can be a laboratory of learning. It offers teachers, administrators, and school food-service personnel opportunities to utilize immediate learning situations to carry out behavioral goals of the curriculum.

### Extent and Quality of Nutrition Curricula, U.S. Schools

There has been little precise information on where, how, and how much nutrition is being taught in schools of the United States and how well it is being done. Three nationwide surveys have been made which furnish some information of this character.

In 1974, Johnson and Butler submitted a survey questionnaire, sponsored by the National Nutrition Education Clearing House, to the superintendents of public instruction in the fifty states and the District of Columbia.[11] This action was taken to assess progress following recommendations of the 1969 White House Conference, that nutrition education be included in the curricula of all U.S. schools. The specific purpose of the survey was to explore the current involvement, in the area of nutrition education, of state departments of public instruction. Forty-two responses were received. Twenty-three states indicated they have a curriculum guide which "includes" nutrition; inspection of a sampling of such guides revealed a wide divergence in the types and significance of material related to nutrition. Several states indicated they were currently developing or revising a nutrition curriculum guide, and others replied that nutrition education was being carried out at local levels through a number of disciplines. States without a specific nutrition policy often reported that nutrition was being covered in such subjects as health and home economics. Ten states had legislated policy concerning nutrition education in their public schools.

In 1975 more recent and detailed information was sought on the status of nutrition education in U.S. schools, this time by the Education Commission of the States under a contract from the U.S. Department of Agriculture.[12] The Commission gathered survey questionnaire data from the U.S. Office of Education (OE), from official state education agencies (SEA), from a sample of local education agencies (LEA), and from more than 1,300 private schools. It examined legislation, grants, and contracts as well as projects, school activities, and curricula. The few highlights reported here chiefly reflect the findings as reported by SEAs. In the main they are more favorable than those from LEA and from the private schools. It was found that thirty-one of the fifty-one SEAs responding to the questionnaire had or were planning to have offices responsible for nutrition education. Thirty percent of the state agencies had programs or projects specifically relating to nutrition education. More than 75% of the SEAs reported sponsoring activities in nutrition education—most of them for school food-service personnel. Seven SEAs reported that nutrition education was mandatory. Two trends in that respect were observed: it was required about twice as often in secondary schools as in elementary schools and more state agencies planned to require nutrition education in the future.

Twenty-six of the fifty-one SEAs reported having nutrition educaton curriculum guides or guides "including nutrition education." Nutrition education was ranked low in priority by SEAs in comparison with other health education subject areas (fourth in elementary, seventh in secondary schools). Only two states reported having requirements in nutrition education for elementary and secondary teacher certification; one reported a requirement for in-service training in nutrition education; only two applied any nutrition education criteria.

In a third survey, Cooper and Go, for the Society for Nutrition Education, assembled and examined seventy-eight curriculum guides in nutrition and related subject areas. Twenty-two of them at the kindergarten through grade 12 level, from a variety of sources and from a broad geographic area, were chosen as representative for in-depth study.[9] To analyze each guide critically for potential effectiveness as a nutrition education tool, an extensive questionnaire was designed and applied as a measuring device. Also, to summarize the results of this device efficiently, a five-point rating scale was developed, corresponding essentially to the questionnaire headings. Curricula were not analyzed in use with students. Ratings were based on specific components of the guides: concepts, objectives, learning activities, and evaluative procedures, as well as organizational format and recognition of social concerns. Some of the strong and weak points of the twenty-two guides are summarized here briefly.

The majority of the nutrition concepts presented in the twenty-two guides corresponded generally with those proposed for school curricula by the 1969 White House Conference. Almost all of the guides presented concepts in a sequential framework. However, concepts in many of the guides were underdeveloped, with the problem ascribed to the weak relationship between concepts, lesson objectives, and learning activities. Fifteen percent of the guides contained lesson objectives that did not correspond to the major concepts; in 41% of the guides, learning activities often were not in agreement with the concepts. More than half of the learning activities did not supply appropriate practice in the behavior outlined in the objective. Many of the activities were merely "busywork," others were inappropriate in character, overly complex or overly simple, or "innovative" but not necessarily effective. Often instructions for the activities were incomplete and confusing. Only 41% of the guides included evaluative procedures on a frequent and consistent basis and only 18% frequently or occasionally measured the ability of students to utilize previously given information in new learning experiences.

As to organization, nearly 80% of the guides were well thought out, simple, and direct. The remainder were frequently cluttered and inconsistent, making it easy to confuse the reader and thus discourage use. About two-thirds of the guides included nutrition information for the teacher, but not all of it was appropriate to the suggested learning activities. A variety of supplementary teaching aids was usually listed but community resources for nutrition education were not always explored thoroughly. In respect to nutrition-related social concerns, the majority of the guides did not integrate socioeconomic and cultural values into the regular lesson activities but treated them in separate units. About three-fourths of the guides did not indicate whether in-service training of teachers was a previous or a concurrent requirement.

The Cooper and Go analysis is more than a mere report of the content of twenty-two existing curriculum guides. The significance of its contribution lies in the identification of roles of separate guide components, and especially their organizational relationship to each other as they affect student learning. In stressing this phase a major purpose of the analysis is served. It was a stated intention to aid nutrition educators and others, charged with selecting or developing school nutrition curricula, to evaluate the factors in guides which determine learner success. The authors make it clear that while a curriculum guide may possess a wealth of nutrition education material (as was true in the case of many of the twenty-two guides analyzed) it may fail of its full purpose if the developers lack understanding of the function and interdependence of its major components.[9] An instrument for use in the analysis of curriculum guides is now available.

It is evident from data available that a considerable amount of activity in the schools can be characterized loosely as nutrition education. An increasing number of schools are including nutrition in their curricula in some manner or degree and many individual teachers are including some nutrition, even when their schools do not recognize nutrition in the curriculum guide. Such efforts are diverse in nature and dispersed widely. The three surveys just reported suggest that relatively few schools have educationally sound curriculum structures in nutrition education and adequate support systems, such as teacher education, to implement effective programs. There is currently no mechanism for coordinating such efforts, nationally.

## Qualified Personnel

A curriculum provides the framework for a school nutrition program, but the personnel involved in its development, interpretation, and implementation can determine its success or failure. The qualifications of those who serve—from policy level to classroom—are deciding factors. Weakness in personnel at any point in the process can jeopardize nutrition education at the school level. Currently, titles and duties are varied and there is no unanimity of judgment as to criteria for selection of those who serve as policy makers, planners, supervisors, and teachers. As a result, individuals with vastly different backgrounds are now serving in positions which call for specific competencies. Many of such individuals are unprepared in both training and experience. There is no concerted effort by the national nutrition education community to develop suitable standards for the different positions. However, attention is being centered on certain types of positions and various suggestions have been made to satisfy interim needs. Some criteria are merely informal projections, others offer concrete guidelines.

### Policy Makers

Policy makers are individuals and groups who serve largely at the federal level in national and international food and nutrition planning. They may be agencies or individuals within the government structure;

national scientific bodies acting in advisory capacities to government; and/or professional consortia, conferences, symposia, or committees which have a voice in establishing policy. Individuals or members of groups must be in a position to make policy decisions themselves or to advise executives or political leaders, lacking expertise in nutrition, who are the authorized policy makers. The advisors should be professionally trained in the science of nutrition with broad understanding in related fields of agriculture, economics, sociology, education.[13-15] They need to recognize and appreciate the importance of trends in food consumption and in population change which eventually influence nutrition practices, at the family level and in nutrition education programs in schools. Finally, they need to demonstrate foresight as to future nutrition needs and expert leadership abilities required to effect change. Such responsibilities indicate the importance of urging high standards of nutrition competence for those in policy-making positions.

### Nutrition Educators

Nutrition educators are relatively new professionals. Increased demand for their services has sharpened the need for selection criteria. Professional groups largely agree that an educator in nutrition must have a strong foundation in the science of nutrition, natural sciences, behavioral sciences, and education. The position calls for planning, directing, and supervising nutrition education programs, usually at state and local levels. Present incumbents represent a confusing variety of titles, training, and experience. Some persons with the commonly used titles *nutrition educator* or *nutrition education specialist* have inadequate training in the science of nutrition; others have little or no knowledge or experience in the field of education. Competence in both is needed.

Johnson and Butler have indicated that a nutrition educator should be competent in nutritional science, applied nutrition, curriculum development, and teaching techniques. They suggest that the background for such a person should include a combination of the following:[11] at least a bachelor's degree in foods and/or nutrition; a master's degree in nutrition education, public health nutrition, or community nutrition; work experience in applied nutrition; teaching certificate and/or teaching experience at the elementary, secondary, or college level; and knowledge of and/or experience in school food service programs.

An ad hoc committee of the California Nutrition Council has described the types of duties a nutrition education specialist would perform and has said that to carry them out a person would require course work in advanced nutrition based on physiology and biochemistry; food composition and preparation; applied nutrition; behavioral sciences; basic education concepts; and curriculum development. He or she should also have a knowledge of school and community organization and experience in schools—preferably coordinated with the course work.[16]

Early in 1976, the California Nutrition Council requested that the Society for Nutrition Education (SNE) establish standards for school nutrition education specialists. As a result a policy was drafted by an ad hoc committee of SNE and the document was published.[17] Member input was invited. The SNE Board considered the member comments, finalized the position paper, and presented it as a resolution for membership vote. When approved it will be published as a society position paper in the *Journal of Nutrition Education*. The resolution, under the title "Nutrition Education Specialists in School Systems (K–12): A Position Paper on Functions and Qualifications," defines the educational qualifications for and the functions of a nutrition education specialist in the elementary and secondary educational systems. The resolution reads, in part:

> There are distinct qualifications for a Nutrition Education Specialist. In order to function effectively, the Specialist must have the following: training in advanced human nutrition based on physiology and biochemistry, in food composition and principles of preparation, in the application of nutritional knowledge; training in basic education concepts including curriculum development, educational psychology, and/or early childhood education; training in the behavioral sciences as they apply to children; knowledge of school and community organization; experience in schools which could be coordinated with course work, such as, but not limited to, classroom teaching.
> These qualifications can be obtained through the successful completion of a Master's degree in one of several areas; nutrition education, nutrition, or public health nutrition, for example. Other Master's level programs may qualify provided they offer the qualifications listed above which are essential to the role of the Nutrition Education Specialist.

In Massachusetts the Bureau of Nutrition Education and School Food Services of the State Department of Education has outlined qualifications of educational specialists in nutrition who serve the state's schools.[18] Positions at four levels of responsibility have been described, ranging from project director, nutrition education, to assistant supervisor, nutrition education. Qualifications differ with the type of position but, in general, there is emphasis at each level on acquiring knowledge in foods and nutrition, institution management, and educational method. A Massachusetts teaching certificate is required at all levels. Paid experience in the field of education with knowledge of food delivery systems is a requisite. Specified substitutions may be made in experience for academic training and vice versa. A bachelor's degree from a recognized college is a basic requirement, with more advanced training indicated for the positions at higher levels of responsibility.

Nutrition leaders in the academic sector also have a stake in establishing qualifications criteria for the position of nutrition educator— or for any other position which requires a background in the science of nutrition.[19] Their failure to propose such standards is perhaps due to delay in reaching an understanding on certain underlying issues. For example, a basic requirement for a nutrition educator is "adequate" training in nutrition. The first question then is, what is "adequate"? The answer must remain inconclusive until certain matters of academic preparation are clarified.

Students receive undergraduate training in nutrition from university departments of nutrition, nutritional science, or food science and nutrition, or from departments of food and nutrition in schools of home economics. The student who takes a series of prescribed courses in nutrition and related subjects may, on graduation, be referred to as a nutritionist. However, at present there is no definition of "nutritionist" in terms of professional training. It has been proposed that professional nutrition societies assume responsibility for such a definition, but so far this has not been done. Meanwhile, certain subject areas are accepted as important to meet scientific qualifications for nutritionists.[19] Requirements and sequences of basic undergraduate core courses for a degree in nutrition differ among recognized universities. For graduate training a student may concentrate on such specialties as public health nutrition, infant nutrition, laboratory nutrition, behavioral nutrition, or community nutrition to which he may or may not have been introduced at the undergraduate level. A person with advanced training in nutrition is often called a "nutritional scientist."

A nutritionist who has, in addition, the required training in education qualifies academically as a nutrition educator. With positions available in nutrition education, universities are planning sequences to satisfy the dual need. Few institutions currently offer a degree in nutrition education although it is rapidly coming to be recognized as a discipline. In that context, Light has recently identified nutrition education as follows:

> It is the specialization which concerns itself with the design, operation and research aspects of systematic efforts directed at intended changes in the way known learners *think, feel* and *act* to meet nutritional needs.[20]

There is concern that universities offer more than merely courses in nutrition *and* in education for the prospective nutrition educator. Training criteria should be based on the knowledge and skills required of the nutrition educator rather than on the completion of specific courses. This theory would envision a university environment to encourage dialogue among various faculty specialists and give students an opportunity for relevant experiences in the different disciplines involved. Cooperative planning would be required on the part of students and university faculty—a faculty well versed in community needs, in educational programs, and in research procedures.

Much more is needed to meet challenges for new methods of approach in nutrition education. "University centers for innovation and evaluation in nutrition education should be designated to initiate, conduct, supervise, assess, and disseminate information about experimental approaches to nutrition education, addressed to the needs and characteristics of different learner groups."[21] Nutrition educators thus trained would be equipped to handle a range of positions from policy making to field level—some with special leadership capacities to project, plan, and initiate; others more specifically to become involved in implementation of programs.[13] There is also need for continuing education. Graduate courses, workshops, and institutes with various emphases in nutrition education are currently not universally available.

---

## Classroom Teachers

Classroom teachers are acknowledged to be the logical ones to teach nutrition to children in the elementary school. Here we have the anomaly of teachers trained as educators who are expected to teach a subject, nutrition, which is rarely included in their preservice training. There is increasing awareness of this inconsistency. Professional individuals and groups have unanimously endorsed some form of basic orientation in nutrition for all teachers. Without it, teachers feel timid and insecure in the nutrition-teacher role. In the judgment of

many there will be no strong thrust forward in school nutrition education until teachers-in-training receive at least one course in the
subject. Preservice education usually results in a comprehension and
appreciation on the part of teachers which influences the quality of
classroom teaching in nutrition and affects the understanding and
attitudes of the children.

## Preservice Education

It is not the purpose of preservice education to make nutritionists of
teachers. It is primarily to give them a simple working knowledge of
practical nutrition, especially as it applies to child learners; to make
them aware of the relation of nutrition to health; to fortify them with
a knowledge of sources of authentic information; to help them discriminate in the selection of sound subject content and effective teaching aids; and finally to give them confidence and the motivation to
teach. The university instructor of such a course should not only be
well grounded in nutrition but should be knowledgeable in modern
approaches to nutrition education as well.

In view of the fact that a nutrition course of this character holds
so much promise for nutrition education in schools, one would expect
such a course to be required of all elementary education majors. This
is not the case. Some university departments of education advise their
elementary education majors to elect a course in nutrition on campus;
for a few it is a high priority. Occasionally it is a course tailored to
the needs of teachers; more often it is a one-semester, general orientation course in nutrition, open to all university students, taught at elementary level. Thus most classroom teachers come to the task without adequate preparation to teach nutrition to children—a striking
example of how unqualified personnel may threaten the success of a
program at a critical point.

Special teachers of such subjects as biology, health education, physical education, or chemistry, in upper grades and high school, who
may devote segments to nutrition, also need a preservice course in
nutrition. Such a course should give particular attention to methods
of integrating nutrition with the subject at hand. School food-service
personnel also have special needs. If school meals are to have their
full impact as aids to nutrition education, personnel must know nutrition subject matter and have some grasp of educational method. This
dual background is particularly indicated if food-service operators
cooperate with teachers in classroom programs, directly or in an advisory capacity.

Despite failure to find a generally acceptable pattern of preservice nutrition education for teachers, the search has continued, due largely to recognition on the part of nutrition educators of its urgent need. A recently completed, three-year experimental program at a teacher's college gives promise of providing such a plan.[22] The School of Education at Eastern Washington State College has demonstrated the feasibility of instructing senior elementary education majors in nutrition and nutrition education and providing an opportunity for them to do their practice teaching in nutrition education. The experiment was made possible by a research grant from the National Dairy Council. The instruction consisted of three, two-credit courses: in nutrition concepts, in nutrition values, and in nutrition teaching methods. Students took the courses on a voluntary basis. The segments were cooperatively planned by the college departments responsible for teaching the courses.

The project was evaluated by an outside agency as well as by faculty and student participants. All student teachers showed an increase in understanding of the subject areas covered by the courses. Student teachers, with their master teachers, developed and taught nutrition units to elementary school pupils under carefully supervised conditions, and sample units were rated positively by teachers not associated with the experimental program. Student-teacher graduates went on to provide nutrition education in their postcollege teaching positions. The faculty at the college evidenced its belief that the experimental program was worthwhile and workable by introducing into the curriculum, on a permanent basis, a minor in nutrition for elementary education majors.

Certain features of the experimental program were believed to contribute importantly to its success. One was the fact that principals and master teachers from the schools where students did their practice teaching attended and became involved in the nutrition and methods courses, along with the college students. Another feature was strong administrative leadership which gave support to the program and provided for joint planning, exchange of information, collaboration, and complete understanding of purposes and procedures, on the part of all participants.

### In-Service Education

For classroom teachers, who enter service without nutrition training, there are several ways to compensate. Class work is available through summer, extension, and home-study courses in nutrition. Such courses should be of the same basic type as suggested for preservice training with emphasis on helping the teacher apply the material in classroom use. A short-term, more informal type of in-service orientation is available through workshops, institutes, symposia and seminars.[18] Members of such groups often participate in establishing objectives and planning procedures. They present nutrition education problems —often those of their own classrooms—for evaluation and solution. Such an approach can prove valuable if the workshop experience is long enough to be really helpful. In-service briefing of a sort can come from within the school itself: planned teachers' meetings, group conferences, and consultation sessions with the nutrition educator.

A community resource, easily overlooked, is the pool of local professionals available. They do not provide in-service nutrition education, as such, but represent a scientific reservoir for teachers attempting to present accurate information. Nutritionists and dietitians, for example, may be asked to answer questions, give advice, or verify points of controversy. Teachers lacking nutrition orientation and groping for teaching material often place reliance on newspapers, popular magazines, television, and other public media for subject content in nutrition.[10] The habit of checking, instead, with persons professionally trained not only can avoid teaching false and misleading material but tends to dignify the subject and reinforce the concept that nutrition is based on a foundation of scientific knowledge. Persons trained in nutrition who may be of service are located in many places: public health departments of many cities and counties and of most states employ nutritionists; the agricultural extension service of each state has at least one nutrition specialist on its staff; there are professional associations such as city and state nutrition councils, dietetic and home economic associations; in addition there are college teachers of nutrition, dietitians in hospitals and other institutions, and nutritionists in local branches of national and state health-related organizations.

A comprehensive effort in behalf of in-service nutrition education for school personnel is that administered by the Food and Nutrition Service (FNS) of the U.S. Department of Agriculture.[23] With the passage of P.L. 91–248, 14 May 1970, federal funding was made possible for the first time for nutrition training of workers, cooperators, and participants in child nutrition programs. Sections 3 and 8 of the law amend Section 6 of the National School Lunch Act (NSLA) and Section 10 of the Child Nutrition Act (CNA) of 1966, respectively. Section 6(3) of NSLA makes available to the Secretary of Agriculture up to 1% of the funds provided for programs under NSLA and CNA, other than Section 3, to supplement the nutritional benefits of the programs through grants to the states and other means.

Objectives in the broad subject area of nutrition training and education are to

1. Provide training to food-service managers at regional, state, and district levels; supervisors and local workers to institute more effective and efficient food service to children. Such training shall include information on nutrition and related school food-service management subjects which shall assist in improving the quality of meals served to children.

2. Educate managers, supervisors, cooperators, that is, teachers, administrators, parents, and children, regarding the relationship of food and nutrition to growth, development, and good health and the role of the child nutrition programs in establishing good eating habits.

To accomplish these objectives, FNS during some years set aside a portion of the available Section 6(3) funds for grants to states for nutritional training and education. Remaining funds for nutritional training and education are expended by FNS via requests for proposals (RFP) resulting in cooperative agreements or other contractual arrangements with states or contracts with nonprofit institutions, universities, or private industry.

In the period since the enactment of P.L. 91–248, a number of projects have been completed.[23] The overall purpose of the projects is four-fold:

To increase participation in school food programs through more effective meal preparation and service (purchasing, preparation, merchandising, nutrition education activities, and so on);

To provide menu flexibility and choice options within Type A pattern;

To determine factors affecting food acceptability (degree of plate waste) in the school cafeteria; and

To utilize to full advantage the USDA basic program aids designed to improve food service management and operations technique.

To this end, in-service programs are designed for training persons in the school setting who are in key positions to help realize this purpose. These persons primarily include personnel associated in various capacities with school food services, and school teachers as well as nutrition educators who provide leadership. Such in-service programs largely take the form of workshops, seminars, class sessions, and demonstrations specifically related to nutrition education in schools. Thus the stated purpose of the projects is served by providing these school personnel with opportunities to upgrade their knowledge and skills in the area of school food-service management as they relate to the ultimate goal of improved food practices in children.

A recently completed nutrition education project holds great promise for achieving this ultimate goal by training teacher/managers to work in pairs as a team. It was a five-state project conducted over a two-year period. The project was based on the premise that the classroom is the logical place for learning about nutrition and the school food-service program is the logical laboratory for practicing nutrition learnings. Therefore, school food-service managers and teachers are jointly responsible for nutrition education. The project identifies competencies (nutrition, interpersonal communications skills, and instructional skills) needed by teachers and by managers to conduct effective nutrition education together. They also developed, tested, and evaluated training modules for this purpose.[24]

## A Coordinated Program for Nutrition Education

It has long been recognized that coordinated leadership at the federal level will be required to bring focus and coherence to food and nutrition policies and programs in the United States.[25] Responsible scientific and governmental groups have proposed various mechanisms to accomplish this objective. While no plan has yet been enacted, there is agreement on some of the issues and approaches: that agricultural and economic policies should be appraised and interpreted in terms of nutritional health; that nutritional status of the people should be known at all times; and that programs should be aligned with indicated nutritional needs. Pertinent in the present context are the benefits to be derived from strong concerted action in the area of nutrition education, largely through the framework of the nation's school systems. This chapter has reviewed important components of school nutrition programs, indicating at certain points where, for lack of coordinated leadership, program effectiveness in nutrition education is sacrificed—notably in the critical areas of curriculum development, selection of qualified personnel, and teacher education.

## References

1   Bosley, B. Moderator of a panel discussion, "Making Nutrition Education Effective." Paper read at the Conference on Education in Nutrition: Looking Forward from the Past, 26 February 1974, at Teachers College, Columbia University, New York.

2   White House Conference on Food, Nutrition, and Health. *Final Report.* Washington, D.C.: U.S. Government Printing Office, Superintendent of Documents, 1970.

3   National Nutrition Consortium, Inc. *Guidelines for a National Nutrition Policy.* Prepared for the U.S. Senate Select Committee on Nutrition and Human Needs. Washington, D.C.: Superintendent of Documents, U.S. Government Printing Office, 1974.

4   U.S. Congress. Senate. *National Nutrition Education Bill of 1974.* S. 3864, 93d Cong., 2d sess., 1974.

5   "National Nutrition Policy: Society for Nutrition Education, Board Statement." *SNE Communicator* 5(1974):4–5.

6   "Position Paper on Child Nutrition Programs." *Journal of the American Dietetic Association* 64(1974):520–21.

7   "Resolutions Approved by Assembly of Delegates." *Journal of the Home Economics Association* 67(1975):46.

8   Griffin, G. A. "Strategies in Curriculum Development." Paper read at the Conference on Education in Nutrition: Looking Forward from the Past, 27 February 1974, at Teachers College, Columbia University, New York.

9   Cooper, K. A., and Go, C. E. "Analysis of Curriculum Guides at K–12 Level." *Journal of Nutrition Education* 8(1976):62–66.

10   Eash, M. J., and Rasher, S. P. *A Needs Assessment of Nutrition Education.* Chicago: University of Illinois, 1975.

11   Johnson, M. J., and Butler, J. L. "Where Is Nutrition Education in U.S. Public Schools?" *Journal of Nutrition Education* 7(1975):20–21.

12   *Nutrition Education Survey of the States, 1975: Final Report.* Washington, D.C.: Food and Nutrition Service, U.S. Department of Agriculture, 1975.

13   Sismanidis, A. "The Preparation of the Nutrition Educator." Paper read at the Conference on Education in Nutrition: Looking Forward from the Past, 26 February 1974, at Teachers College, Columbia University, New York.

14   Berg, A. "Fear of Trying." *Journal of the American Dietetic Association* 68(1976):311–16.

15   "Orrea F. Pye Symposium: The Educator's Response to World Hunger." *Journal of the American Dietetic Association* 68(1976):309–10, 317–29.

16   Peck, E. B. "Nutrition Education Specialists: Time for Action." *Journal of Nutrition Education* 8(1976):11–12.

17 "Draft of School Nutrition Education Specialist Policy Statement." *SNE Communicator* 7(1976):6–7.

18 Callahan, D. L. "Inservice Teacher Workshops." *Journal of Nutrition Education* 5(1973):233–36.

19 Briggs, G. M. "Undergraduate Training in Nutritional Science." *Journal of Nutrition Education* 4(1972):129–31.

20 Light, L. "The Role of the University in Preparing Educators for the Future." Paper read at the Conference on Education in Nutrition: Looking Forward from the Past, 26 February 1974, at Teachers College, Columbia University, New York.

21 Pye, O. F. *Recommendations for Nutrition Education Policies, Strategies and Plans: National Nutrition Policy: Nutrition and the Consumer: II.* Washington, D.C.: Senate Select Committee on Nutrition and Human Needs, Superintendent of Documents, U.S. Government Printing Office, 1974.

22 Schults, V. "Relationships of Teachers' Motivations and Attitudes to Pupil Learning in Nutrition Education." Submitted to the *Journal of Nutrition Education* for publication.

23 Food and Nutrition Service mimeographed reports of completed nutrition education and training projects status: 1974, pp. 1–31; 1975, pp. 1–31; 1976, pp. 1–35. Washington, D.C.: U.S. Department of Agriculture.

24 *Five-State Nutrition Education Project, 1975: Final Report.* Washington, D.C.: Food and Nutrition Service, U.S. Department of Agriculture, 1975.

25 Select Committee on Nutrition and Human Needs of the U.S. Senate. *Nutrition and Health.* Washington, D.C.: Superintendent of Documents, U.S. Government Printing Office, 1975.

# Chapter Ten

## Nutrition Education of Children

## Learning Principles Applied to Curricula

This chapter is concerned mainly with the learning process and how it may be utilized in interpreting the school nutrition education curriculum at the instructional level. We are told that we do not teach children, that they learn for themselves. Educators have studied the elements of the learning process and have identified major principles involved in learning.[1-3] There is not full agreement on these principles, nor on their relative importance, but certain of them have rather wide acceptance. They include the following:

*Focus on the Learner*: When focus is on the learner, rather than on the thing to be learned, learning proceeds more readily. The process is centered on a child's interests, his problems, his concerns, and his motivations. Learning must relate to the learner's perception of tasks to be accomplished and his ideas, values, and goals. There is no real learning in the abstract. Children, provided with opportunities, materials, and effective teachers, will demand to learn. "Learning is an inherent feature of being a human being."[2]

*Relate Learning to Life*: Learning must relate to life situations in a child's world—his home, his school, his community. Gordon says that when we separate school from life, "we sterilize the former, we make it a place where academic games are played, in which what should be relevant is irrelevant and in which what should be studied is eliminated."[2] Children are motivated to learn when their needs, problems and interests are channeled into life-related experiences. A child acquires knowledge and develops skills rapidly when he needs them to accomplish self-imposed tasks which relate to his own living.

*Personal Involvement*: Active, personal involvement speeds learning. Children must have the opportunity to learn through real experiences, not alone through contrived class exercises. Such experiences challenge children to create, organize, compare, draw conclusions. The more closely experiences are related to their own environment, the better they serve as steps in learning. Also, the more actively a child participates rather than merely observes, the more does the experience contribute to learning.

*Problem Solving*: Genuine involvement in life-related experiences proceeds to the ultimate in the learning process, that of problem solving. Following the development steps enumerated above for such experiences, comes the further challenge for marshaling the facts, weighing the evidence, considering alternatives, exercising judgment, and making decisions. For persons and groups who go through this problem-solving process, behavior changes can be expected in line with decisions made.

If these principles are to be useful in the schoolroom, they require translation to terms of program procedures. The definition of nutrition education (see p. 249) refers to it as "planned . . . it requires . . . a knowledge of the learning process and a good understanding of appropriate techniques to be employed. . . ." It is pertinent therefore to examine elements of the nutrition education curriculum as they serve as instruments to achieve learning through the human components who guide the learning process.

## Human Components of the Learning Process

Teachers are assumed to be the chief contributors to child learning because the process takes place in the formal learning environment of the school. But parents are the earliest and a continuing factor in learning, and perhaps the most potent influence. The community and the people who live there are added resources for learning and help relate a child's school and family experiences to a broader sphere of living. The process starts with the learner himself.

## Child Learners

"Learning is a change in human disposition or capability which can be retained and which is not ascribable to the process of growth."[1] It consists of a series of experiences which gradually becomes more complex as a child grows. What is learned depends on the stage of his growth. That means that he is ready for different experiences at different times. Real learning basically implies a change in behavior and behavior is influenced both by the stage of development and the factor of learning. It is learning that accounts for the fact that he can choose between a good and a poor lunch, but the fact that he is now capable of learning *any* meal pattern is influenced by the factor of growth. Experiences must be kept at a learner's level of maturity if maximum learning is to take place. If primary level children, for example, are exposed to nutrition information beyond their understanding, not only does learning fail to take place, but it may interfere with the effective use of the material at more advanced levels.

Individual children learn at different rates and in different ways and there are conditions under which a child learner makes maximum progress. His nutritional status and health are important factors (chapter 6). An active, vigorous, well-nourished child usually approaches learning with enthusiasm. He enjoys people and things around him and is in a receptive mood for learning. Any child responds best when he is motivated to pursue his own goals. This happens most consistently when he is encouraged to be observant and curious about the things in his environment and to feel concern about how and why things happen and what can be expected as outcomes.[4] This attitude of inquiry is fostered in a relaxed atmosphere which permits uninterrupted study of problems and arrival at well-considered conclusions. It requires a free exchange of ideas with others, consultation with resource persons, and careful planning periods, exempt from anxieties and distractions which often clutter a child's schedule. A child also makes more rapid strides in learning if, in the process, he has minmum but understanding guidance that gives him a sense of direction as he proceeds.

## Teachers Guide Child Learners

In the school setting, teachers are probably the single greatest influence on child learners. They can create situations in which children, in a rich environment, can learn largely through their own discoveries. Such learning assumes adult leadership at its best, an essential element of which is a warm personal relationship between teachers and children. Teachers who listen to children and who are aware of their needs, interests, and problems are in the best position to establish a favorable learning climate.[5] Unfortunately all teaching, including nutrition teaching, does not meet these qualifications.

The nature and quality of classroom nutrition teaching varies greatly. Reasons for poor performance are often attributed to unconcern on the part of administrators and/or lack of preparation and motivation on the part of teachers. Also, teaching methods are uneven and often fruitless. Too many teachers continue to assume the traditional role of teller or lecturer and place emphasis on students' memorization of nutrition facts found in their health education textbooks. In these circumstances teachers and children are indifferent or negative to nutrition, and little learning takes place.

A vastly different situation can exist when teachers make nutrition education a vital part of the total school curriculum. They use the nutrition curriculum guide to structure the processes of their teaching around children's life concerns.[6] Adaptations are made, in individual classrooms, to recognize such factors as learning level of the children, economic status of the population, ethnic origins, locale—rural or urban, interests and occupations of the community. The curriculum guide starts with the concepts to be embodied. These become the unifying threads in carrying forward the program. Subconcepts serve as supporting ideas and give direction in choosing and arranging subject matter. Concepts also serve as bases in selecting learning objectives and give direction to choice of learning experiences and to planning evaluative procedures. These elements of the nutrition curriculum guide are closely related. When one is out of line with the others, the effectiveness of the program is in jeopardy. They are considered here separately.

### Concepts

A concept is a major thought or idea on which instruction is built. It is sometimes defined as a generalization or an identification of related information. An example of a major nutrition concept is *Food selection and eating patterns are determined by physical, social, mental, economic, and cultural factors.*[7] A subconcept might be stated as follows: *Choice of foods determines nutritional balance.* In turn, other subconcepts could be developed and classified by physical, mental, and social dimensions. In the school's nutrition curriculum guide, concepts are usually stated in general terms, as are those in the examples above. It is expected that teachers and students will interpret and personalize them in terms of needs in their own situation.

### Learning Objectives

Learning objectives belong primarily in three areas: (1) cognitive, (2) affective, and (3) action or psychomotor, characterized loosely as knowledge, attitudes, and practice. The cognitive domain is concerned largely with what a child is expected to achieve in the way of mastery of facts, comprehension, and interpretation. The affective domain relates to beliefs, attitudes, awareness, and value judgments. The action or psychomotor domain deals with manipulative skills which are attained as a result of applying cognitive and affective learnings. All three have behavioral implications, but some educators believe that behavioral objectives, as such, presuppose learning processes which are too controlled and regimented toward specific goals; that such objectives should be reserved for basic skills such as reading and mathematics which can be easily measured. They consider that nonbehavioral learning is the self-directed, unstructured type that many advocate as true learning.

Behavioral objectives are precise statements of what students will be able to do after they have engaged in certain learning experiences. They are developed in sequence, in line with learning experiences, and at different school progression levels, to take into account age and abilities of children. Table 10.1 provides an example of how objectives can grow in substance and complexity from levels 1 through 4, with the numerals representing unspecified school grades from lowest to highest. The categories A through D suggest logical sequences for objectives at the different levels. The table is adapted from a curriculum design developed under the concept stated above: *Food selection and eating patterns are determined by physical, social, mental, economic, and cultural factors.*[7] The purpose of the table is to demonstrate a method of handling the progression-sequence problem, not to advocate the approach used or the objectives, as stated.

Because of their general nature, objectives as presesented on curriculum guides usually represent long-range goals of comprehensive programs rather than immediate objectives of shorter units of work. For example, a guide may establish the following general goals: to comprehend that the choice of foods determines the nutritive balance vital to growth and development throughout life; to be aware of similarities and differences in nutrient content and value among foods;

**Table 10.1**  Food Selection and Eating Patterns:  Behavioral Objectives:  Progression and Sequence for Teaching-Learning Experience

| Progression Level* | SEQUENCE | | | |
| --- | --- | --- | --- | --- |
| | A | B | C | D |
| 1 | Distinguishes among a wide range of foods | States reasons for eating a variety of foods | Is aware of factors that detract from or enhance eating certain foods | Identifies ways that types of foods and patterns of eating may be related to different cultures |
| 2 | Describes food nutrients and their functions as they relate to health | Develops acceptable criteria for food selection and patterns of eating | Cites examples of social and emotional influences on nutritional behavior | Relates different eating patterns to circumstances of living |
| 3 | Explains how personal experiences and concerns influence food choices | Compares ways that nutritional status enhances or deters physical, mental, and social attainments | Discusses temporary and long-lasting health problems resulting from quality of food selection and eating patterns | Illustrates how nutritional requirements vary in relation to such factors as heredity, age, sex, activity, and state of health |
| 4 | Analyzes physical, mental-emotional, social, and economic factors that affect an individual's diet | Interprets relationships between nutritional status and disease | Assesses the interrelatedness of diet, activity, and other factors to the control of weight | Develops a plan of nutritional behavior that promotes health for himself and his family |

SOURCE: Excerpts from table reprinted with permission from *Food Selection and Eating Patterns*. Teaching-Learning Guides, St. Paul: Minnesota Mining and Manufacturing Co., 1972 © 1967 by School Health Education Study, Inc.
*Four progression levels; no grades specified therein.

and to demonstrate nutritional behavior reflecting knowledge of the nutritive values of foods.[7] The more immediate corresponding objectives, reflecting needs of children in the classroom, may be to learn to like and eat regularly certain dark leafy green and deep yellow vegetables, to recognize and choose more nutritious snacks, to eat a good breakfast daily before coming to school.

Thus many objectives may be attained in a nutrition education program. Children may acquire certain information about foods; become more aware of the importance of nutrition to health; and they may learn to assemble foods in nutritionally adequate meals. But, if they fail to apply such information routinely in terms of improved food practices, a significant objective of the learning is lost. "It is a false assumption that learning, knowing and behaving are the same process."[8]

## Learning Experiences

Learning experiences are the means by which objectives are achieved. The more closely experiences relate to objectives, the better is learning facilitated. Broadly conceived, learning experiences include the acquiring of suitable background information as well as the specific activities in which students engage, as part of the learning process. One potential source of nutrition information for students is health textbooks. They can be useful if the facts are sound and if they are geared to the learning level of the children. Currently there are several health series designed for elementary schools which include some timely, reliable nutrition information, suitably presented. Unfortunately, for many classrooms no health texts are available; fewer still have access to the up-to-date attractive books. Those often found in classrooms contain little or nothing on nutrition, or the nutrition content is obsolete, erroneous, or misleading. Frequently they are drab and uninviting in format. Accurate and timely reference material for teachers is also essential if they are to guide learning experiences effectively. Nutrition curriculum guides should, and sometimes do, provide certain relevant nutrition information. The ability of teachers to choose, interpret, and apply nutrition material appropriately depends largely on the extent and quality of their preservice or in-service nutrition education.

Learning experiences should offer new and challenging concepts as a child proceeds through school. In general the types of nutrition activities suitable are those comparable to learning levels of subject areas in which nutrition is integrated. Those activities too difficult or too simple fail to meet objectives. When familiar topics recur, at advancing levels, they must take into consideration the greater understanding of students and their superior ability to interpret and apply more complex material. Children in a first grade, for example, might explore and discuss taste and textures of starches and sugars as items in their daily foods, while at higher levels they might apply tests to identify starches and sugars chemically and consider carbohydrate foods as components in national and international food supplies. How can individual teachers, at specific grade levels, find their niche and contribute effectively to this progressive learning process?

Obviously, a sequential nutrition education curriculum guide offers a basis for selecting suitable learning experiences at each level. Its reliability depends on the skill and knowledge with which it is developed. At its best, it should help teachers identify subject boundaries for their own class levels and grasp their function to provide background for learning at higher levels. It should be particularly helpful in meeting problems of repetition when nutrition topics (as dental health) normally appear at regular intervals throughout the elementary school period. Under such circumstances, the curriculum guide would be expected to differentiate between the approaches to be made at each new entry. The challenge is to provide new information at a higher level which will offer greater insights into a more advanced situation. Reintroduction of topics, without suitable sequence, results in repetition, and undue repetition has proved to be a deterrent to nutrition learning. Overuse of the Basic-Four food guide in elementary schools is often cited as an example of this error. It seems likely that the fault lies not in the concept of a simple pattern for choosing meals but in its continuous, unvarying application in nutrition teaching. Procedure more compatible with modern learning theory would call for planned emphasis on the pattern at suitable grade intervals, always with new learning objectives and more involved learning experiences, relevant to the higher learning level. Such an approach would relieve tedium in early school years and forestall rejection of such a pattern at upper grade levels.

Another problem of suitable learning experiences relates to the question of the level at which to introduce individual food nutrients and their technical names. A sequential nutrition education curriculum guide should offer teachers basic direction in this respect, but the question of placement is not completely resolved among nutrition educators and there may be occasions for legitimate variation in practice. In early years of nutrition education programs, recommendations largely favored delay in common use of nutrient names until students reached upper grades or high school. This was on the theory that "mouthing" the words did not signify understanding and that habitual use of the terms had the same negative effect of repetition, just discussed, before the time came for meaningful application. More recently there has been a tendency to introduce individual nutrients at an earlier school level in the belief that children are now more conversant with such terms, as a result of television programs and advertisements, and are curious about them. Since interest and curiosity create conditions for learning, an opportunity is thus presented. Curriculum guides, in the main, take a somewhat conservative position on the question of nutrition terminology placement, in line with general interests among children. It has been suggested that teachers meet the challenge for more advanced and specific information when children themselves ask for it. However, elementary school teachers, untrained in nutrition, should not be expected to handle questions involving nutrients and their functions. They should be prepared to call upon scientific staff in their schools or professional members of the community to answer technical questions raised, or to assist in directing learning experiences which may arise as a result of such questions.

In upper grades and high school, students should investigate, explore, experiment—in the classroom, in the laboratory, at home, and in the community. Experiments should be entered into seriously with a view to satisfying the genuine curiosity and interest of students with respect to nutrition. Students should be encouraged to initiate their own activities and carry them through, individually and in groups, with considerable independence, but with competent consultation always available. Nutrition learning activities in subjects such as biology, health, and home economics can take many different forms and directions compatible with the original subject.[9-11]

Students at all development levels enjoy food experiences. They vary from identifying and tasting individual foods or putting together simple snacks to planning, shopping for, cooking, and serving meals. Inherent nutrition learning situations are many.[9,12,13] It is important to apply the principles of learning in selecting and implementing food experiences. Purposeful effort and genuine involvement are essential. If children in a fourth grade, for example, with proper guidance, take chief responsibility for direction and preparation of a breakfast at school, and if all of the children perform tasks commensurate with their abilities, the activity provides many learnings. If, on the other hand, high school home economics students or mothers prepare and serve the meal or assume major responsibility for it, learning opportunities are greatly lessened. Improved food practices are a natural outcome of food experiences if objectives have been properly established and serve as goals of the learning activities.

Increasingly students are finding learning experiences in the school lunchroom (chapter 9). School food-service personnel are serving as resources for elementary school classrooms and for specialized subject areas at upper grade levels. They strive for student acceptance of foods in lunchrooms by working with committees of children to plan meals that meet both student approval and government lunch specifications. Students become involved in other related learning experiences: taste panels to judge when a new dish has met criteria for general service on the cafeteria counter; food preference surveys among student patrons; plate waste studies after introduction of new foods; and explorations with flavors of unfamiliar foods, by trying typical dishes of countries of the world currently under classroom study.

### Learning Aids

Just what qualifies as a learning aid? Any resource or device used as a tool to make nutrition education more effective. These may be persons, places, or things found in the school, the home, the community, or the outside world. Teachers and students are literally surrounded by potentially effective resource materials that often are neither recognized, as such, or utilized. Such materials, found in the school setting are legion—reference books, food models, the school lunch, school garden. Homes are also a rich reservoir of resources: family pets, the home orchard, animals, and crops in a farm setting; family members—fathers, mothers, grandparents—who may be called upon to teach a skill, explain a process, or supervise the building of equipment needed in the program. Resources of the community include those persons and things that make nutrition education a reality. Grocers, policemen, nurserymen, naturalists, dairymen, beekeepers, bakers, and the places where they work can bring classroom experiences to life.

Such resources can stimulate and broaden the scope of nutrition education and facilitate learning. Because of the vast number of aids available, teachers have responsibility to choose those which give greatest promise of helping achieve objectives. In the main, teachers tend to use too many different aids and often apply them in ways which are unproductive in the learning process. Learning aids should be just that—with emphasis on strengthening the learning process, not dominating it. Ready-made devices should not overshadow teachers' and learners' own efforts.

The importance of properly chosen instructional aids can scarcely be overestimated. Aids which help students visualize and understand a problem help them solve it. Learning to eat good lunches can best be taught in the school lunchroom; learning to like vegetables is encouraged most successfully when, with teachers and peers, they are tasted at school. Mere contact with a resource may be stimulative but unless it contributes to problem solving, it fails of its major purpose.

In addition to nontraditional types of resources cited, there are an overwhelming number of formal instructional aids designed for nutrition education.[14] These include printed books and leaflets, posters, charts, flannel graphs, films, film strips, slides, records, tape recordings, games, and devices for self-teaching. The very number of such resources available heightens the problem of selection. Their use in a given learning situation should meet stringent tests of relevance. Following are some of the ways they may function at different points in nutrition teaching:

> To create interest, to stimulate thinking and questions: photographs, posters, slides, films
>
> To work toward the stated objectives: textbooks, readers, records, plant growth experiments, role playing
>
> To make learning experiences contribute to understanding: field trips, photographs, animal feeding demonstrations, television programs, slide films
>
> To summarize a unit: recordings, dramatizations, graphs, scrapbooks, exhibits, homemade films or slides, dioramas

When the choice of resources is to be made, two criteria are paramount: reliability of subject matter and effectiveness as an educational tool. Selection of materials calls for standards that can be applied to judging their worth. If the following questions can be answered in the affirmative, the aid gives promise as a useful resource.[9]

> Is the nutrition subject matter sound, free of bias and food fads? (Teachers should check this question with a nutritionist if the content is in doubt.)
>
> Is it suited to the learning level, the interests and needs of the children?
>
> Does it provide pertinent, timely, up-to-date information that contributes to the solution of the problem at hand?

Sometimes suggestions dealing with the use of teaching aids can best be stated negatively. The following are examples of practices to be avoided:

Avoid adopting resources that are being widely publicized before making a careful analysis of their potential value as learning tools. Nutrition games are a case in point. Games based largely on skill in memorizing and utilizing prescribed nutrition facts fail to apply the principles of learning. Individual students or groups may well devise their own games with the purpose of making the project a learning experience.

Avoid repeating dramatic animal feeding demonstrations without checking scientific consultants on their validity. Especially to be avoided are tests of nutritious foods, fed as sole items of diet. They yield misleading results and can lead to erroneous conclusions with respect to using wholesome foods in an ordinary mixed diet.[15]

Avoid using classroom films, film strips, slides, television programs, unless they make specific contributions to the subject under study. Do not show films and other visual aids without previews.

One of the most valuable resources for classroom teachers is the assistance available from specialists in nutrition, health, and education in the locality (chapter 9). If school programs are to embody correct concepts of nutrition and nutrition education, professional assistance in these fields must be available to teachers on a continuing basis.

### Evaluation of Learning

Evaluation is gathering evidence on the extent to which objectives are achieved. In discussing this concept, Wolf has this to say on the scope of evaluation:

The term of "gathering evidence" includes not only tests that we would give to students or learners to find out what they know, but also observations we would make about what they are doing, what they are feeling, what they are interested in and thinking about, as well as a variety of other formal and informal procedures—so that "evaluation" is much broader than "testing" or "measurement". Evaluation has to deal with the gathering of all kinds of evidence that will give us some indication of the extent to which our objectives are being attained.[16]

Evaluation is an integral part of the curriculum and instructional process. It is considered here particularly to emphasize its importance in the development and operation of a nutrition education program. Almost continuous evaluation serves as a rudder for keeping a program on course as it moves toward its learning objectives. When this is done evaluation itself becomes an aspect of learning experiences and adequate time is allowed for teachers and students to engage in it together. Curriculum content should be subject to constant adjustment and modification in response to current needs of pupils. Evaluation reveals where changes should be made, and their nature.

*Evaluating Behavior Change.* The influence of learning is measured by comparing what behavior was possible before an individual was exposed to a learning situation and what behavior was possible afterward. Many types of evidence are sought in evaluating nutrition education programs. One type is largely cognitive and usually employs paper and pencil tests such as multiple-choice, true-false, and essay. They call for specific knowledge of nutrition facts and principles as well as ability to apply the principles, their complexity depending on the grade level where used. A common example of such tests is to require a child to show on paper how to assemble from a given list of assorted foods, meals which conform to specific patterns. It is conceded that knowledge of *what* to do is basic to doing it correctly; therefore a good showing in such tests would be acceptable as one way to measure behavior.

Attitude change is another type of evaluative evidence sought. Attitudes are in the affective domain and involve such characteristics as awareness, appreciation, tolerance, and development of a value system. Attitudes are more difficult to measure than knowledge, but progress is being made in devising authenticated evaluative tools for the purpose.[17] Informal probings are valuable for supplementing the more objective measures, if they are made with affective goals in mind. Once nutrition activities are under way in the classroom, teachers can note how children react to nutrition concepts and utilize them in planned learning experiences, how they approach and deal with nutrition problems that arise. Do students exhibit increasing leadership in group activities? Are they assuming more responsibility for their own food practices? Similar evidence can be provided by parents and by anecdotal records and diaries kept by teachers and/or students.

The most challenging aspect of evaluation of nutrition education lies in measuring performance in terms of objectives sought. Various observational procedures are used as evaluative techniques to determine whether the learner actually performs differently as a result of his new knowledge of nutrition and his changed attitudes. It goes beyond the behavioral objective of showing *how* to do it to the stage of accountability which implies adopting the practice. Demonstrated improvement in food practices of children is the most coveted evidence of the benefits of nutrition education. The importance of this evidence makes the discovery and application of accepted evaluative techniques a critical concern. To obtain evidence of changed eating practices, teachers should employ every valid means. It is not easy. The inherent weakness of any self-reporting device is the basic problem. Experience has shown that people do not remember well what they have eaten and that postprogram reports are apt to reflect what the child learner has been taught, rather than what he does.

An alternative is to observe children in free-choice situations, when they are in a position to select foods at will and are not under the direct scrutiny of adults at the point of selection. Choices in the school lunchroom can provide such a setting if there is a free-choice lunch or, in lesser degree, if there is leeway for substituting foods in the Type A lunch formula. The acceptance of certain foods in the lunch, once rejected, can likewise be an indication of learning. In situations where children are permitted to choose between the school lunch and less desirable meals on the outside, the mere choice of the school lunch may represent progress. Examination of packed lunches is a legitimate evaluative measure if a lunch represents a child's own choice. Improvement is indicated when it includes nutritious foods, once spurned. Reduction in plate waste can likewise be used as a measure if it can be related to increased acceptability of food, as a result of nutrition education. School tasting lessons offer an evaluative device if they reflect the extent to which desired foods have added to the variety and nutritive value of meals.

There are ways to collect bits of information, informally, chiefly from parents, which may contribute indirectly to the general picture of improved patterns of eating. Children may be helping more with family marketing, packing their own lunches, assisting with preparation of home meals. Children themselves may volunteer information on their home food practices if the atmosphere of the classroom is one of candor.

The effort continues to obtain measurable indications of improvement in food practices of schoolchildren as an outcome of nutrition education, but there are those who maintain that full satisfaction in that respect is impossible. They point out that most meals are eaten outside the school under conditions which defy efforts to apply evaluative techniques. Evidence gathered today largely indicates not what children have learned but what they are practicing in a parent-controlled situation. Others postulate that the benefits of nutrition education are often delayed, that children practice, years later, what they have learned in the present. In support of this theory, in a nationwide survey of private households, more homemakers reported they learned about nutrition in high school than from any other source.[18] There are still others who believe the benefits most to be sought from nutrition education lie in a broader but intangible area which cannot be measured, that is, the diffusion of favorable attitudes toward foods and nutrition throughout school, home, and community. Some, like Passow, imply that we are perhaps too concerned with evaluating specific activities and neglecting those which are more fundamental to eventual understanding. He says our concern for nutrition education needs to be thought of in terms not just of curriculum or content instruction but rather how nutrition education pervades the entire educational process, directly and indirectly, "by the way we educators behave, by our own attitudes, by our own interactions and relationships." The challenge for nutritionists, Passow says, is "to think of nutrition education in terms of how it permeates the lives of our children and our youth."[19]

*Evaluating Nutritional Environment.* One logical objective of the nutrition education program may be to improve the school environment in behalf of better food practices of children. Issues include availability of sweets and "junk" foods on school premises and failure to use the school lunch to its full educational potential. Evaluative techniques are simple, direct questions: Have candy, soft drinks, and unwholesome snack foods been excluded from sale on school premises? Have changes been made in the school's schedule to permit sufficient time for a lunch period free from pressure? Have efforts been made to further the influence of the school lunch as a nutrition teaching tool? Are there arrangements to prevent children from spending all or a portion of their lunch money for miscellaneous other foods, thus making it impossible to buy the full planned lunch?

The ultimate in evaluation of nutrition education is the nutritional health of the children themselves. Teachers may have a part in the measuring procedures. The school physician, nurse, dentist, and others are involved. Progress in health status may be real even though evidence is inconclusive due to the evaluative devices used by the school. Better school attendance and fewer minor illnesses may have some significance as indicative of the effectiveness of the program. In schools which keep a visual record of children's growth throughout school life, teachers may plot height and weight curves which indicate whether they move upward consistently. Some such records show also which children maintain their positions in corresponding zones for height and weight (chapter 4). In cases of deviation, a physician may look for possible causes which, in some cases, may be nutritional in nature and will respond to educational procedures.

Thus, there are many methods of evaluation of nutrition education: formal and informal, objective and subjective, simple and complex. All make some contribution in the effort to assess what has been accomplished by a nutrition education program.

## Parents of Child Learners

The home has been aptly called "the hidden curriculum." Groundwork for children's food practices, good or bad, is laid in their homes. Their eating habits are inseparable from family food practices and the latter, in turn, are rooted in generations of racial and religious customs. The sooner teachers realize that programs to improve food practices of young children must extend beyond classrooms into homes, the sooner will they try to involve parents in the process. Teachers cannot fully understand their students' needs and how to meet them until they know parents and the homes from which the children come. They must know, for example, the types of meals served in homes, what influences family meal patterns, the attitudes of parents toward food, and have some comprehension of the family's problems, economic or other, with respect to food. However, there is little evidence that teachers take advantage of the extraschool learning opportunities offered them.[20] Teachers should make a conscious effort to bring parents into the learning arena and parents should respond to teachers and children more actively in broadening the base of learning. Regular contacts and meaningful participation from curriculum construction to classroom experiences have proved to be effective collaborative procedures.

Changes taking place in homes have a direct effect on food practices of families and indirectly implicate nutrition education in schools. Children today see less of their parents and spend less time in their homes than formerly. They start to school at an earlier age and more of them leave home for college in their teens. Also more mothers are employed outside their homes than before and more meals and snacks are eaten away from the family table. These facts suggest that the home's influence on children's food practices is changing. Obviously such a situation requires a new perspective and a different approach— not an abdication of responsibility. Parents need to recognize and analyze the new conditions created and take practical steps to deal with them. They are still key factors in children's nutrition learning.

Older children are already responding. It is estimated that fourteen million teenagers prepare an average of eleven family meals per week and shop for what they cook. Such children need parental training in planning, buying, cooking, and serving home meals. School nutrition programs should be geared to give maximum support. Also, with more meals and snacks eaten away from home, children need help in choosing meals and snacks from a menu and instruction on how to evaluate prices in terms of nutritive values. Personal guidance and consultation on the part of parents and assumption of responsibility on the part of children constitute a team effort which can result in growth in nutrition learning. Here are the inherent needs and problems which provide motivations for learning. While this approach is a departure from the traditional parent-child relationship, with respect to food and meals in homes, it offers rewarding learning opportunities for both parents and children.

## The Community: Setting for Learning

If the purpose of education is truly to prepare children for living, the community—in the sense of the broader world beyond school and home—must be fully utilized as settings.[3,20,21] Education, at all levels, is closely bound to social, economic, and political forces and their change. Classrooms must be extended literally to encompass the community—people and objects to provide the subject matter; the entire community to be the educator. Examples of traditional ways children may relate school nutrition experiences to the community have been cited earlier but educators are looking beyond that to a more sophisticated type of community involvement. So strongly do some educators believe that children learn what they live that they envision a work-study program for students from the time they enter school.[22] The curriculum of the school would provide for active participation in the real world. Programs would be planned and sequential. Students would carry on much of their educative activities at locations in the community where special resources are available, such as industries, hospitals, restaurants, stores. The school would have essentially a coordinating function. Such a philosophy of learning may have special significance for nutrition education.

Currently some secondary schools carry on work-study programs routinely. A few high schools offer a "rich variety of participatory experiences" in the world of work.[22] Some exploratory projects of the more adventurous and comprehensive type have obtained financial support from foundations for further experimentation. Thus far there are very few examples at the lower grade levels. Meantime all schools are attempting to extend their boundaries beyond the school walls.

Involvement of the community in child learning is a two-way street. The school staff and students need to reach out to learn about the community, its organization and its offerings. The community through its citizens needs to acquaint the school with its resources. In some school districts a community representative is a member of the curriculum planning committee. He is in a position to interpret community needs to the school and to suggest community resources which can become part of the school curriculum.

It seems clear that the more completely the school, the home, and the community are integrated into one continuous environment favorable to the child learner, the more is learning facilitated. It is through conscious and coordinated effort on the part of those functioning in these three areas that the environment can be made to exert a consistent and unified influence on the learning of children.

## References

1  Gagne, R. M. *The Conditions of Learning.* New York: Holt, Rinehart & Winston, 1970.

2  Gordon, I. J. *On Early Learning.* Washington, D.C.: Association for Supervision and Curriculum Development, 1971.

3  Murphy, L. B., and Leeper, E. M. *Conditions for Learning.* Publication (OCD) 74–1034. Washington, D.C.: U.S. Department of Health, Education, and Welfare, 1974.

4  Gross, D. W. "Curiosity in Context." *Childhood Education* 51(1975): 242–43.

5  Trubowitz, S. "The Listening Teacher." *Childhood Education* 51(1975): 319–22.

6  Gross, D. W. "Encouraging the Curious Mind through the Curriculum." *Childhood Education* 51(1974):5–7.

7  *Food Selection and Eating Patterns.* Teaching-Learning Guides, School Health Education Guides. St. Paul: Minnesota Mining and Manufacturing Co., 1972.

8  Kneller, G. F. "Behavioral Objectives? No!" *Educational Leadership* 29 (1972):397–400.

9  Martin, E. A. *Nutrition Education in Action.* New York: Holt, Rinehart & Winston, 1963.

10  Mills, E. R. "Applying Learning Theory in Teaching Nutrition." *Journal of Nutrition Education* 4(1972):106–7.

11  Picardi, S. M., and Pariser, E. R. "Food and Nutrition Minicourses for 11th and 12th Grades." *Journal of Nutrition Education* 7(1975):25–29.

12  McAfee, O.; Haines, E. W.; and Young, B. B. *Cooking and Eating with Children: A Way to Learn.* New York: New York Association for Childhood Education, International, 1974.

13  Goodwin, M. T., and Pollen, G. *Creative Food Experiences for Children.* Washington, D.C.: Center for Science in the Public Interest, 1974.

14  Catalog listings: *Index of Nutrition Education Materials.* Washington, D.C.: Nutrition Foundation, 1974; *Nutrition Education Materials: Annual Catalogue.* Rosemont, Ill.: National Dairy Council; *Publications List, 1977.* Chicago: Chicago Nutrition Association, 1977.

15  Hegsted, D. M., and Ausman, L. M. "Sole Foods and Some Not So Scientific Experiments." *Nutrition Today* 8(1973):22–25.

16  Wolf, R. D. "Evaluation of Techniques in Education." Paper read at the Conference on Education in Nutrition: Looking Forward from the Past, 26 February 1974, at Teachers College, Columbia University, New York, 1974.

17  Lake, D.; Miles, M.; and Earle, R. *Measuring Human Behavior.* New York: Teachers College Press, 1973.

18  *Homemakers' Food and Nutrition Knowledge, Practices and Opinions.* Home Economics research report no. 39. Washington, D.C.: U.S. Department of Agriculture, 1975.

19  Passow, A. H. "Today's Challenges in Education." Paper read at the Conference on Education in Nutrition: Looking Forward from the Past, 27 February 1974, at Teachers College, Columbia University, New York.

20  Gross, D. W. "Balancing Basics: Quality Settings for Learning." *Childhood Education* 50(1974):122–24.

21  Irwin, M., and Russell, W. "Let's Begin with the Real World." *Childhood Education* 51(1975):187–89.

22  Foshay, A. W. *Curriculum for the 70's: An Agenda for Invention.* Washington, D.C.: National Education Association, 1970.

# Appendixes

# Appendix 1

## Recommended Dietary Allowances

Designed for the maintenance of good nutrition of practically all healthy people in the United States

| | Age (years) | Weight | | Height | | Energy | Protein | Vitamin A Activity | | Vitamin D | Vitamin E Activity[e] |
|---|---|---|---|---|---|---|---|---|---|---|---|
| | | | | | | | | **Fat-Soluble Vitamins** | | | |
| | | (kg) | (lbs) | (cm) | (in) | (kcal)[b] | (g) | (RE)[c] | (IU) | (IU) | (IU) |
| Infants | 0.0-0.5 | 6 | 14 | 60 | 24 | kg × 117 | kg × 2.2 | 420[d] | 1,400 | 400 | 4 |
| | 0.5-1.0 | 9 | 20 | 71 | 28 | kg × 108 | kg × 2.0 | 400 | 2,000 | 400 | 5 |
| Children | 1-3 | 13 | 28 | 86 | 34 | 1300 | 23 | 400 | 2,000 | 400 | 7 |
| | 4-6 | 20 | 44 | 110 | 44 | 1800 | 30 | 500 | 2,500 | 400 | 9 |
| | 7-10 | 30 | 66 | 135 | 54 | 2400 | 36 | 700 | 3,300 | 400 | 10 |
| Males | 11-14 | 44 | 97 | 158 | 63 | 2800 | 44 | 1,000 | 5,000 | 400 | 12 |
| | 15-18 | 61 | 134 | 172 | 69 | 3000 | 54 | 1,000 | 5,000 | 400 | 15 |
| | 19-22 | 67 | 147 | 172 | 69 | 3000 | 54 | 1,000 | 5,000 | 400 | 15 |
| | 23-50 | 70 | 154 | 172 | 69 | 2700 | 56 | 1,000 | 5,000 | | 15 |
| | 51+ | 70 | 154 | 172 | 69 | 2400 | 56 | 1,000 | 5,000 | | 15 |
| Females | 11-14 | 44 | 97 | 155 | 62 | 2400 | 44 | 800 | 4,000 | 400 | 12 |
| | 15-18 | 54 | 119 | 162 | 65 | 2100 | 48 | 800 | 4,000 | 400 | 12 |
| | 19-22 | 58 | 128 | 162 | 65 | 2100 | 46 | 800 | 4,000 | 400 | 12 |
| | 23-50 | 58 | 128 | 162 | 65 | 2000 | 46 | 800 | 4,000 | | 12 |
| | 51+ | 58 | 128 | 162 | 65 | 1800 | 46 | 800 | 4,000 | | 12 |
| Pregnant | | | | | | +300 | +30 | 1,000 | 5,000 | 400 | 15 |
| Lactating | | | | | | +500 | +20 | 1,200 | 6,000 | 400 | 15 |

[a] The allowances are intended to provide for individual variations among most normal persons as they live in the United States under usual environmental stresses. Diets should be based on a variety of common foods in order to provide other nutrients for which human requirements have been less well defined.

[b] Kilojoules (kJ) $= 4.2 \times$ kcal.

[c] Retinol equivalents.

[d] Assumed to be all as retinol in milk during the first six months of life. All subsequent intakes are assumed to be half as retinol and half as $\beta$-carotene when calculated from international units. As retinol equivalents, three-fourths are as retinol and one-fourth as $\beta$-carotene.

| Water-Soluble Vitamins | | | | | | | Minerals | | | | | |
|---|---|---|---|---|---|---|---|---|---|---|---|---|
| Ascorbic Acid (mg) | Folacin[f] (µg) | Niacin[g] (mg) | Riboflavin (B₂) (mg) | Thiamin (B₁) (mg) | Vitamin B₆ (mg) | Vitamin B₁₂ (µg) | Calcium (mg) | Phosphorus (mg) | Iodine (µg) | Iron (mg) | Magnesium (mg) | Zinc (mg) |
| 35 | 50 | 5 | 0.4 | 0.3 | 0.3 | 0.3 | 360 | 240 | 35 | 10 | 60 | 3 |
| 35 | 50 | 8 | 0.6 | 0.5 | 0.4 | 0.3 | 540 | 400 | 45 | 15 | 70 | 5 |
| 40 | 100 | 9 | 0.8 | 0.7 | 0.6 | 1.0 | 800 | 800 | 60 | 15 | 150 | 10 |
| 40 | 200 | 12 | 1.1 | 0.9 | 0.9 | 1.5 | 800 | 800 | 80 | 10 | 200 | 10 |
| 40 | 300 | 16 | 1.2 | 1.2 | 1.2 | 2.0 | 800 | 800 | 110 | 10 | 250 | 10 |
| 45 | 400 | 18 | 1.5 | 1.4 | 1.6 | 3.0 | 1200 | 1200 | 130 | 18 | 350 | 15 |
| 45 | 400 | 20 | 1.8 | 1.5 | 2.0 | 3.0 | 1200 | 1200 | 150 | 18 | 400 | 15 |
| 45 | 400 | 20 | 1.8 | 1.5 | 2.0 | 3.0 | 800 | 800 | 140 | 10 | 350 | 15 |
| 45 | 400 | 18 | 1.6 | 1.4 | 2.0 | 3.0 | 800 | 800 | 130 | 10 | 350 | 15 |
| 45 | 400 | 16 | 1.5 | 1.2 | 2.0 | 3.0 | 800 | 800 | 110 | 10 | 350 | 15 |
| 45 | 400 | 16 | 1.3 | 1.2 | 1.6 | 3.0 | 1200 | 1200 | 115 | 18 | 300 | 15 |
| 45 | 400 | 14 | 1.4 | 1.1 | 2.0 | 3.0 | 1200 | 1200 | 115 | 18 | 300 | 15 |
| 45 | 400 | 14 | 1.4 | 1.1 | 2.0 | 3.0 | 800 | 800 | 100 | 18 | 300 | 15 |
| 45 | 400 | 13 | 1.2 | 1.0 | 2.0 | 3.0 | 800 | 800 | 100 | 18 | 300 | 15 |
| 45 | 400 | 12 | 1.1 | 1.0 | 2.0 | 3.0 | 800 | 800 | 80 | 10 | 300 | 15 |
| 60 | 800 | +2 | +0.3 | +0.3 | 2.5 | 4.0 | 1200 | 1200 | 125 | 18+[h] | 450 | 20 |
| 80 | 600 | +4 | +0.5 | +0.3 | 2.5 | 4.0 | 1200 | 1200 | 150 | 18 | 450 | 25 |

[e] Total vitamin E activity, estimated to be 80 percent as α-tocopherol and 20 percent other tocopherols.

[f] The folacin allowances refer to dietary sources as determined by *Lactobacillus casei* assay. Pure forms of folacin may be effective in doses less than one-fourth of the recommended dietary allowance.

[g] Although allowances are expressed as niacin, it is recognized that on the average 1 mg of niacin is derived from each 60 mg of dietary tryptophan.

[h] This increased requirement cannot be met by ordinary diets; therefore, the use of supplemental iron is recommended.

SOURCE: Food and Nutrition Board. *Recommended Dietary Allowances,* 8th ed. Washington, D.C.: National Academy of Science-National Research Council, 1974.

# Appendix 2

## Current Guidelines for Criteria of Nutritional Status for Laboratory Evaluation

| Nutrient and Units | Age of Subject (years) | Deficient | Marginal | Acceptable |
|---|---|---|---|---|
| *Hemoglobin (gm/100ml) | 6-23 mos. | Up to 9.0 | 9.0- 9.9 | 10.0+ |
| | 2-5 | Up to 10.0 | 10.0-10.9 | 11.0+ |
| | 6-12 | Up to 10.0 | 10.0-11.4 | 11.5+ |
| | 13-16M | Up to 12.0 | 12.0-12.9 | 13.0+ |
| | 13-16F | Up to 10.0 | 10.0-11.4 | 11.5+ |
| | 16+M | Up to 12.0 | 12.0-13.9 | 14.0+ |
| | 16+F | Up to 10.0 | 10.0-11.9 | 12.0+ |
| | Pregnant (after 6+ mos.) | Up to 9.5 | 9.5-10.9 | 11.0+ |
| *Hematocrit (Packed cell volume in percent) | Up to 2 | Up to 28 | 28-30 | 31+ |
| | 2-5 | Up to 30 | 30-33 | 34+ |
| | 6-12 | Up to 30 | 30-35 | 36+ |
| | 13-16M | Up to 37 | 37-39 | 40+ |
| | 13-16F | Up to 31 | 31-35 | 36+ |
| | 16+M | Up to 37 | 37-43 | 44+ |
| | 16+F | Up to 31 | 31-37 | 33+ |
| | Pregnant | Up to 30 | 30-32 | 33+ |
| *Serum Albumin (gm/100ml) | Up to 1 | — | Up to 2.5 | 2.5+ |
| | 1-5 | — | Up to 3.0 | 3.0+ |
| | 6-16 | — | Up to 3.5 | 3.5+ |
| | 16+ | Up to 2.8 | 2.8-3.4 | 3.5+ |
| | Pregnant | Up to 3.0 | 3.0-3.4 | 3.5+ |
| *Serum Protein (gm/100ml) | Up to 1 | — | Up to 5.0 | 5.0+ |
| | 1-5 | — | Up to 5.5 | 5.5+ |
| | 6-16 | — | Up to 6.0 | 6.0+ |
| | 16+ | Up to 6.0 | 6.0-6.4 | 6.5+ |
| | Pregnant | Up to 5.5 | 5.5-5.9 | 6.0+ |
| *Serum Ascorbic Acid (mg/100ml) | All ages | Up to 0.1 | 0.1-0.19 | 0.2+ |
| *Plasma vitamin A (mcg/100 ml) | All ages | Up to 10 | 10-19 | 20+ |
| *Plasma Carotene (mcg/100 ml) | All ages | Up to 20 | 20-39 | 40+ |
| | Pregnant | — | 40-79 | 80+ |
| *Serum Iron (mcg/100 ml) | Up to 2 | Up to 30 | — | 30+ |
| | 2-5 | Up to 40 | — | 40+ |
| | 6-12 | Up to 50 | — | 50+ |
| | 12+M | Up to 60 | — | 60+ |
| | 12+F | Up to 40 | — | 40+ |
| *Transferrin Saturation (percent) | Up to 2 | Up to 15.0 | — | 15.0+ |
| | 2-12 | Up to 20.0 | — | 20.0+ |
| | 12+M | Up to 20.0 | — | 20.0+ |
| | 12+F | Up to 15.0 | — | 15.0+ |
| **Serum Folacin (ng/ml) | All ages | Up to 2.0 | 2.1-5.9 | 6.0+ |
| **Serum vitamin $B_{12}$ (pg/ml) | All ages | Up to 100 | — | 100+ |

* Adapted from the Ten State Nutrition Survey
** Criteria may vary with different methodology.

*Adapted from the Ten State Nutrition Survey.
**Criteria may vary with different methodology.

| Nutrient and Units | Age of Subject (years) | Criteria of Status | | |
|---|---|---|---|---|
| | | Deficient | Marginal | Acceptable |
| *Thiamine in Urine (mcg/g creatinine) | 1-3 | Up to 120 | 120-175 | 175+ |
| | 4-5 | Up to 85 | 85-120 | 120+ |
| | 6-9 | Up to 70 | 70-180 | 180+ |
| | 10-15 | Up to 55 | 55-150 | 150+ |
| | 16+ | Up to 27 | 27- 65 | 65+ |
| | Pregnant | Up to 21 | 21- 49 | 50+ |
| *Riboflavin in Urine (mcg/g creatinine) | 1-3 | Up to 150 | 150-499 | 500+ |
| | 4-5 | Up to 100 | 100-299 | 300+ |
| | 6-9 | Up to 85 | 85-269 | 270+ |
| | 10-16 | Up to 70 | 70-199 | 200+ |
| | 16+ | Up to 27 | 27- 79 | 80+ |
| | Pregnant | Up to 30 | 30- 89 | 90+ |
| **RBC Transketolase-TPP-effect (ratio) | All ages | 25+ | 15- 25 | Up to 15 |
| **RBC Glutathione Reductase-FAD-effect (ratio) | All ages | 1.2+ | — | Up to 1.2 |
| **Tryptophan Load (mg Xanthurenic acid excreted) | Adults (Dose: 100mg/kg body weight) | 25+(6 hrs.) 75+(24 hrs.) | — — | Up to 25 Up to 75 |
| **Urinary Pyridoxine (mcg/g creatinine) | 1-3 | Up to 90 | — | 90+ |
| | 4-6 | Up to 80 | — | 80+ |
| | 7-9 | Up to 60 | — | 60+ |
| | 10-12 | Up to 40 | — | 40+ |
| | 13-15 | Up to 30 | — | 30+ |
| | 16+ | Up to 20 | — | 20+ |
| *Urinary N'methyl nicotinamide (mg/g creatinine) | All ages | Up to 0.2 | 0.2-5.59 | 0.6+ |
| | Pregnant | Up to 0.8 | 0.8-2.49 | 2.5+ |
| **Urinary Pantothenic Acid (mcg) | All ages | Up to 200 | — | 200+ |
| **Plasma vitamin E (mg/100ml) | All ages | Up to 0.2 | 0.2-0.6 | 0.6+ |
| **Transaminase Index (ratio) | | | | |
| †EGOT | Adult | 2.0 + | — | Up to 2.0 |
| ‡EGPT | Adult | 1.25+ | — | Up to 1.25 |

\* Adapted from the Ten State Nutrition Survey
\*\* Criteria may vary with different methodology
† Erythrocyte Glutamic Oxalacetic Transaminase
‡ Erythrocyte Glutamic Pyruvic Transaminase

\*Adapted from the Ten State Nutrition Survey.
\*\*Criteria may vary with different methodology.
†Erythrocyte glutamic oxaloacetic transaminase.
‡Erythrocyte glutamic pyruvic transaminase.

SOURCE: Reprinted, with permission, from Christakis, G., ed. "Nutritional Assessment in Health Programs." *American Journal of Public Health* 63(1973[suppl.]):34–35.

# Appendix 3

## Food Intake: Form A—
## Twenty-Four-Hour Recall

Name _____

Date & Time of Interview _____

Length of Interview _____

Date of Recall _____

Day of the week of Recall

      1–M    2–T    3–W    4–Th    5–F    6–Sat    7–Sun

"I would like you to tell me about everything your child ate and drank from the time he got up in the morning until the time he went to bed at night and what he ate during the night. Be sure to mention everything he ate or drank at home, at school, and away from home. Include snacks and drinks of all kinds and everything else he put in his mouth and swallowed. I also need to know where he ate the food, but now let us begin."

What time did he get up yesterday?_____

Was it the usual time?_____

What was the first time he ate or had anything to drink yesterday morning? (list on the form that follows)

Where did he eat? (list on the form that follows)

Now tell me what he had to eat and how much?

(*Occasionally the interviewer will need to ask:*)
    When did he eat again? or, is there anything else?
    Did he have anything to eat or drink during the night?

Was intake unusual in any way? Yes _____ No _____

(If answer is yes) Why? _____

               In what way? _____

_____

What time did he go to bed last night? _____

Does he take vitamin and/or mineral supplements?

             Yes _____ No _____

(If answer is yes) How many per day?_____

                   Per week?_____

What kind? (Insert brand name if known)

Multivitamins_____

Ascorbic Acid_____

Vitamins A and D_____

Iron_____

Other_____

## Suggested Form for Recording Food Intake

| Time | Where Eaten* | Food | Type and/or Preparation | Amount | Food Code** | Amount Code** |
|------|--------------|------|-------------------------|--------|-------------|---------------|
|      |              |      |                         |        |             |               |
|      |              |      |                         |        |             |               |
|      |              |      |                         |        |             |               |

SOURCE: U.S. Department of Health, Education, and Welfare. *Screening Children for Nutritional Status: Suggestions for Child Health Programs.* Washington, D.C.: Superintendent of Documents, Government Printing Office, 1971.

*Code

H—Home

R—Restaurant, drug store or lunch counter

CL—Carried lunch from home

CC—Child care center

OH—Other home (of a friend, babysitter, or relative)

S—School

FD—Food dispenser

**Do not write in these spaces

# Appendix 3

## Food Intake: Form B— Dietary Questionnaire

Name_____

Date_____

1. Does the child eat at regular times each day?_____

2. How many days a week does he eat—
    a morning meal?_____
    a lunch or mid-day meal?_____
    an evening meal?_____
    during the night*_____

3. How many days a week does he have snacks—
    in mid-morning? _____
    in mid-afternoon?_____
    in the evening?_____
    during the night*_____

4. Which meals does he usually eat with your family?
    None ___ Breakfast ___ Noon Meal ___ Evening Meal ___

5. How many times per week does he eat at school or child care center or day camp?
    Breakfast _____ Lunch _____ Between meals _____

6. Would you describe his appetite as Good? _____ Fair? _____ Poor?_____

7. At what time of day is he most hungry?
    Morning _____ Noon _____ Evening _____

8. What foods does he dislike?_____
    _____

9. Is he on a special diet now? Yes _____ No _____

    If *Yes*, why is he on a diet? (check)
    _____for weight reduction (own prescription)
    _____for weight reduction (doctor's prescription)
    _____for gaining weight
    _____for allergy, specify _____
    _____for other reason, specify _____

298

If *No*, has he been on a special diet within the past year?
Yes _____ No _____
If *Yes*, for what reason? _____

10. Does he eat anything which is not usually considered food? Yes___ No___
    If *Yes*, what?_____ How often?_____

11. Can he feed himself? Yes___ No___
    If *Yes*, with his fingers? _____ with a spoon? _____

12. Can he use a cup or glass by himself? Yes___ No___

13. Does he drink from a bottle with a nipple? Yes___ No___
    If *Yes*, how often?_____ At what times of day or night?
    _____

14. How many times *per week* does he eat the following foods (at any meal or
    between meals)?
    Circle the appropriate number:

    Bacon ......................... 0 1 2 3 4 5 6 7 >7, specify_____
    Tongue ........................ 0 1 2 3 4 5 6 7 >7, specify_____
    Sausage ....................... 0 1 2 3 4 5 6 7 >7, specify_____
    Luncheon meat ................. 0 1 2 3 4 5 6 7 >7, specify_____
    Hot dogs ...................... 0 1 2 3 4 5 6 7 >7, specify_____
    Liver—chicken ................. 0 1 2 3 4 5 6 7 >7, specify_____
    Liver—other ................... 0 1 2 3 4 5 6 7 >7, specify_____
    Poultry ....................... 0 1 2 3 4 5 6 7 >7, specify_____
    Salt pork ..................... 0 1 2 3 4 5 6 7 >7, specify_____
    Pork or ham ................... 0 1 2 3 4 5 6 7 >7, specify_____.
    Bones (neck or other) ......... 0 1 2 3 4 5 6 7 >7, specify_____
    Meat in mixtures (stew, tamales,
      casseroles, etc.) ........... 0 1 2 3 4 5 6 7 >7, specify_____
    Beef or veal .................. 0 1 2 3 4 5 6 7 >7, specify_____
    Other meat .................... 0 1 2 3 4 5 6 7 >7, specify_____
    Fish .......................... 0 1 2 3 4 5 6 7 >7, specify_____

15. How many times *per week* does he eat the following foods (at any meal or between meals)?
    Circle the appropriate number:

    Fruit juice ....................  0  1  2  3  4  5  6  7  >7, specify____
    Fruit ........................  0  1  2  3  4  5  6  7  >7, specify____
    Cereal-dry ....................  0  1  2  3  4  5  6  7  >7, specify____
    Cereal-cooked or instant ........  0  1  2  3  4  5  6  7  >7, specify____
    Cereal-infant .................  0  1  2  3  4  5  6  7  >7, specify____
    Eggs .........................  0  1  2  3  4  5  6  7  >7, specify____
    Pancakes or waffles .............  0  1  2  3  4  5  6  7  >7, specify____
    Cheese .......................  0  1  2  3  4  5  6  7  >7, specify____
    Potato .......................  0  1  2  3  4  5  6  7  >7, specify____
    Other cooked vegetables .........  0  1  2  3  4  5  6  7  >7, specify____
    Raw vegetables ...............  0  1  2  3  4  5  6  7  >7, specify____
    Dried beans or peas ............  0  1  2  3  4  5  6  7  >7, specify____
    Macaroni, spaghetti, rice, or
       noodles ...................  0  1  2  3  4  5  6  7  >7, specify____

    Ice cream, milk pudding, custard
       or cream soup ..............  0  1  2  3  4  5  6  7  >7, specify____
    Peanut butter or nuts ...........  0  1  2  3  4  5  6  7  >7, specify____
    Sweet rolls or doughnuts ........  0  1  2  3  4  5  6  7  >7, specify____
    Crackers or pretzels ...........  0  1  2  3  4  5  6  7  >7, specify____
    Cookies ......................  0  1  2  3  4  5  6  7  >7, specify____
    Pie, cake or brownies ..........  0  1  2  3  4  5  6  7  >7, specify____
    Potato chips or corn chips .......  0  1  2  3  4  5  6  7  >7, specify____
    Candy .......................  0  1  2  3  4  5  6  7  >7, specify____
    Soft drinks, popsicles, or Koolaid ..  0  1  2  3  4  5  6  7  >7, specify____
    Instant Breakfast ..............  0  1  2  3  4  5  6  7  >7, specify____

16. How many servings *per day* does he eat of the following foods?
    Circle the appropriate number:

    Bread (including sandwich), toast,
       rolls, muffins (1 slice or 1
       piece is 1 serving) ...........  0  1  2  3  4  5  6  7  >7, specify____
    Milk (including on cereal or other
       foods) (8 ounces is 1 serving) ..  0  1  2  3  4  5  6  7  >7, specify____
    Sugar, jam, jelly, syrup (1
       teaspoon is 1 serving) .........  0  1  2  3  4  5  6  7  >7, specify____

17. What specific kinds of the following foods does he eat most often?

Fruit juices _____

Fruit _____

Vegetables _____

Cheese _____

Cooked or instant cereal _____

Dry cereal _____

Milk_____

SOURCE: U.S. Department of Health, Education, and Welfare. *Screening Children for Nutritional Status: Suggestions for Child Health Programs*. Washington, D.C.: Superintendent of Documents, Government Printing Office, 1971.

*Include formula feeding for young children

# Appendix 4

## Obesity Standards in Caucasian Americans

Minimum Triceps Skinfold Thickness
Indicating Obesity (mm)

| Age (yr) | Males | Females |
|---|---|---|
| 5 | 12 | 14 |
| 6 | 12 | 15 |
| 7 | 13 | 16 |
| 8 | 14 | 17 |
| 9 | 15 | 18 |
| 10 | 16 | 20 |
| 11 | 17 | 21 |
| 12 | 18 | 22 |
| 13 | 18 | 23 |
| 14 | 17 | 23 |
| 15 | 16 | 24 |
| 16 | 15 | 25 |
| 17 | 14 | 26 |
| 18 | 15 | 27 |
| 19 | 15 | 27 |
| 20 | 16 | 28 |
| 21 | 17 | 28 |
| 22 | 18 | 28 |
| 23 | 18 | 28 |
| 24 | 19 | 28 |
| 25 | 20 | 29 |
| 26 | 20 | 29 |
| 27 | 21 | 29 |
| 28 | 22 | 29 |
| 29 | 22 | 29 |
| 30–50 | 23 | 30 |

SOURCE: From Seltzer, C. C., and Mayer, J. "A Simple Criterion of Obesity." *Postgraduate Medicine* 38(1965): A101–7.

NOTE: To normalize skewness to the right, logarithmic means rather than arithmetic means were used. The figures represent logarithmic means plus one standard deviation.

# Appendix 5

## Milestones in the History of the School Lunch in the United States

| | |
|---|---|
| Early 1900s | Supplementary feeding of children in poor sections of New York, Philadelphia, Chicago; some of it through the schools. |
| 1915–20 | Several urban high schools and rural consolidated schools introduced a hot noon meal when students lived too far away to go home at noon. Schools arranged for cooking and serving the food. |
| 1925 | Up until about 1925, little or no thought was given to the lunch as a nutrition education experience. Gradually, lunchroom managers with home economics or dietetic training were employed to plan and supervise the preparation of the school lunch. |
| 1933 | Federal loans were made to several communities to pay labor costs of preparing and serving school lunches. |
| 1935 | Under P.L. 320, federal food assistance to schools began; donated surplus foods were distributed for use in free school lunches. |
| 1943 | USDA provided cash reimbursements to schools to partially cover the cost of foods purchased locally through regular commercial channels. |
| 1946 | (4 June) P.L. 396, the National School Lunch Act, was passed by Congress "to safeguard the health and well-being of the Nation's children and to encourage the domestic consumption of nutritious agricultural commodities and other food, by assisting the States, through grants-in-aid and other means, in providing an adequate supply of foods and other facilities for the establishment, maintenance, operation, and expansion of nonprofit school lunch programs." |
| 1960s | The National School Lunch Program was operating in public and private schools in all fifty states, the District of Columbia, Puerto Rico, the Virgin Islands, and Guam. |
| 1962 | National School Lunch Week was established to annually promote, in the second week of October, the nutritional values of the school lunch. |

303

| | |
|---|---|
| 1966 | Passage of the Child Nutrition Act strengthened and expanded the NSLP. |
| 1970 | (14 May) P.L. 91–248 was signed. It provided greater assistance than previously to needy children, by assuring every child from a low income home the right to be provided with a meal at school. National standards based on family income were established to determine individuals eligible for free or reduced-price lunches. |
| 1971–72 | Amendments were made to P.L. 91–248 authorizing major changes in funding procedures for school lunches. Funds were allocated to states to reimburse participating schools on a performance basis; that is, the more students served, the more federal assistance rendered. |
| 1972 | The federal reimbursement rate for all lunches was increased to 8 cents per lunch, an increase of 2 cents compared with the 1971 rate but still 1 cent less than the 9-cent rate paid in the late 1940s. Additional funds were made available to pay for free and reduced-price lunches. |
| 1973 | (7 November) P.L. 93–150 was signed. It increased the federal reimbursement rate from an average of 8 to 10 cents per lunch with an additional 45 cents average for free lunches. This law also contained an escalator clause which required USDA to review rates twice annually in accordance with the food-away-from-home index, and make adjustments as necessary. Rates were adjusted upward from 10 to 10.5 cents; 45 to 47.25 cents. (The escalator clause also applied to the breakfast program.) |
| 1975 | (7 October) P.L. 94–150. National School Lunch Act and Child Nutrition Act of 1966, amendments of 1975. |
| | Amendments were made in order to extend and revise the special food service programs for children and the school breakfast program, and for other purposes related to strengthening the school lunch and child nutrition programs. |

# Index

Abbott, O. D., 85
Adipose tissue
  in adolescence, 139
  growth of, 57–58
  in obesity, 171–75
  subcutaneous, measurement of, 37, 39–40, 79
Adolescence
  anemia in, 163–65
  growth in, 76–87, 141
  nutrition in, 138–48
  pregnancy in, 146, 148
Agency for International Development (AID), nutrition services of in developing countries, 233, 234, 236
Agricultural Experiment Station cooperative study, 144
American Academy of Pediatrics, 162, 232
American Diabetes Association, 211
American Dietetic Association, 215, 231, 252
American Home Economics Association, 215, 232, 252

American Institute of Nutrition, 231
American Medical Association
  participation in enrichment programs, 183, 189
  policy of regarding formulated foods, 193
American Nurses Association, 232
American Public Health Association, 15, 18–19, 216, 232
American Red Cross, 214, 227
American School Food Service Association, 231
American Society for Clinical Nutrition, 231
Anderson, J., 68
Anemia, iron-deficiency
  in adolescence, 163–65
  in pregnancy, 119, 160–61
  in surveys, 35–43
  symptoms of, 21
  in young children, 161–63
Anemia, megaloblastic, in pregnancy, 125
Anthropometric measurements, selection of, 22–23, 54–55

Nutrition Canada National Survey, 13, 25, 41–43
Nutrition committees in the United States, state and local organizations, 228
Nutrition counseling for diabetic children in group
in a clinic environment, 209–10
in a diabetic camp, 211
Nutrition education of children
as applied to schools, 252–68
curriculum development for, 252–56
definitions of, 248–49, 263
elements of learning process in, 271–72
factors which favor progress in, 273
influence of teachers in, 273–74
participation of parents in, 286–87
relationship of community to, 287–88
Nutrition Education Specialist in School Systems, resolution defining functions and qualifications for, 261
Nutrition educators
at policy-making level, 259–60
efforts to define qualifications of, 260–63
qualified personnel as, 259–68
training for, 262–63
variations in titles for, 260
Nutrition Foundation, 226
Nutritionists
number of in service, 215
qualifications of, 215–20
services of in United States, 214–15
Nutrition policy making, agencies, organizations, and groups in United States involved in, 230–32
Nutrition programs
concerned with nutrition policy in United States, 221, 229, 230–32
domestic in the United States, 221, 222–28
functioning internationally through U.S. agencies, 229, 233, 234–35
functioning through the United Nations, 236, 237–38, 240–45
functioning through foreign-based voluntary service organizations, 245–46
throughout the world, 220–45

Nutrition services, priorities for in-state health agencies, 219–20

Oakland Growth Study, 69, 71, 81
Obesity in children, 20, 129, 171–76
Office of Economic Opportunity, 154–55
Organs, growth of, 58–60
Overweight children, nutrition program in camp for, 207–9. *See* Camp for overweight children

Passow, A. H., 285
Pearson, W. N., 13
Peckham, C. W., 62, 64
Percentiles, calculation of, 95–96
Physique, classification of, 107–8
Placenta, 118–19
Porter, W. T., 62, 64–65
Pregnancy
anemia in, 119, 125, 160–61
fetal growth in, 73–74
nutritional needs in, 117–25
in teenage girls, 146–48
weight gain in, 121–23
Preschool child
growth of, 75–77
nutritional needs of, 134–37
Preschool Nutrition Survey (PNS)
anemia in, 137, 162–63
clinical findings in, 15, 36–38
dietary assessment in, 30
food expenditures of families in, 154
growth retardation in, 165–66
infant feeding in, 126
Protein in diet
of adolescent, 143, 146
in childhood, 116
in lactation, 128–29
in pregnancy, 117–18, 120–22, 124
in teenage pregnancy, 148

Qualifications of nutritionists
historical development of since 1930s, 215–17
recent revision of guidelines for, 216–18
special consideration of in maternal and child health services, 217–18

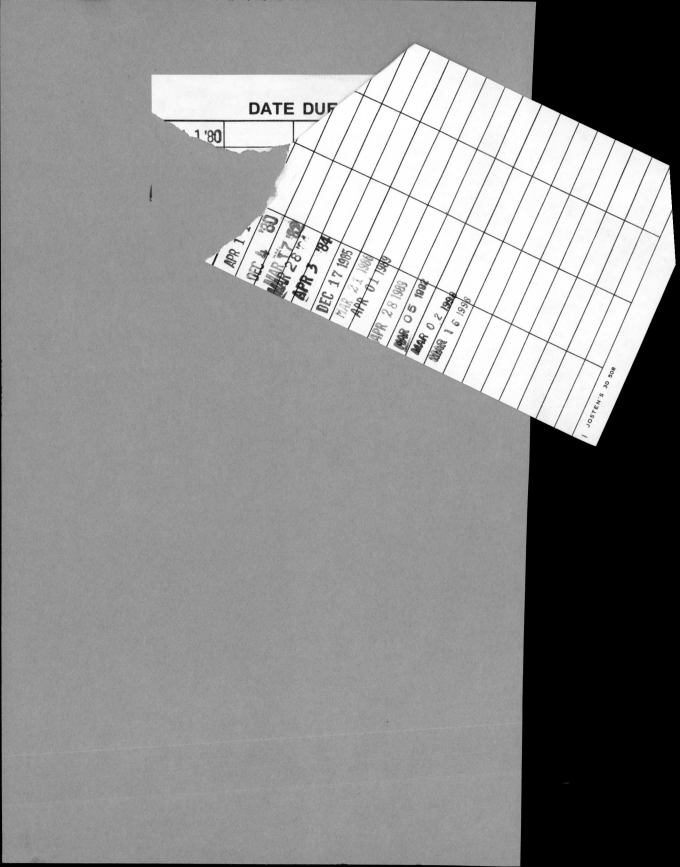